VETERINARY CLINICAL MEDICINE

NIPA GENX ELECTRONIC RESOURCES & SOLUTIONS P. LTD.
New Delhi-110 034

VETERINARY CLINICAL MEDICINE

Ramesh Chandra Patra, PhD

NAVS Fellow, ISVM Fellow, IAAVR Fellow
BOYSCAST Fellow (USA), DBT CREST Fellow (UK)
DBT Overseas Associate and Endeavour Research Fellow (Australia)
Professor and Head, Department of Veterinary Clinical Medicine
Former Dean, College of Veterinary Science & Animal Husbandry and
Former Dean of Research, Odisha University of Agriculture & Technology
Bhubaneswar, Odisha-751003, India

S.K. Panda, PhD

Fellow IAVP, and Diplomate ICVP
Professor and Head
Department of Veterinary Pathology
College of Veterinary Science & Animal Husbandry
Odisha University of Agriculture & Technology
Bhubaneswar, Odisha-751003, India

NIPA GENX ELECTRONIC RESOURCES & SOLUTIONS P. LTD.
New Delhi-110 034

NIPA GENX ELECTRONIC
RESOURCES & SOLUTIONS P. LTD.
101,103, Vikas Surya Plaza, CU Block
L.S.C.Market, Pitam Pura, New Delhi-110 034
Ph : +91 11 27341616, 27341717, 27341718
E-mail:newindiapublishingagency@gmail.com
www: www.nipabooks.com

For customer assistance, please contact
Phone: + 91-11-27 34 17 17 Fax: + 91-11- 27 34 16 16
E-Mail: feedbacks@nipabooks.com

ISBN: 978-93-90591-79-4

Composed and Designed by NIPA.

Preface

The veterinary profession has made tremendous strides over the years in the field of clinical practice for both the large and small animals. The profession has helped for livelihood for creation and nutrition security. The veterinarians have played a major role in serving the speachless animals and controlling diseases. Our main aim has been to publish an easy-to-understand and concise text book for Undergraduate Veterinary students, and Post graduate students with clinical interest.

Introduction of Minimum Standard of Veterinary Education (MSVE) by Veterinary Council of India (VCI) and partitioning of Veterinary Medicine into 'Veterinary Clinical Medicine' and 'Epidemiology and Preventive Medicine' in the year 2008 ignited the first author to write a reader friendly concise book on Veterinary Clinical Medicine by referring standard books, research articles and utilizing writing and teaching skill, knowledge and experience gained from clinical practice for more than two decades. This book contains chapters on General and Systemic states and Production and Deficiency Diseases in the line of course curriculum in MSVE of VCI.

The first author of this book, Dr R C Patra had initial exposure to poultry farming in a rural set up during his school days from where he got interest in veterinary profession. He was admitted to undergraduate veterinary course in the year 1984, in the state of Odisha. Subsequently, he pursued his master and doctoral degree in the discipline of Veterinary Medicine in the premier national institute, Indian Veterinary Research Institute. He started his professional career as a grassroot level field veterinarian for improving animal production and health. His academic career started with joining Indian Council of Agricultural Research as Agricultural Research Scientist. During this period he availed BOYSCAST fellowship to pursue post-doctoral research in John Hopkins University, USA. He moved to his Alma-matter as Professor of Veterinary Medicine after serving for almost one and half decade in ICAR.

The second author of the book, Dr S K Panda, a nationally reputed Veterinary Pathologist, and a Diplomat, Indian College of Veterinary Pathology with towering experience in both domestic animal and wildlife pathology, was invited to contribute to the book as a co-author at a later stage to improve overall standard of the book in general and pathological section of each chapter, in particular. Dr Panda worked as a Farm Manager in Central Poultry Development Organization, Bhubaneswar and Junior Veterinary Officer in Govt. of Odisha after completion of post-graduation in the year 1992 in Veterinary Pathology from Odisha University of Agriculture & Technology. Then, he switched to teaching profession in the year 1995. Presently, he is continuing as Professor and Head, Veterinary Pathology, and has excelled in rendering diagnostic services to the diseased animals and birds.

As a senior author, I extend my gratitude and profuse thanks to my beloved teachers, loving students and my colleagues and friends whose constant inspiration and support helped to complete this noble job in publishing this text book on Veterinary Clinical Medicine. I hope this publication will be liked by the students pursuing career in veterinary science as well as by the veterinary practitioners.

Authors

Contents

1

History and Scope of Veterinary Medicine

Veterinary Clinical Medicine is a subset of Veterinary Medicine, and refers to study on animal diseases at the patient bed side for diagnosis, monitoring, prognosis and treatment of the disease. The Veterinary Medicine is that branch of veterinary science that deals with diagnosis, treatment, prevention and control of diseases, disorders and injury in domesticated, pet, wild, zoo, captive, free-living animals and birds. Thus, the discipline covers and deals with all aspects of disease in animals including examination of patient, and its environment, laboratory investigation, diagnosis of disease, differential diagnosis from other related diseases, prognosis of disease, treatment, monitoring of disease process, control and prevention of diseases.

The word Medicine has come from Latin word "Medire" means heal. Thus, Medicine is the art and science of healing. Therefore, a Veterinary Medicine specialist engages his knowledge, skill and past experience for the relief of animals' suffering and for control and prevention of animal diseases. He has to interact with the animal owners for the collection of history of the disease, examines the animals and their environment, and provides animal healthcare services for the cure form of the disease. Disease diagnosis, herd health management, care of newborns, issues related to veterinary public health, creation of public awareness about zoonotic diseases, epidemiological studies on animal diseases, animal welfare, extension activities in the field of livestock health are some of the important facets of veterinary medicine. An expert in veterinary medicine should have sufficient knowledge on animal physiology, ecology, anatomy, biochemistry, pharmacology and pathology for investigation of the disease and subsequent measures for ameliorating the suffering of the animal and for cure and control of the disease.

In India, the Veterinary Medicine is a clinical discipline of Veterinary Science and Animal Husbandry, where subjects such Veterinary Medicine, Animal welfare, Ethic and Jurisprudence, Wild and pet animal healthcare are being covered. The course curriculum has been extensively designed by the Veterinary Council of India (VCI) with some liberty given to different colleges, institutions to revise the courses as per the regional needs. Thus, VCI in its regulation (2008) enforces to maintain minimum standard of veterinary education for award of B.V.Sc and AH degree. In western countries, Veterinary Medicine refers to whole gamut of Veterinary Science and most of colleges are named as College of Veterinary Medicine.

History of Veterinary Medicine

The history of veterinary medicine that is having expertise on animal healing practice, dates back of 3000 BC. Urlugaledinna in Mesopotamia is considered as an expert in animal healing. Subsequently, there has been reference to veterinary practice and veterinarian in the literature. The practice of veterinary medicine is believed to exist in the Temple Cities of Babylon of Egypt. Archaeological evidences also suggest that the ancient Egyptian nearly over 4 millennia ago had the well-developed veterinary profession. Veterinary and animal husbandry practices are considered to be well developed in ancient India, and there are mentions of animal healing practices in *Rigveda* and *Atharvaveda.* The ancient Indians also had distinction to establish the first state funded well-equipped veterinary hospital during the period of the Great *Ashoka* (238 BC). The treatment of animal diseases has been described in books written by *Salihotra* (1800 BC), *Charak* (2300 BC), and *Palikapaya* (1000 BC). *Nakula* and *Sahadeva*, during the period of Pandavas as mentioned in great epic, Mahabharat, had expertise in treatment and management of horses and cattle, respectively. *Shalihotra* is considered to be the first known veterinary doctor in the world who lived around 1800 BC in Northern India. Hippocrates is known as the Father of Medicine. During these periods, veterinary profession has only one facet that is to render animal healing. The involvement of microbes in disease process as suggested by Pasteur, Koch, and others, and identification of many different kinds of bacteria and protozoa by the end of the nineteenth century with the research work of Lewis Pasteur, Robert Koch and many other scientists helped to better understand the disease in animals. In 1898, Löffler and Frosch reported that the hoof and mouth disease is caused by “a previously undiscovered agent of disease”. The use of the term “virus” evolved gradually, and viruses could be detected by electron microscopes by 1940s.

The veterinary profession can be said to have started with the establishment of Veterinary School in Lyon, France by a veterinarian Claude Bourgelat in 1971. Subsequently, London Veterinary College started in 1791, thus giving scope for creation of dedicated professional group in the area of animal medicine. Treatment of horses remained a focus for many years to meet the need of the Army. Then, the interest of the profession spilled to cattle, other livestock and poultry. This was followed by interest in treatment of dogs, cats and other companion and exotic animals.

In India, a veterinary training school started at Pune in the year 1862. Subsequently, Veterinary colleges were established in different parts of India such as Mumbai (1884), Madras (1892), Bengal (1893), Bihar (1930), and Orissa (1954). The last one century has witnessed tremendous progress in the field of veterinary science, and the period from 1945 to 1985 is considered as the golden age for veterinary profession. The advances in bio-medical tools for use in clinical veterinary practice such as endoscope, ECG, ultrasound, and modern molecular techniques have assisted in prompt and reliable diagnosis of animal health problems in a non-invasive or semi-invasive way. Development in vaccine production, newer drug discovery, and understanding of disease process added a fillip for better management of diseases in livestock, pet and wild animals. Eradication of once dreaded disease, Rinderpest – the second viral disease to be eradicated from the whole world, and effective control of several infectious diseases including the control of African horse sickness outbreaks in 1960s, Equine influenza in 1980s and recently, the bird flu are the notable examples of implementation of advanced animal healthcare practices. Veterinary Medicine in the 21st Century has several facets besides primary job of animal healthcare.

Scope of Veterinary Medicine

The veterinary medicine has wide scope covering all species of domesticated and wild animals and birds. The veterinary medicine has been extensively practised with or without the professional supervision. There has been increasing demands of veterinarians to meet the rising demand for animal health and animal production related sectors such as public health, animal welfare, disease diagnosis, quarantine and research on biomedical and veterinary subjects, more particularly on infectious agents having potential to spread the disease to human beings. Bioterrorism with use of microbes, pathogenic to both human and animals, necessitated the expertise of veterinary professionals to deal with the subjects and to control the spread of pathogens. Strict biosecurity has been enforced in several laboratories and firms with technical support of veterinary professionals. Over the years, the responsibilities of veterinary profession have become multi-dimensional and demand driven. India has made steady progress in livestock sector with index of meat and milk production rising to about 170 in 2005 from the base of 100 in 1991, a sustained annual growth rate of more than 3.5 percent.

India has 15% and 57% of total cattle and buffalo population in the world and ranks number one in milk production, 4th in egg production and 6th in broiler meat production. The country produced about 198.4 million tons of milk in the year 2019 an increase of 6.5% over the previous year. The dairy industry is growing at an annual growth rate of 5%. However, the productivity of cattle is very low because of poor genetic make up, environmental stress, and poor feeding and healthcare facilities. The lower per capita animal production from livestock in India also reveals a great scope of the profession to increase the productivity with implementation of efficient feeding, breeding and healthcare measures. There are about 65 thousands veterinary instutions including hospital, veterinary dispensaries (37, 647), and veterinary-aid-centres (28, 168) in the year 2019 as per Annual Report (2019-20) of Department of Animal Husbandry and Dairying, Ministry of Fisheries, Animal Husbandry and Dairying, Government of India.

The increased demand for food of animal origin, use of animals as sentinels for environmental monitoring, security screening, generation of animal draught power, control measures for existing and emerging diseases, use of animals for biomedical research, drug trials and issues related to animal welfare have broaden the scope of veterinary medicine. The profession of animal or veterinary science is now expected to contribute substantially to national growth, to provide food security, safe food for human consumption and food free from drug residues and contaminants, and to ensure animal welfare.

The world enjoys negative status for Rinderpest, the second infectious disease to be eradicated. However, Indian livestock and poultry industry is still threatened with economically important diseases like foot and mouth disease, brucellosis and infectious bovine rhinotracheitis (IBR) in bovines; sheep pox, PPR, enterotoxaemia and blue tongue in sheep; goat pox, contagious ecthyma and contagious caprine pleuropneumonia in goats; swine fever, swine pox, gastroenteritis in pigs; herpes virus and *Salmonella Abortus equi* abortions, glander and strangles in equines, and Ranikhet disease, fowl pox, Gumboro disease, egg drop syndrome and Marek's disease in poultry. Besides these, there are number of wasting diseases such as tuberculosis, Johne's disease and parasitic infections and infestations, and non-infectious diseases like gastro-intestinal disorders, metabolic and deficiency diseases, and plant and chemical poisoning, which adversely affect the productivity of various livestock species. Thus, there is a need for better animal healthcare support system for livestock, particularly for high yielding animals and crossbred cows.

Veterinary practices do not normally have numerous veterinary technologists, laboratory staff, interns, residents, and highly trained personnel, with various levels of expertise. The differences between human and animal hospitals as regards personnel, equipment, testing capabilities, fees, operating expenses, and the required private investment involved in operating a veterinary facility, are not well understood and appreciated by the public users of veterinary services. So, the veterinarians in practice have a duty to their clients and the public, as well as themselves, to inform their clients and the public, generally and up front, about their facilities and its policies. This information should include choices concerning hospitalization, various methods and personnel for patient monitoring, after hours and emergency services, and the use of emergency clinics where available. In the changing scenario of veterinary practice "One world and one health approach" OIE (Office International des Epizooties) has taken some initiatives to practice good veterinary governance. Evaluation of veterinary services through use of Performance of Veterinary Services (PVS) tool, PVS gap analysis, and PVS follow up evaluation is under progress in different states and OIE Member countries including India. The OIE performance evaluation tool is designed to assist Veterinary Services to establish their current level of performance, to identify gap and weakness regarding their ability to comply with OIE international standards, to form a shared vision with stakeholders and to establish priorities and carry out strategic initiatives.

In spite of several challenges for the veterinary students and practitioners, there are many newer options for veterinarians to choose a career within the profession. The veterinarians are also now trained for their roles that perhaps the public are not so familiar with. Some roles played by the today's veterinarians include ensuring food safety, border control and quarantine, pet and sports animal practice, animal production and health, animal welfare, research and technical services, wildlife health and environmental protection. A postgraduate degree in veterinary medicine is the minimum qualification for teaching and research jobs in India. However, PhD degree in concerned subject is preferred for such jobs. Veterinarian with the B.V.Sc. and A.H qualification can serve as veterinary surgeon in government hospitals and in private run institutions for animal healthcare. Hospitals in cities provide scope to veterinarians to practise on both domesticated livestock and pets. The posting in rural areas increases the responsibilities of veterinarian towards cattle, sheep, goat, and poultry and, in some regions, horses. Veterinarians in urban areas can set up private practice and such practice involving companion animals can be quite profitable, especially in big cities. Dairy sector also employs large number of veterinary doctors for increased healthcare support and breeding of dairy cattle. The spectacular growth of poultry sector in India has also widen the scope of veterinarians to work in poultry farms to maintain health of poultry birds and to develop strains with high egg productivity and increasing poultry production for meat consumption. Veterinarians also work as extension officers at block levels to educate farmers, encourage livestock rearing and production, and to advise on animal farm management and animal health problems.

Veterinary Medicine and its practice must remain relevant to the changing needs of the society. Veterinary medical education is required to meet changing needs through creating areas of professional focus. Academic veterinary medicine should reflect the existing and anticipated diversity in the society. Veterinary medicine should seek greater collaboration and cooperation with human health in the public health area, with veterinarians playing a lead role in the management of zoonotic diseases, public health and ecosystem health.

2

Concept of Animal Disease

The deviation from normal health is defined as disease. Health refers to the very absence of the disease. Therefore, health is a state where all the body systems function normally and the activities continue within the physiological limits. So, the disease can be defined as the inability to perform physiological functions at normal levels even when nutrition and other environmental requirements are provided at adequate level. The above definition includes both clinically ill animals as well as animals not performing as expected. However, the disease frequencies in epidemiological studies are calculated considering that the disease is binary. That is the animal is either suffering from the disease or it is free from disease or in good health. But such situation is not always true due to varied sensitivity and specificity of disease tests used for identification of the disease, and manifestations of the disease are not that discrete or binary in all diseases. The concept of the health and disease can be described in following five categories.

Health as normality: The animal should have normal features, appearance and behaviours including posture and gait, rumination, alertness, body coat conditions etc. to be considered as healthy. Under such categorization, health refers to soundness of the body and absence of the disease. This definition of health is not the actual description of health but serves as an operational definition of clinical health.

Health as homeostasis: The concept of homeostasis refers to maintenance of delicate balance within the individual or within the processes of an individual. In holistic term, the word "health" implies to the concept of a mind and body together in harmony with the environment. As per this concept, health is defined as a state where all organs are in a delicate balance within the individual and with the surrounding world.

Health as biological function: The disease is considered as a state where there are structural and functional alterations in the cells within the body of the living beings. As per this definition, disease is the disturbance in proper performance of the body functions. Functional disturbances are manifested by physical signs which are being detected in a diseased animal.

Health as physical and psychological wellbeing: As per this categorization, health is defined as a state of physical and psychological wellbeing. But there are problems associated with applying this definition to all animals. Domestic animals are more or less subordinate to human interests and this is more obvious in farm animals. Health definition linked to psychological well-being can be misleading in relation to the general purpose of livestock production.

Health as productivity including reproduction: The health in animals is the same as productivity from animals. The animal is considered to be in good health, if it is with normal production and reproduction. A slight modification of health definition related to health has been introduced as positive health. It refers to optimal production with the provision of a complete diet, an environment that is optimal for the animals' physiological needs, comfortable to animal senses, in which animal is secure and is free from fear, and with no undue challenge by pathogenic microorganism or predator.

Classification of the disease: The following parameters or criterion are being used for classification of the disease.

Criterion		Disease	Manifestations/ Characteristics
Clinical signs	1	Subclinical	No visible abnormality is recognized/ No apparent signs of illness unless the profiles of milk production, performance or growth rate are monitored regularly, or biochemical or haematological tests are being performed
	2	Clinical	Manifestation of overt and recognizable clinical signs like fever, breathing difficulty, convulsions, lameness etc.
Duration of illness /Course of the disease (period from first appearance of clinical signs till recovery or death)	1	Peracute	The course of the disease is too short and may be in hours. In many instances, animals are found dead without any visible clinical signs being observed by the owner or the veterinarian. Example Peracute form of anthrax, HS, snake bite
	2	Acute	The course of the disease is in days
	3	Subacute	The course varies from one to several weeks
	4	Chronic disease	The disease persists for months
Disease aetiology	1.	Infectious disease	Diseases caused by infectious agents like bacteria, virus, protozoa, helminths etc.
	2.	Non-infectious	The disease is caused by factors, other than infectious agents. Example the Metabolic diseases, Deficiency diseases, Diseases caused by allergens and toxicants

Severity	1	Sever	disease involves high risk with poor prognosis (expected outcome) and treatment may not have positive outcome
	2	Moderate	moderately sever and the prognosis of the disease is also favourable
	3	Mild	The disease process is slow, the ill effects produced are minimal and the prognosis is favourable.

3

Concept of Diagnosis, Differential Diagnosis and Prognosis

The term "diagnosis" is derived from Greek words *dia* (between) and *gignoskein* (to know). It literally means to recognizing a disease and knowing difference between the two diseases or conditions. Therefore, diagnosis includes – determination of specific cause, abnormality of structure and function produced by the causative agents and clinical manifestations associated with the abnormality. Prompt and reliable diagnosis plays a key role for successful therapeutic management and favourable outcome of the disease. Some commonly used terms for making a diagnosis are given below.

Signs: It is the manifestation of a particular disorder in an animal which is observed by the clinician, attendant or owner.

Symptoms: Manifestation of disease or disorder that is noticed/ felt by patient himself or herself.

Pathognomonic signs: It is the specific sign observed in a particular disease that provides sufficient clues for making a diagnosis. Roaring sound in laryngeal paralysis

Pathognomonic lesions: It is the gross or histological alteration that is very specific to a particular disease. Abomasal ulcers in theileriosis

Syndrome: A group or combination of clinical signs that forms a distinct clinical feature indicating a particular disease or disorder. Eg. Downer Cow Syndrome, Metritis-Mastitis-Agalactia Syndrome in recently whelped pig

Prognosis: It refers to forecasting of outcome of the disease. It is based on clinical observations of the animals and clinicopathological alterations in a disease process and response to continuing treatment.

Differential diagnosis: This is a process of confirming a particular disease from other diseases producing almost similar clinical signs. This is carried out by specific test or group of test that identify a particular disease from other diseases. Example: Differentiating lead poisoning from other causes of laryngeal paralysis as seen in rabies.

Making a diagnosis of the disease involves a detailed clinical examination that consists of three different components: examination of the animals including physical examination of the patient and few relevant laboratory investigation, history taking and examination of the environment. History taking or anamnesis comprises of three parts – patient data (name of the animal and owner, address etc), disease history (present and past disease) and management history (floor space, housing, vaccination, feeding habits and breeding etc). Such information are collected through interrogation with the client and make the entire process easier to arrive at a conclusion. Certain changes in appearance/ attitude are being recorded by the animal owners or non-veterinary personnel and are collected during history taking. Besides, the clinician has to look into the environment for possible cause of the disease. A schematic representation on clinical examination is given below that helps to arrive at diagnosis.

Clinical Examination

Physical and Laboratory Examination	History taking	Examination of the Environment
• General and physical Examination including	• Patient data	• Outdoor environment
• Examination from a distance	• Disease history including past disease, present disease, distribution of the disease	• Stocking rate
• Examination using palpation, percussion and auscultation	• Management history including nutrition, reproductive management, housing etc	• Feed and water supply
• Examination of body parts		• Waste disposal
• Laboratory examination of the body fluids and other biosamples		• Indoor environment including sanitation, hygiene, floor space and ventilation

Examination of animal includes observation of clinical signs from a distance followed by physical examination at close quarters, collection of biosamples, laboratory investigations etc. Respiration or breathing movements are examined from a distance, preferably with the animal on standing posture. The respiration rate may be counted by observation of nostril movement or by feeling the nasal air movements by placing palm about 2-3 cm in front of nostrils. During the process of making a diagnosis and more particularly during examination of the patient from a distance, some of the following changes may be noticed by the clinician. Even, the animal attendant or the owner may provide some idea of such changes during history taking those were be further investigated by the clinician.

Behaviour: The changes in behaviour include Separation from group or following the group, sluggish, dull or indifferent response, anxiety, restlessness, yawning, hyper-excitation including abnormal movement with vigour, violent licking of own body or eating and licking of other inanimate objects, jumping, and kicking etc.

Voice: Altered voice includes hoarse voice as in rabies, soundless bellowing, and continuous lowering of voice.

Appetite may be partial (inappetance) to complete loss (anorexia) of food intake. This is one of the foremost signs in diseased animals. There may be painful or difficulty in prehension, mastication, swallowing, regurgitation or rumination.

Rumination: Rumination is observed as jaw movement for re-mastication of regurgitated feed. Rumination is reduced or completely absent in certain conditions, and is mostly seen in fever and oesophageal or rumen disorders.

Faecal characteristics: Frequency of defaecation, volume and consistency of faeces provide indications of the possible problem in the diet or diseases of gastrointestinal system.

Urination: Change in colour, volume, frequency of urine gives idea about the disease condition, particularly involving kidney and associated organs. Dribbling of urine is a common sign of partial obstruction of the urethra. Painful urination occurs in cystitis and urethritis.

Posture and Gait: Abnormal posture (when animal is in stationery state), gait (movement), bodily conditions (obese, thin or emaciated), shape and size of different body regions, etc. point to the unhealthy state of animals.

Skin coat: Skin is a true reflection of health and its abnormalities such as alopecia, discolouration of hair or wool, itching and bleeding can be noticed from a distance.

The body temperature, respiration and heart rate are commonly examined to identify the underlying problem during physical examination of the patient. Increase in body heat coupled with dryness of the muzzle is the common complaints of the animal owner during history taking. As the normal body temperature of most of the domesticated livestock and pets is higher than that of human beings, only touching the body coat may give a misleading conclusion that the animal is having fever. So, accurate recording to body temperature by a semi-skilled person helps in asserting the temperature. Body temperature of domestic animals is generally taken per-rectally using a rectal thermometer. A conventional clinical thermometer for human use may be used for animals. The bulb end of the thermometer is lubricated and gently inserted with a rotary through the anus into rectum. The thermometer is tilted slightly to make contact of the bulb with mucous membrane of the rectum and held for two minutes. Pulse is taken on the middle coccygeal or facial arteries in cattle, facial artery in horses and mules, and femoral artery in sheep and goat. The pulse rate depends on heart rate but may or may not entirely represent heart rate because of pulse deficit, difference between heart rate and pulse rate.

Methods of Diagnosis

***Syndrome / Pattern recognition*:** The diagnosis is made by correlating the exhibited signs in past cases with similar signs and symptoms. The past experience of the clinician helps in making diagnosis in this method of arriving at diagnosis. Bloody diarrhoea with typical odour of the faeces may indicate parvo viral infection in dogs. Ascending posterior paralysis is a good indication of rabies in domesticated animals. But, confirmatory diagnosis of the disease requires laboratory investigation.

***Hypothetico-deductive reasoning*:** List out all the diseases those produce the exhibited clinical signs, and deduct the disease one by one by specific reasoning based on presence or absence of disease specific clinical sings.

***Algorithm/ Arborization*:** Short list the suspected diseases and diagnose the disease through clinic-pathological tests and examination of biosamples one after another

Key abnormality method: The system involved is identified first. Then what are the organs involved and then investigation is carried out to find out the location and type of lesions followed by specific diagnosis.

Data-base method: This is a computer based method where inference is drawn after feeding the information to the computer programme.

Physical Examination

A careful physical examination of the patient may result in arriving at identification of the problem, making a diagnosis of the disease and institution of the therapeutics for successful management. Following distant examination and a close visual inspection of the body, physical examinations involving audiovisual inspection, palpation, auscultation, percussion, ballottement and tactile percussion are conducted to investigate the abnormality associated with the disease. The skill of an experienced veterinarian helps to identify the problem with the use of some of these techniques. Others examinations such as temperature, pulse, respiration, state of hydration/ dehydration, and ruminal movement can be monitored by a trained para-veterinary personnel or animal owners. The common methods for physical examination include palpation, percussion, and auscultation.

Palpation

The guiding principle behind this physical examination method is sense of touch. It reveals the information regarding body temperature, pain, oedema, fluid accumulation, consistency and contour of the organ. Palpation includes direct palpation consisting of handling the tissue by means of fingers for which one or both the hands may be used. Indirect palpation is done through probe, catheters, probing (stomach tube) instruments. Palpation of internal organs is very difficult in small and medium sized animals. But in animals like cattle, buffalo and horses, palpation of some internal organs through per rectal examination has got some advantages. Animals should be kept in standing position while undergoing palpation. The clinician should approach the animal very patiently and slowly, otherwise the animal may react before palpation. Palpation and demarcates the location of the organ provides the following information.

- Presence of pain, if any, and the intensity of pain
- Shape, size, and consistency of any part of the body
- Cutaneous thermal response: Hypo/Hyperthermia
- Consistency of different organ such as doughy, hard, fluctuating, emphysematous, fluctuating, or resilient

Doughy: The palpation finding is said to be doughy when the soft tissues retains figure impression for few seconds during palpation as seen in oedema and impaction of rumen.

Resilient: It is a condition where tissue appears solid-like muscles and moves with palpation. E.g. neoplasm and abscesses.

Hard: The feeling of bone like consistency E.g. ossification of cartilage

Fluctuating: The soft tissue is soft and elastic and undulates on pressure. It doesn't retain figure impression as the case with doughy feeling i.e. hematoma.

Emphysematous: - The palpation of the affected area produces crepitating and crackling sound on pressure E.g. B.Q. in calves and malignant oedema in bullocks.

Palpation of external and internal body parts

Pharyngeal region: In large animals, palpation of pharyngeal region is usually performed with both the hands. In small animals, a similar technique is applied by using one or two finger to detect pain, swelling and stenosis on pharyngeal region. The internal palpation of this region in cattle can be done using a mouth gag.

Oesophagus and trachea: The cervical region of oesophagus and trachea can be palpated by one hand on one side of neck and feeling along the jugular groove starting from the pharynx downwards. It gives valuable information regarding pain, local swellings deformities, if any. Internal palpation of oesophagus is done by indirect method with the use of probang or stomach tube to diagnose obstruction, stricture or dilatation.

Thorax: Palpation of chest wall corresponding to lungs area has limited value in large animals.

Cardiac area: Palpation is done by pressing the palm of left hand against the cults inside left elbow at the fourth intercostal space. The animal suffering with traumatic pericarditis may elicit sever pain response with deep and strong palpation.

Abdominal organs: Rumen can be palpated through abdominal wall on left side, particularly over the paralumbar fossa. The rumen motility can be detected in the upper part of left flank or at the paralumbar fossa. In case of bloat, the rumen is tense and bulging. In case of impaction, the rumen palpation gives a doughy and firm feeling. External palpation of reticulum is not possible due to its anatomical position on the right side of the rumen. But by applying pressure at the lower end from 6th to 8th intercostal space may produce a reticular grunt in case of TRP. Pressure on lower part of right costal arch or in the area from 7th to 9th intercostal space may produce pain in case of omasal impaction. Normally, it is difficult to palpate abomasum, spleen and liver. However, enlarged liver can be palpated on right dorsal arch.

Lymph node: Mandibular, prescapular, prefemoral or supramamary lymph nodes are normally palpable. The parotid, pharyngeal, cervical and inguinal lymph nodes are palpable when they are enlarged.

Palpation of internal organs through rectum: Per rectal examination of the abdominal and pelvic organs are more helpful in large animal practice, particularly in livestock. Palpation of pelvic cavity organs becomes easy by rectal palpation. The examination through rectum must be carried out carefully to prevent any damage to organs. In cattle, the rumen is distended in bloat and vagus indigestion. In ruminal acidosis, the fluid content of fore stomach can be palpated. In right side abomasal displacement, a large balloon like structure occupies the right dorsal sac of right peritoneal cavity. In left abdominal displacement, the abomasum can be felt only when it is exceptionally displaced. It will be felt like a tense, oval, balloon on the left of the dorsal sac of rumen. In rectal examination, caecal volvulus or caecal dislocation can be detected. Normally, the peritoneum is smooth and not painful on palpation. In peritonitis, it becomes rough and nodular and produces pain on palpation.

Percussion

This is a physical method of examination of animal wherein audible sound is produced from the underlying organ with the use of finger or instrument. The nature of the sound produced gives a clue about the underlying organ. Depending on whether only fingers (direct/ immediate percussion) or plexor or pleximeter (indirect/mediate percussion) are used, percussion is divided into two categories. Direct percussion is mainly used on thin and small animals using the middle finger to strike on the left hand over the organ to be percussed. This is called as finger to finger percussion. The information obtained by this method is very limited in buffalo and fatty animals. Indirect palpation is done by putting an oval or circular plastic plate (pleximeter) directly on the body surface and a stroke is applied with plexor or percussion hammer. However, percussion has limited application and output in animal practice due to presence of excessive subcutaneous fat in pigs and thick wool in sheep, thick bones in large animals. In large animal practice, percussion is done for two reasons. Acoustic percussion is used for areas of lungs, reticulum, rumen, liver, caecum and spleen where the effect extends up to a depth of only 7 cm. However, problem existing deeper to this cannot be identified. Pain seeking percussion is very useful in cattle and buffaloes and is aimed at localization of pain. Deep percussion was used over the reticular area in suspected cases of traumatic reticular peritonitis (TRP) and over abomasal area for torsion or impaction. Very brief strike is applied on the suspected area and the strength is gradually increased. The area of the lesion is identified wherever percussion elicits maximum pain. The best percussion results can be obtained when following points are taken into consideration.

- An empty closed room is suitable for percussion.
- Suitable instrument is very important.
- Animal must be in standing position and at rest.
- The percussion hammer should be held at a high level compared to pleximeter.
- The pleximeter must be placed firmly and flat on the area to be percussed
- Percussion stroke should be perpendicular to pleximeter, must be sharp, clear and decisive and should not be too close.

- Corresponding parts of either side of body should be compared
- The stroke should not be heavier than necessary.

The types of sound produced by percussion can be described as follows.

Tympanic: It is loud sound produced by organs filled with gas under pressure, like sound generated while beating a drum. It is heard in case of ruminal tympany, and left and right displacement of abomasum. Tympanic lung sound is seen in early or late stage of pneumonia, pneumothorax and pulmonary emphysematous condition.

Resonant/ringing sound: This type of sound is produced when large volume of air/gas is present beneath the site of percussion. *Eg.* Normal lung sound produced during percussion of normal lung area.

Dull sound: This type of sound is produced from on organ not filled with gas or by percussing a solid organ. The dull sound itself indicates that the particular part has tissue with reduced or no gas in it.

Metallic ring sound: It is similar to tympanic sound but its sound character is more pronounced. This sound is very high pitched and resembles with the striking of an empty metallic jar. Example – Ping sound produced in abomasal displacement while tapping at the 9th intercostal space on left side in left side displacement of abomasum.

Empty muscle sound/ absolute damping sound: This type of sound is produced over large muscle, or from liver in cases of hepatitis, heart affected with pericarditis etc.

Tactile percussion: It is a modified form of percussion consisting of both palpation and percussion to know the consistency and boundaries of deeply situated organs. This is accomplished by firm pushing the organ back with the fist of the hand and allowing the organ to rebound on finger tips. It is done normally for ballotment of foetus and fluid ballotment in ascites, exudative peritonitis, rumen acidosis and rupture of urinary bladder to notice the fluid thrill. This method of physical examination also helps in pregnancy diagnosis. In case of dog and cat, the palm of one hand is placed firmly against one side of abdomen and on the opposite side, percussion of various intensities is applied to palpate with the hand placed on the body surface. The impact of fluid wave can be detected by finger tips. In large animals, an assistant is required to generate the wave or fluid thrill by strong percussion.

Percussion area for lungs: The area of percussion is more or less triangular in shape on either side of the chest. In cattle, the superior upper border is formed by an imaginary line drawn from posterior angle of scapula to the tubercoxae.

The anterior border forms the posterior angle of the scapula to the olecranon process of ulna. The left side posterior border is formed starting from the 11th rib or 11th intercostals space goes to the 9th rib in the middle of ends at lower part of 5th intercostal space. So it is very important to examine the lungs border between 5th and 9th rib. When there is enlarged reticulum, the lungs border will be pushed upward to the 7th or 8th rib. It is better to percuss the lungs at right side. In case of horse, the superior border is formed by a line joining the posterior angle of scapula and last second intercostal space. The anterior border is formed from posterior angle of scapula to olecranon process of ulna. The posterior border is formed by extending upward and backward from olecranon process of ulna to join the dorsal end at the second largest intercostal process. In case of dog and cat, the area available for lung percussion is similar to horse.

Percussion of heart: Heart gives a complete non resonant sound as it is a muscular organ and air free. Heart is located approximately in the lower 2/3rd of thoracic cavity between the 3rd to 6th pair of ribs. Anterior part of the heart is covered by muscles of shoulder area. So it is difficult to percuss. An increase in the area of cardiac dullness occurs in case of cardiac enlargement i.e. cardiac hypertrophy or dilation, pericarditis and lateral displacement of heart. Reduction of cardiac dullness occurs in case of over distension of lungs i.e. emphysematous condition. Tympanic sound is produced when there is presence of gas in the pericardial sac. However, it is very difficult to reach at a conclusion particularly in large animal practice.

Auscultation

The word auscultation is derived from Latin word "*auscultare*" which means to listen. Auscultation is the process by which various functional and pathological sounds produced by different organs of the body can be heard. This physical method of examination is used to hear the sounds emitted by internal organs for the purpose of assessing mainly the circulatory, respiratory and gastrointestinal system. Previously it was practised with the help of naked ear. Later stethoscope is used. "Stethos" means chest and "scope" means to examine. In veterinary practice phonendoscope is very common which can amplify even the minute pathological sounds. Auscultation should be made in a calm and quite place to avoid the sounds of surrounding environment. There are two methods of auscultation.

Direct/ immediate auscultation is carried out by putting the ear directly on the body surface to listen the sounds. There are some disadvantages of this method. It is difficult to keep the ear in contact with the animal body where it is restless or vicious. The skin coat of the animal may be soiled or dirty with faeces, secretion and various discharges. Skin may be in fected with ectoparasites like fleas, mites, ticks, etc or may be infected with bacterial and fungal infection which may be transmitted to the clinician while keeping the ear in contact with the body.

Indirect auscultation is performed by means of stethoscope in small animals and phonendoscope in large animals. In clinical practice, a flexible stethoscope is used. It consists of sound-detecting device (chest piece), flexible tube or conduction tube and two ear pieces at the other end. The sound-detecting device has a thin plastic sheet on one side and a bell shape with a hole in on the other. There may be a rubber ring in the chest piece to avoid friction with the hairs of the animal. In small animals, auscultation can be performed with chest piece of 5 cm diameter, surrounded by a hard plastic diaphragm.

***Heart area of Auscultation*:** Careful auscultation of heart gives valuable information about the functional status of the heart than any other clinical procedure. The cycle of cardiac activity is divided into two phases, systole and diastole. The cycle is measured from the onset of one ventricular contraction to the beginning of succeeding contraction. Auscultation of heart is performed in large animals on standing position. It is better when the left foreleg is drawn forward. The small animal should be placed on a table of convenient height for clear heart sound and the mouth of the animal may be closed for few minutes. The purpose of auscultation is to determine the character of heart sound and to detect the presence of any abnormal sounds. The best site to auscultate heart is 4th and 5th intercostal spaces.

Heart sounds: Cardiovascular sounds are classified into two groups, transient and murmur. Transient heart sounds are the normal heart sounds. Loud heart sounds are produced in case of cardiac hypertrophy and anaemia. Increased heart sounds are produced in early stage of febrile condition. The heart sounds are reduced in case of cardiac insufficiency and congestive heart failure. The heart sounds are weaker when heart is displaced from thoracic wall or fluid is present in pleural or pericardial cavity like anasarca, hydropericarditis, exudative and proliferative pericarditis, hydrothorax etc. Abnormal heart sound or murmur or adventitious heart sound may originate from the cavities of heart or pericardium. Cardiac murmur may produce hissy, humming, or whirring sounds. Stenosis or narrowing of valvular orifices may also produce humming or whirring sound. Incomplete closure of valves may also produce hissing sound. The functional murmur is produced when there is no structural alternation of the valve of the heart. Pericardial rubbing sound is produced from the pericardium.

Auscultation of lungs area: Normal respiratory sound is consisted of two sounds; 1) Vesicular (lung) sound, 2) Tubular (bronchial) sound. Vesicular sounds are audible when the air rushes through small alveoli and bronchi. These sounds are audible only in case of normal lungs. The vesicular sound resembles the sound produced when the letter "V" is pronounced. This sound is normally heard throughout the respiratory area except in the area where it is masked by the bronchial sound. The vesicular sounds are clear during inspiration. During expiration, it may change its character and resembles the sounds produced when letter "F" is pronounced. In resting large animals, the rate of air movement is reduced and therefore, the respiratory vesicular sound is poorly or hardly audible. In case of dog, cat and other small animals, the vesicular sounds are very clear. Vesicular sound is reduced, when the chest wall is thick and the air content of the lungs is reduced as seen in early stage of pneumonia, passive congestion of lung or the lungs are compressed by the fluid of pleural sac. The tubular / bronchial sounds are produced while air passes through large bronchi and trachea. It resembles the sound produced when the letter "H" is pronounced. Normally, it is audible over trachea and larynx.

Diseases of bronchi, lungs, pleura and diaphragm result in production of abnormal respiratory sounds, and include different types of rales, emphysematous sounds, friction sounds etc. Moist rales are produced by the presence of fluid or mucous of relatively low viscosity within the alveoli or bronchi or both. It is better audible during inspiration than expiration. These rales are classified as fine or coarse moist rales. Prognosis for presence of fine rales is more unfavourable than coarse rales. Moist rales are found in case of lobar pneumonia, bronchopneumonia, pulmonary oedema, and pulmonary haemorrhage. Dry rales are heard when air is being forced through a bronchial tube which is partially constricted either by dry mucous or by severe swelling of the mucous membrane. Dry rales vary in pitch according to the diameter of the bronchial tube. These produces humming, rattling, whistling, crackling sounds. It occurs in early stage of acute bronchitis, spasm of bronchial mucosa, pulmonary neoplasm and tuberculosis. Crepitating rale is produced by separation of sticky walls of alveoli and bronchioles. This type of sound is produced when the bronchial mucosa is sufficiently swollen or exudation has affected the alveoli so that the opposing wall becomes adherent to one another and separated by incoming air. The sudden separation of the adherent mucous membrane causes a low pitched crackling sound. It is also called as fine moist rales. It is clear in later part of inspiratory phase. Care should be taken to avoid friction between chest piece of the stethoscope and body coat of the animal, that adds confusing sounds.

Auscultation of Abdominal Area

It gives an idea about the functional status of the rumen and reticulum. The contraction of the rumen produces gargling sound and booming gassy sounds due to the movement of the fluid and solid material on which a gas layer is superimposed. Reduction in rumen activity is accompanied by a decrease in frequency and volume of the sounds. A soft fluid sound may be heard at approximately 7 cm behind the point of elbow at the costochondral junction of the left side when ruminal contents move into reticuloruminal fold. A similar type of sound is produced when fluid returns to the reticulum by the contraction of ventral sac of the rumen.

Temperature Recording

Temperature varies in different species of animals. Body surface temperature is usually lesser than the visceral organs. Temperature in animal is generally taken from the rectum by inserting a thermometer through the anus. In case of female animals, vaginal temperature may be considered. But, vaginal temperature remains higher during approximately, normally 1°F higher than rectal temperature in healthy animals. The following precatution should be taken for accurate recording of the temperature.

- Animals should be in an isolated area away from herd with minimum excitation.
- It should be restrained properly with minimum disturbances
- It should be kept away from hot exposure prior to recording the temperature.
- It should be given 20-30 minute rest if it has travelled long distance especially in hot summer.
- Temperature should not be recorded after prolonged working, walking, race or ploughing.
- Animal should not be offered hot or cold water at least 20-30 minutes prior to recording the temperature.
- Thermometer should be kept in contact with mucous membrane to obtain correct temp.

Temperature of healthy animals may vary during day time. Morning and evening hour's temperature differs slightly. In a healthy animal, the lowest temperature is recorded in morning and the highest in the evening hours. This type of variation is called diurnal variation. Critical temperature is the highest level beyond which, it is considered as abnormal. The temperature of the animals also varies with respect to age, sex, breed, environment and body weight.

- Age: -Temperature of young animal is 1 °F higher than adults of same species.
- Sex: - Temperature of female animal is higher than male animal.
- Breed: -Temperature of purebred & cross breed is little higher than indigenous breed.
- Body weight: - Temperature is inversely proportional to body weight.
- Feeding: -The body temperature, increases during the process of ingestion, mastication, digestion etc.
- Infection: - Any infection or inflammation process causes rise i n temperature.
- Environment: - Body temperature goes up in day time during summer and goes down in night time. This variation does not exceed 2-3 °F.

The normal body temperature, pulse and respiration rate in livestock are given in the below table 1.

Table 1: Normal values of temperature, pulse and respiration rate in domestic animals

Animal	Body temperature		Pulse	Respiration
	Normal	Critical	(per minute)	(per minute)
Cattle/ buffalo	38⁰C (100.5⁰F)	39⁰C (102)	60-72	20-30
Calf	38.5⁰C (101.5⁰F)	39.5⁰C (103⁰F)	80-120	24-36
Sheep	39⁰C (102⁰F)	40⁰C (104⁰F)	70-90	20-30
Goat	39.5⁰C (103⁰F)	40⁰C (104⁰F)	70-90	20-30
Horse	38 ⁰C (100.5⁰F)	39⁰C (102⁰F)	28-46	10-16
Camel	35⁰C (95⁰F)	37⁰C (99⁰F)	25-32	6-12
Pig	39⁰C (102⁰F)	40⁰C (104⁰F)	60-90	10-20

Physical Examination of Eye

Examination of the eye from a distance and at close quarters gives valuable clue for diagnosis of the disease. The unilateral discharge from the eye suggests localized infection. Bilateral eye discharge is seen in systemic infection. The type of discharge also provides information regarding the associated disease.

Watery discharge: It can be due to obstruction of lacrymal duct or gland

Serous discharge: Early stages of inflammation

Purulent discharge (Pus discharge): Later stage of inflammation due to pus forming bacteria.

Bloody discharge: Unilateral trauma, injury etc.

Movement of eyelid: The abnormal movement of eyelid is noticed in CNS disorder, and it is painful in acute conjunctivitis, acute keratitis, and deranged nervous function. Excess movement of eyelid is noticed in canine distemper, hypomagnesemia, lead poisoning, encephalitis, and prolapse of 3rd eyelid in tetanus in horses.

Physical examination of the conjunctiva gives very good indication of the physical state of an animal: pale colour in anaemia, icteric (yellowish) in jaundice, mud colour in toxaemia, and cyanotic in anoxia, particularly when the oxygen saturation is low.

There are different methods to test blindness. Those include menace reflex, obstacle test etc

Similarly, different organs and body parts are required to be examined one after another for identification of the problem and associated changes in behaviour, posture, gait, reflexes and reaction to physical examination.

Diagnostic Techniques in Veterinary Clinical Medicine

The process of diagnosis of a disease involves general physical examination to determine abnormality of function. Special examination of the suspected organ or system(s) reveals the problem, and locate lesion. Special examination of the lesion specifies the kind of lesion, and examination of specimen determines the cause of lesion. The first two aspects of disease diagnosis are effectively completed by an experienced clinician with the help of routine diagnostic aids. The other steps however, require specific bio-medical tools to perform diagnostic tests such as endoscopy, ECG, EEG, angiography, phonocardiography, ultrasonography, radiography, tomography, image intensification and scintigraphy. These modern techniques permit better evaluation of functional profile of different internal organs. However, all these techniques have limitation in its application particularly while examining the large animal with heavy body mass and thick layer of subcutaneous tissue.

***Endoscopy*:** Endoscopy (Greek - *endon* = within; *skopion* = to look at) is a tubular instrument used to examine interior of body cavity or a hollow organ. The advent of fiberoptic endoscope in 1957 made this technique a valuable tool in veterinary medicine particularly in canine and equine practice. Besides examination of respiratory system *(Bronchoscopy),* the endoscopy is also used to examine esophagus *(Esophagoscopy) to* determine diverticulum, foreign body, fistula, meso-oesophagus, rupture, stricture and ulceration; stomach *(Gastroscopy)* for gastric ulcers, pyloric stenosis, squamous cell carcinoma, and presence of parasitic (*Gastrophilus, Draschia*) larvae in horses; small intestine *(*Enteroscopy*)* for duodenal conditions, ulcers, mucosal lesions; large intestine *(Colonoscopy)* for the presence of whip worms, brush cytology, foreign body and mucosal lesions and peritoneal cavity *(Laparoscopy)* for abdominal tumor and abscess, evaluation of peritonitis, chronic colic and abdominal metastatic lesions, location of cryptorchid testes and in ovarian and urogenital disorders.

Electrocardiography: This has mainly been used to identify cardiac abnormalities that limit performance of heart and to evaluate heart size. In equine, change in ECG such as absence of P waves, irregular R-R interval and baseline F and S waves are generally indicative of arterial fibrillation, a common cause of poor performance Phonocardiography is used for recording cardiac sounds and murmurs using chest surface microphone. Phonocardiography and telemetric ECG is used to measure cardiac function during exercise in horses.

Ultrasonography: It is a safe non-invasive diagnostic technique, which has wide application in canine and equine practice for identifying cystic structure and to distinguish dense masses within organs. Contractile organs can be evaluated by ultrasonography without using contrast medium. Oscillometry and ultrasonography are considered reasonably accurate techniques for indirect blood pressure measurement. Ultrasonography is also an excellent method for early detection of pregnancy in equines for which portable ultrasound units are available.

Computed Tomography: Computed Tomography (CT Imaging) is also known as CAT (Computed Axial Tomography) scanning. The computed Tomography is based on the X-ray principle. As X-rays pass through the body, they are absorbed or attenuated at different levels creating a matrix or profile of X-ray beam of different strength, which is registered on a banana shaped detector. This measures the X- ray profile. The CAT scan differs from the radiograph in that the former consists of a very thin beam of X-ray, which passes through a cross section of the body in a rotational manner, whereas, the latter is a cross section of the body in a rotational manner. The radiograph is one dimensional image where the overlying organs present deep in the area are superimposed.

Magnetic Resonance Imaging (MRI): It is a sophisticated computerized imaging technique, which has been a clinical diagnostic tool since 1980. The distribution of hydrogen nuclei (Protons), found in cellular water, depends on the tissue type and whether or not the tissue is healthy or diseased. The MRI uses radio waves and strong magnetic fields to create images. The MRI machine produces images by creating resonance (vibrations) in the water found in the body. This causes a radio signal to be emitted from the water in the body, which can be interpreted by receptor called a coil. The coil produces a cross sectional image of body water content found in the tissues. These methodologies can pick up very minute differences in water density that is missed by other methods.

Scintigraphy or Nuclear medicine: Scintigraphy was introduced in veterinary medicine in 1970s. Its principal use is in orthopaedic conditions. It is highly sensitive and can detect bone damage well before radiological identification. The techniques are also being applied to evaluate vascular perfusion, pulmonary ventilation and muscle damage, to measure cardiac output and in intra-thoracic pathology. The scintigraphy involves the production of images following internal administration of radioactive pharmaceuticals to a patient. The two-dimensional image obtained by sophisticated 'gamma camera' indicates the distribution of radioactive material in the body. Using advanced computer technology, these images can then be analysed to provide both qualitative and quantitative information. In this procedure, the principle of X-ray and radioactivity are combined. The advantage of scintigraphy is that it allows to detect sub clinical signs of damage.

Diagnosis of Chemical Toxicity

Chemical toxicity or poisoning with wild plants, organophosphate, organochlorine compounds and agrochemical and environmental contaminants is not uncommon in livestock and pet practice. These chemicals produce more of less similar kind symptoms. The symptoms and illness are noticed at the same time in a group of animals having access to the toxicant. Diagnosis of chemical toxicity in isolated case is more difficult. It is only the acquaintance with the syndrome produced by the common toxicants and environmental evidence such as distribution of poisonous plant in a particular locality, recent use of pesticides in the agricultural field, particular industrial enterprise in the locality that give clue for diagnosis of the toxicity in animals. So, while investigating the cause of disease in a group of animals, it is highly essential to thoroughly examine the animal's immediate environment in addition to clinical and physical examination of the animals. The confirmatory diagnosis of toxicity in animals also poses a serious problem and, thus, majority poisoning cases are symptomatically treated but not with specific antidote.

4

General Systemic States

The general systemic states are generalized in nature and involve whole body systems. They are common to many diseases and contribute to the pathogenesis of the disease. Pathogenesis is defined as the changes in functioning at the cellular level and establishment of disease process. Hyperthermia, hypothermia, fever, toxaemia, septicaemia, bacteraemia, shock, dehydration, acid-base imbalance, hyponatremia, hypokalemia etc. are some examples of general systemic states.

Hyperthermia

Hyperthermia is defined as elevation of body temperature beyond the critical temperature due to high environmental temperature, in absence of circulating toxin in the blood vascular system, and results from failure of thermoregulation by the hypothalamus. Hyperthermia differs from fever in the mechanism that fever is associated with change in the body's temperature set-point in the hypothalamus. Thus, body tries to gain heat and reduce heat dissipation to increase the body temperature to an elevated set-point level.

Neurons in both the preoptic anterior hypothalamus and the posterior hypothalamus receive two kinds of signals. The peripheral nerves transmit signals from warmth/cold receptors in the skin. The temperature signals are also received from blood-bathing regions. These two types of signals are integrated by the thermoregulatory center of the hypothalamus to maintain normal temperature. However, the body temperature rises above the set point due to failure of the thermoregulation and is associated with production of excess heat in the body through metabolism or absorption of more heat from the environment and failure to dissipate it. The common examples are heat stroke and adverse drug reaction. In heat stroke, the regulating mechanisms eventually become overwhelmed and unable to effectively deal with the absorbed heat when the body is exposed to excessive heat in a humid climate for a prolonged period causing the body temperature to climb uncontrollably. Hyperthermia is relatively a rare side effect of many drugs, particularly those that affect the central nervous system. Malignant hyperthermia is a rare complication of some types of general anesthesia. Severe muscular exhaustion, especially when humidity is high, fatty animals with heavy hair coat, and confinement in an inadequately ventilated area are some of the factors for hyperthermia. Hyperthermia can be created artificially by drugs or medical devices. Hyperthermia therapy may be used to treat some kinds of cancer and other conditions, most commonly in conjunction with radiotherapy.

Hyperthermia is a medical emergency and requires immediate therapeutic measures to prevent disability and death when the body temperature is sufficiently higher than the critical temperature. Hyperthermia is associated with increased thirst due to dryness of the mouth. The heart rate increases due to rise in blood temperature but the blood pressure falls due to peripheral vasodilatation. Respiratory rate and depth increases due to the effect of increased temperature on respiratory centre. The formation of urine and urinary output decrease due to reduced renal blood flow. High rise in body temperature may lead to depression of nervous system activities and that of respiratory centres leading to death of the animal. Circulatory failure may also occur due to myocardial weakness, fast and irregular heart rate. The body endogenous metabolism increases and extensive degenerative changes are set in the different parts of the body in prolonged hyperthermia.

Clinical findings: An increased body temperature above the critical limit is the primary sign observed in affected animal. The heart and respiration rate increases, and the pulse is weak. Sweating and salivation are recorded initially as a compensatory mechanism of heat dissipation, but not later when the sweating is almost absent. In the early stage, there is increased thirst and animal search for cool places and often prefer to lie in water. But, when the body temperature goes above 106°F, the respiration becomes laboured and general distress is evident. Beyond this point, respiration becomes shallow and irregular with rapid and weak pulse, and this is accompanied by convulsion, coma and collapse. The death occurs in most species when the temperature reaches 106°F to 108°F.

Hyperthermia for a longer period may be associated with high incidence of embryonic mortality in 3 to 6 weeks pregnant animals, and abortion. Breeding efficiency is adversely affected by prolonged heat stress and number of litter born to a ewe may be reduced. The conception rate reduces and there is increased incidence of anoestrus in adult animals.

Necropsy finding: There will be peripheral vasodilatation, blood clotting is slow, rigor mortis and putrefaction sets early.

Diagnosis: Examination of the environment gives an ideal impression for hyperthermia in animals. As rise in body temperature above the critical level is the primary manifestation in other systemic states, it has to be differentiated from fever, toxaemia and septicaemia. However, temperature in fever seldom exceeds 106°F. In toxaemia, fever is not a significant clinical picture. In septicaemia, petechial haemorrhage of mucous member and skin can be observed and blood culture for microorganism may come positive.

Treatment: Slow intravenous administration of fluid, cold application including cold pack, immersion and spraying may help in reducing the body temperature. Adequate amount of glucose and protein may be given to compensate increased utilization and deficient intake. Animal should be provided with adequate drinking water and air movement inside the shed should be ensured. Shelter alone is a most important factor in maintaining comfort of livestock. If animals are to be confined to environment of high temperature and humidity, tranquilizing drugs such as chlorpromazine may be administered to reduce body activity.

Hypothermia

Hypothermia occurs when the body cannot maintain a normal temperature and it drops below the level that is required for normal metabolism. Hypothermia is caused by prolonged exposure to low temperatures and is considered as a medical emergency requiring immediate treatment. It results from excessive loss of heat or the body heat is insufficiently produced. Decreased muscular tone as seen in parturient paresis, acute ruminal impaction, during anesthesia and sedation, profuse diarrhoea, peripheral vasodilatation in shock, reduction of metabolic activities in terminal stage of many diseases result in hypothermia. It may be a significant cause of post-shearing mortality in sheep due to loss of hair coat that gives protection against inclement weather, particularly in cold weather.

During a protracted period of hypothermia because of very low environmental temperature, the digestibility is reduced, and animal consumes more food to achieve a similar digestible energy intake. The thermoregulatory mechanism of neonates are of particular importance especially in piglets, lambs and calves, as they fail to maintain the body temperature in low environmental temperature, and neonatal mortality rate increases in an organized herd. Cold region pigs have lower blood glucose level and low glycogen content of the liver and muscles than those maintained in hot region. Cold region pigs huddle more and neglect their food.

Signs and symptoms of hypothermia vary on the severity and some of those include gradual loss of mental and physical abilities, shivering, cold extremities, listlessness, lethargy, drowsiness, decreased rectal temperature, slow and shallow breathing and reduced heart beat. Severely hypothermic patients may collapse, and goes into coma leading to death.

The following protocol should be used to examine a hypothermic animal

1. Attention to ABCD: A. Airway; B. Breathing; C. Circulation; D. Degrees. One should make sure that the animal has an open airway, is breathing, and has a heart beat
2. Brief history on animal (e.g. duration of exposure, regarding circumstances in which animal was found etc.) should be collected.
3. Brief physical examinations including a) feel of body temperature, and rectal temperature, b) level of consciousness and neurological examination. c) cardio-pulmonary examination, d) associated trauma and e) weight of animal should be assessed. Depending upon the availability of staff and equipment, chest x-ray, urinalysis, complete blood examination, and arterial blood gas analysis are also recommended.

Factors Responsible for Increased Susceptibility to Hypothermia

- Poor body condition
- Very young or aged animals
- Calves with lower birth weight
- Ewes/ sow with higher litter number
- Young ones delivered prematurely
- Breed susceptibility: Body coat condition, length of the wool or hair
- Climatic conditions, particularly windy, low environmental temperature associated with rain fall
- Food intake, particularly milk intake during the early post natal life

Treatment: Early detection, and treatment of new born can improve the condition and survival rate. Provision of warm and dry environment and injection of 20% glucose solution through intra-peritoneal route increases the body temperature through conservation of heat and heat production by elevation in body metabolism. When temperature comes to near normal the animal should be provided with warm food and young ones with mother's milk or colostrums.

The primary objectives in the treatment and handling of a hypothermic animal are to keep the animal alive by warming, to avoid any further exposure to cold, and to transport the animal to a site of complete veterinary care. The following precautions are to be observed while treating a hypothermic animal

The hypothermic animal may appear to be beyond help because of skin and membrane colors, pupil dilatation and depressed vital signs, but a positive attitude works.

However, direct application of hot objects or excessive pressure should be avoided. Ensure that items such as oxygen and fluids coming into contact with the animal are warmed. Severely hypothermic animal should not be kept in a shower or bath.

Drug treatments are not useful in treating severe hypothermic animals since the cold heart will not respond as expected. If administered, drugs will not be metabolized normally by the liver and kidneys; instead these will accumulate in the body and become active as it warms. Lactated Ringers solution should not be used as the hypothermic liver may not be able to metabolize the lactate normally. Cold fluid administration must be avoided.

Fever

Fever refers to an increase in internal body temperature to levels above critical body temperature and is most accurately characterized as a temporary elevation in the body's thermoregulatory set-point, usually above the normal body temperature. It is also known as pyrexia, and is derived from the Greek word *pyretos* meaning fire, or a febrile response, from the Latin word *febris*, meaning fever. This is a general systemic state of the body associated with feeling of cold despite an increased body temperature, and increases in heart rate, muscle tone and shivering, all of which are caused by the body's attempts to counteract the newly perceived hypothermia and to reach the new thermoregulatory set-point. Although hyperthermia, associated with increased body temperature, is not associated with elevated set point in thermoregulatory center, unlike fever, but results from excessive heat production or insufficient thermoregulation, or both.

Fever is considered as body's immune mechanism to counter perceived threat inside the body, be it bacterial, viral or endogenous pyrogen. So, increased body temperature (hyperthermia) associated with toxaemia is termed as fever. Fevers are of two types (septic & aseptic). Septic fever, a more common type, is associated with infection with bacteria, virus, protozoa or fungi resulting from generalized or localized infection. On the contrary, aseptic fever is caused due to non-infectious reasons such as injection of foreign protein such as vaccine, some chemicals like dinitrophenol, break down of tissue as occurs in surgical procedures, tissue necrosis and immune reactions due to anaphylaxis.

Pathogenesis: Pyrogens are the substance responsible for inducing fever. These can be either internal (endogenous) or external (exogenous) to the body. The lipopolysaccharide (LPS) present in the cell wall of all Gm -ve bacteria is an example of an exogenous pyrogen. Pyrogenicity can vary, some bacterial pyrogens are known as superantigens that can cause rapid and dangerous fever.

Endogenous pyrogen includes cytokines, especially interleukin 1, that is a part of the innate immune system of the body and are produced by phagocytic cells. Other examples of endogenous pyrogens are interleukin 6 (IL-6), and tumor necrosis factor-alpha (TNF α). These cytokines are released into general circulation, from where they migrate to the brain and bind with endothelial receptors on vessel walls, or interact with local microglial cells. Interaction of cytokine with the microglial cells leads to activation of the arachidonic acid pathway and production of PGE2. Exogenous pyrogen like LPS binds with an immunological protein called lipopolysaccharide-binding protein (LBP). The LBP–LPS complex then binds to the CD14 receptor of a nearby macrophage. Such binding results in synthesis and release of various endogenous cytokines such as IL-1, IL-6 and TNF α. In other words, exogenous factors cause release of endogenous factors, which, in turn, activate the arachidonic acid pathway.

PGE2 release comes from the arachidonic acid pathway. This pathway is mediated by the enzymes phospholipase A2 (PLA2), cyclooxygenase-2 (COX-2), and prostaglandin E2 synthase. These enzymes ultimately mediate the synthesis and release of PGE2, the ultimate mediator of the febrile response. The temperature set-point of the body will remain elevated until PGE2 is no longer present. The brain ultimately orchestrates heat effector mechanisms via the autonomic nervous system. They include increased heat production by increased muscle tone, shivering and hormones like epinephrine, and prevention of heat loss, such as vasoconstriction. Thus, fever can be differentiated from hyperthermia by the circumstances surrounding it and its response to anti-pyretic medications.

Clinical symptoms: Fever is associated with the combined effects of toxaemia and hyperthermia. There is increased body temperature, pulse rate, respiration rate, wasting, oliguria, increased thirst, anorexia, constipation, depression and muscle weakness. In farm animal practice, most common cause of fever is presence of an infectious disease such as peritonitis, pnuemonia, mastitis, encephalitis, septicemia etc. The fever may be classified as follows depending on nature of occurrence.

Simple fever: Temperature rises and remains high with variation of less than 1 to 2°F for several days

Transient fever: Fever subsides within 24 to 48 hr after its onset as seen in bovine emphemeral fever.

Continuous fever: The temperature remains high for a longer period as in. Tick borne fever

Intermittent fever: It is a type or pattern of rise in body temperature in which there is an interval where temperature drops to normal.

Recurrent fever: It takes the form of relatively prolonged attack with non-febrile periods of about similar duration.

Atypical fever: The fever runs an irregular course

Biphasic fever: The temperatures shoots to a new height and drops down to normal and again shoot to the new height. It is seen in diseases like Canine distemper, louping ill, strangles, swine erysipelas.

Classification of Fever on the Basis of Etiology

Septic fever it is caused due to bacteria, virus, protozoa or fungi, localized infection, abscess, cellulitis, empysema.

- Intermittently systemic as in bacteremia
- Consistently systemic as in septicemia

Aseptic fever

- Chemical fever is caused by injection of foreign protein, intake of dinitrophenols.
- Surgical fever occurs due to breakdown of tissues and blood
- Fever from tissue necrosis eg. breakdown of muscle after injection of necrotizing material
- Severe hemolytic crisis
- Extensive infarction
- Extensive necrosis in rapidly growing neoplasm
- Immune reaction-anaphylaxis, angioneurotic edema
- Drug induced-prolonged use of antimicrobials may cause cryptic fever

Clinical Classification of Fever

1. Acute fever- Sudden sharp elevation of body temperature as seen in acute viral or bacterial diseases. E.g. Acute Pneumonitis, Acute peritonitis
2. Subacute fever- Temperature does not rise too high and remain below of 103° F. It is seen in mild inflammatory conditions like nephritis, cystitis, metritis etc.

3. Chronic fever- Temperature persists for a prolonged period.

   E.g. Pulmonary tuberculosis, chronic pyometritis, surra in horse etc.

Types of Fever

1. Simple fever- It is the type of fever where the temperature does not exceed 2° F in 24hrs. This type of fever is seen in lobar pneumonia, enteric fever etc.
2. Remittent fever – Temperature does not touch the normal limit in 24hrs and variation of temperature is more than 2° F in 24hrs. This type of fever is observed when diurnal variation is exaggerated. Observed in septicemia, broncho pueumonia, urinary tract infection.
3. Intermittent fever- It is a type of fever where the rise of temperature persists for a few hours of the day, as seen in human malaria, chronic surra & canine distemper. It is further classified as;
   a. Quotidian-daily rise and fall of temperature eg; E.coli infection, pyelitis
   b. Tertian - temperature appears and disappears every alternate days eg; malaria in human
   c. Quartan - temperature comes and goes every 4th day
   d. Hectic - sudden rise of temperature daily with chillmor rigor, profuse sweating when temperature falls
4. Irregular fever (Atypical fever)- Daily fluctuation of temperature does not following a regular pattern eg; louping ill, canine distemper, swine erysepelas, strangle in horses
5. Transient fever- Fever subsides within 24 hrs without any diurnal variation eg; Ephemeral fever
6. Continous fever- Plateau of temperature remains for a longer period eg; Tick borne fever
7. Periodic fever-Periodic attack of fever alternating with a febrile and non-febrile period.
8. Sthenic fever - High rise of temperature is accompanied with a strong bounding pulse as observed in acute inflammatory conditions eg; acute laminitis in horses
9. Asthenic fever- Moderate temperature accompanied with weak but quick pulse, eg, fever in pulmonary tuberculosis
10. Pel-ebstein fever- Special kind of fever associated with Hodgkin's lymphoma, being highest for 1 week and low for next week

11. Neutropic Fever Febrile Neutropenia- It occurs in the absence of normal neutrophils, commonly seen in immune –suppressing chemotherapy

Stages of Fever

First stage; (Initial stage , stadium incrementii)

- Body temperature rises as the result of spasms of blood vessels in the skin
- The phase of rapidly rising temperature is accompanied by chills due to stimulation of cutaneous nerve endings following fall of temperature caused by spasm of superficial blood vessels

Second stage (Hot stage, stadium fastigii)

- This is the period of maximum temperature which remains more or less constant
- There is cessation of shivering

Third stage (Stadium decrementii, stage of defervescence)

- This is the satage of decline of temperature.
- Heat loss is ensued as a result of profuse sweating due to dilatation of peripheral blood vessels
- Body regains its normal temperature.

Clinical signs of fever

First stage

- Dullness, drowsiness, disinclination to move
- Inappetance, errection of hair, arched backs rapid respiration
- Shivering
- Deep colored urine

Second stage

- Profound dullness, drooping of ears
- Lowering of head, frequent respiration, rapid pulse
- Congested mucus membrane, hot breath
- Dry muzzle, anorexia
- Drop in milk production
- Increased thirst
- Constipation, scanty urine

Third stage

- Respiration less frequent
- Regain of appetite
- Muzzle is moist and urine turns normal

Clinico pathology

- There is no clinico pathologic changes which are specific to fever
- The hemogram will reflect the changes associated with the cause of fever
- Inflammation is characterized by marked changes in total leukocyte count (TLC) in blood picture

Diagnosis

- Microbiological testing of blood samples
- Analysis of serous fluid from body cavity
- CSF analysis
- Milk sample analysis
- Reproductive tract secretion analysis
- Joint fluid analysis
- Biopsy
- Explorative laparotomy

Treatment

Antimicrobials

Antimicrobials are indicated to treat bacterial infection. The selection of antibiotics depends on cause, severity and accessibility of the drug to the lesion. In on canes of fever of unknown origin broad spectrum antibiotics used.

Antipyretics

If the fever is high enough to cause discomfort, the use of Non-Steroidal Anti-Inflammatory Drugs (NSAIDs) may be considered. Most NSAIDS like Phenylbutazone, flunixin meglumine, Acetyl Salicylic Acid, Sodium Salicylate are inhibitors of prostaglandin synthesis that lower the thermoregulatory set point . If required, fluid and electrolyte therapy should be given.

Toxaemia

It is a generalized clinical state characterized by circulation in the blood stream of the toxin produced by bacteria, parasites and/or body cells. However, it does not include the diseases caused by plants or insects or ingested organic or inorganic poisons. Theoretically, the diagnosis of toxaemia can be made only if the toxin is present in the blood stream, but in many cases, there is contributory evidence of antigenic toxin, or a probable source of toxin which in many cases, are virtually impossible to isolate or identify.

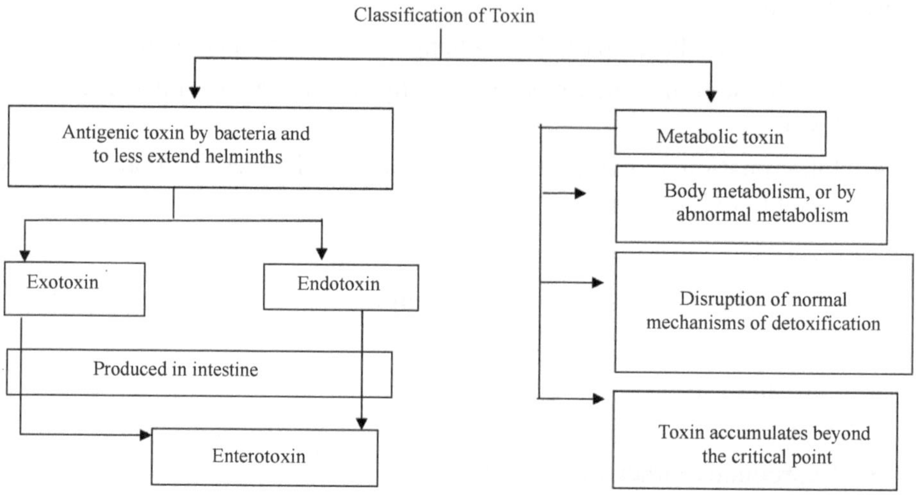

Exotoxin is protein in nature and is produced by living Gm +ve organisms. The toxin diffuses to the surrounding medium and has specific site of action. Example: tetanus toxin acts at motor end plate. The exotoxin produced in the intestine is called enterotoxin. Example: Toxin produced by *Clostridium perfrigens* in the gastrointestinal tract. Endotoxins are lipopolysaccharide in nature, found within the cell as a part of cell wall of Gm -ve organism, and are liberated into the media or surrounding upon destruction of the cell wall. *E. coli, Salmonella* sp *and Pasteurella species* are the important pathogenic organisms in livestock that produce endotoxins. Endotoxaemia is also one of the important causes of death in horses affected with gastrointestinal disorders in which there is physical obstruction causing strangulation and ischaemia. Endotoxins are not ordinarily absorbed through the intestinal tract unless it is injured as in case of enteritis or more commonly acute intestinal obstruction. Generally, a small amount of endotoxin that is absorbed from the intestinal tract into the circulation is detoxified in the liver. A state of endotoxaemia is produced only when the endotoxin are produced in larger quantity and are being absorbed or the liver fails to detoxify it as in case of hepatic insufficiency. Endotoxins may also be produced in large amount in case of server mastitis, peritoneal abscess or from other septic foci or large areas of injured traumatised infracted tissue. Best known endotoxins are those of *E. coli* which are used extensively as a model for experimental endotoxaemia.

In case of obstruction of lower alimentary tract, there may be increased absorption of toxic substance such as phenols, cresols, and amines which are normally excreted in the faeces, resulting in development of syndrome called autointoxication. Production of toxins by abnormal metabolism enhances production of histamine and histamine-like substances in damaged tissue. Ketonemia, due to an improper fat metabolism and lactic acidemia due to acute ruminal impaction are common examples of toxins produced by abnormal metabolism.

Pathogenesis: Toxaemia affects metabolism of carbohydrate, protein and minerals, and also damages vital organs including liver and kidney parenchyma. Fall in blood sugar level, sever drop in liver glycogen, increased level of blood pyruvate and lactate are some of the outcome of toxin effects on carbohydrate metabolism. Toxins also produce effects on protein metabolism, and include increased tissue break down, rise in blood non-protein nitrogen level, increased total serum protein, and enhanced serum protein as a result of increase in antibody production and alternation in relative proportion of animo acids in blood. Hypo ferremia, hypozincemia, hypocupraemia, due to increased blood ceruloplasmin, have been recorded in patients. Weakness of myocardium with reduced response to cardiac stimuli, damage to renal tubules and glomeruli leading to albuminuria, loss of musclular tonicity, depression of hematopoiesis with increased leukocytes count, hypersensitivity reactions are seen in toxaemia.

Clinical Findings

The clinical symptoms vary with the species and severity of toxic process. In acute toxaemia, depression, anorexia, and muscular weakness are common. Lethargy, separation from group, inappetance, failure to grow or produce, weak, rapid but irregular pulse are the characteristic findings. Heart rate is increased, but the sounds are reduced. There may be albuminuria. Fever may be present if toxaemia is associated with infections. The rise in temperature may normal in early stage, but later the termperature may become subnormal. Terminally, there is muscular weakness, convulsion, coma, and death occurs in coma or during convulsion.

Clinical Pathology

It may be possible to isolate and identify the specific toxin and determine the source. Low blood glucose level, increased level of urea, total serum protein, decreased A/G ratio, albuminuria, and aplastic anaemia are the common clinic-pathological findings. Leukocyte count shows leukopenia, neutropenia and lymphopenia in severe cases of endotoxaemia. However, leukocystosis along with neutrophillia is recorded in mild cases of endotoxaemia.

Necropsy finding: Microscopically, liver and kidney parenchyma shows degenerative changes. Glomeruli and tubules of the kidney, myocardium and adrenal gland may show degenerative necrosis.

Treatment: Identification of toxin and administration of specific antitoxin reduces the severity of the disease. But in many cases, it is impossible to pinpoint the toxin. Intensive fluid and electrolyte therapy should be given through intravenous route to improve the excretion of the toxin and to prevent shock due to fall in peripheral circulatory volume. Parental nutrition is indicated in anorexic patients till the animal eats and drinks normally. Glucose, amino acids and fat emulsion may be added to fluid therapy for parental nutrition. Glucocorticoids are given at the dose rate of 1 mg/kg body weight intravenously at every 24 hours. Non-steroidal anti-inflammatory drugs such as acetylsalicylic acid, phenyl butazone (15 mg/kg body weight initially and 10 mg/kg body wt at 6-12 hrs internal) are administered to reduce inflammation and pain. In acute infection, the administration of antimicrobial drugs will usually control the infection and the animal will recover.

Septicemia

Septicemia is a general systemic state of the body where toxaemia is compounded with hyperthermia and presence of large numbers of infectious microorganisms including viruses, bacteria or protozoa in the blood stream. The presence of bacteria in the blood stream for only a transitory period unaccompanied with clinical signs is called bacteraemia. In septicaemia the causative agent is present throughout the course of the disease and is directly responsible for the appeared clinical signs.

Causes of septicaemia in all species

Anthrax, Pasteurellosis, Salmonellosis, Pseudomonas, Rift valley fever, Leptosporidia, Sarcosporidia.

Cattle, Sheep, Pig

Pasteurella multocida, Pasteurella haemolytica, Pasteurella (yersinia) *pseudotuberculosis*

Sheep

Histophilus ovis, Hoemophilus agni.

Horse

Pasteurella haemolytica.

Pig

Hog cholera, African swine fever, *Streptococcus zeoepidemicus*, *Erysipelothrix insidiosa*

The exotoxins or endotoxins produced by infectious agents produce a profound toxaemia and high fever: This is due to the rapidity by which they multiply and the rapid spread to all body tissues. The microorganism also localizes in many organs and may cause direct endothelial damage and haemorrhages into tissues. In viremia, the same general principles also present the except that toxins are not produced by virus. The general clinical signs are caused by the products of tissue cells killed by the multiplying virus. Septicaemia may also result from loss of leukocyte production because of injury to bone marrow as seen in radiation injury. Immuno incompetence due to congenital defect in the immune system, and immuno suppression resulting from treatment with corticosteroid in adult animals leads to septicaemia due to poor body resistance. Disseminated intravascular coagulation occurs in fatal septicaemic diseases. Circulation of foreign materials such as bacterial cell walls, antigen-antibody complexes and endotoxins brings about vascular injury with partial disruption of the endothelial lining, subsequent platelets adherence, and formation of platelet thrombi. The symptoms produced in septicaemia are those of toxaemia and hyperthermia. Submucosal and subepidermal petechial or ecchymotic haemorrhages are seen under the conjunctiva, mucosa of mouth and vulva.

Treatment: The animal should be treated with antibacterial drugs, sera and antitoxin as soon as possible. The body temperature should be reduced with the use of antipyretic drugs. If the animal is anorectic, parenteral nutrition reduces starvation. Hygienic precautions and prophylactic measures are to be taken to prevent the spread of the disease.

Shock

Shock is a condition that results from a depressed state of many vital body functions caused by a lack of effective circulation, decreased arterial blood pressure, inadequate supply of oxygen to the tissues, or an inability of the tissues to properly use oxygen. The state is manifested by clinical sings such as acute depression, coldness, a weak rapid pulse, fast breathing. Regardless of cause, shock is life-threatening and requires immediate attention and treatment. Decreased blood volume as occurs after internal or external haemorrhage, dehydration, burn and severe vomition and diarrhoea, reduced activity of heart, peripheral vasodilatation of veins – reduction in effective circulatory blood volume, so there is insufficient blood to fill heart during distole

Classification of Shock

Hypovolemic Shock: Reduced blood volume due to dehydration or hemorrhage, and fall in blood pressure leads to hypovolemic shock. It occurs when the volume of circulatory fluid is significantly reduced, where there is severe haemorrhages with acute loss of 35% or more of total blood volume, and in dehydration from severe diarrhoea, intestinal obstruction, especially if fluid loss is severe and over a short period.

Cardiac output is the amount of blood that the heart can pump out in one minute. It is calculated as the stroke volume (how much blood each heart beat can push out) multiplied by the heart rate (how fast the heart beats each minute). If there is less blood in the system to be pumped, the heart speeds up to keep its output steady, resulting tachycardia. So, increased heart rate is a compensatory mechanism to prevent hypovolemic shock.

Vomiting and diarrhoea due to gastroenteritis and excessive sweating due to heat exhaustion and heat stroke, and infectious disease condition, diabetic ketoacidosis lead to significant loss of water, and create a situation of hypovolemic shock. In hypovolemic shock, the animal fails to replenish the amount of lost fluid by taking in enough water, and the body is unable to maintain blood pressure and cardiac output. In all shock states, when cells start to malfunction waste products build up, a downward spiral of cell death begins, increased acidosis occurs, and a worsening body environment leads to further cell death - and ultimately organ failure.

Hemorrhagic Shock: It is a subset of hypovolemic shock and occurs due to significant bleeding that occurs relatively quickly. So, the total blood volume is reduced. Trauma is the most common example of bleeding. Blood loss has two effects such as loss of volume within blood vessels to be pumped and a reduced oxygen carrying capacity because of the loss of red blood cells.

Maldistributive shock: During severe trauma or burn injury, following major surgery, after prolapse of uterus, rapid withdrawl of ascitic, fluid and severe colic pain in horses, the distribution of thrid is disorganised leading to shock.

Cardiogenic Shock: This occurs as a result of an acute reduction of cardiac output due to myocardial damage or myocardial asthenia with loss of muscular power which causes failure of tissue perfusion.

The loss of ability of heart to pump blood to the rest of the body results in fall in blood pressure, and cardiogenic shock is produced although there is enough red blood cells and oxygen and adequate blood volume. The myocardium itself requires blood supply for its functioning. The resultant decrease in stroke volume leads to fall in cardiac output.

Neurogenic shock: The involuntary muscles within blood vessel walls maintain the squeeze so that the volume within the vessels stays constant even if the body position changes. The squeeze is maintained by signals from nerves in the sympathetic trunk, a long bundle of fibers running from the skull to the tail alongside the vertebral column. The sympathetic trunk stops working in brain and spinal cord injury and blood vessels get dilated resulting in blood pooling away from the heart. Since there isn't enough blood returning to the heart, the heart has a hard time pumping blood into the body. This situation looks like hypovolemic shock, but there is enough blood but effective blood volume is reduced.

Hypoglycemic Shock and Hyperglycemia: The brain is very susceptible to low blood sugars. High or low blood sugars are almost associated with diabetes in pet animals. When blood sugar levels spiral high out of control, there is risk of significant dehydration due to glycosuria. If there is not enough insulin in the blood stream, cells cannot use the glucose and instead turn to an alternative anaerobic metabolism to generate energy. Since glucose can't enter cells to be used, hyperglycemia occurs as the glucose level build in the blood stream. The kidneys try to excrete excess sugar, but because of chemical concentration gradients between blood and urine, significant amounts of water are lost as well. The body quickly becomes dehydrated and blood pressure drops, decreasing blood flow to cells. Cells which are now lacking glucose inside them are now starved of oxygen and turn to anaerobic metabolism, causing acid waste product to build up. Excess acid in the body changes the metabolism for all organs, making it more difficult for oxygen to be used. This downward spiral will continue until insulin and significant fluids are given.

Anaphylactic shock: Shock may be caused by presence of bacteria or their toxin in the blood stream. Severe allergic reaction (anaphylactic shock), overdoses with drug such as certain anaesthetic or acute stress may lead to shock. In some cases, a combination of above causes may be involved. Anaphylactic shock is an extreme generalized allergic reaction in which widespread histamine release causes bronchial constriction leading to respiratory distress, dilation of veins, circulatory collapse and possibly death.

Toxic/Septic shock: It can occur when endotoxin and micro organisms get assess to the circulation and act on vascular system either directly or via mediation released by their interaction with host cells. Endotoxin is oviously important in the development of shock in G-ve bacterial sepsis.

Clinical signs of Shock

Early Signs of Shock

The animal may be either excited or subdued.

Rapid heart rate

Pulse not difficult to find

Gums may be normal or pale

Late Signs of Shock

Gums extremely pale or show a bluish discoloration.

Heart rate is probably elevated and irregular, but may be normal or below normal as heart muscle begins to fail.

The pulse will be weak and either difficult or impossible to locate.

Coldness to touch and rectal temperature is below normal.

Respiration may be slow or rapid, shallow or deep.

The eyes may take on a glazed appearance and appear not to focus normally.

Mental condition deteriorates from depression to stupor to coma.

Diagnosis

1. Clinical signs.
2. Estimation of arterial blood pressure is one of the best methods of measuring the severity of shock. In severe shock, the systolic blood pressure falls from normal of approx .120 mm Hg to bellow 60 mm Hg which indicates a fatal outcome.
3. Shock should be anticipated in septicaemic diseases especially in neonates in acute localized infection with intestinal diseases, severe trauma, severe fluid loss of any reason and in major surgery.

Treatment: If signs of shock are recognized, or a serious injury has taken place, supportive care, such as intravenous fluids, oxygen and other measures can help reverse shock and prevent permanent organ damage. The key to successful treatment is prompt professional care. The treatment of hemorrhagic shock depends on finding and controlling the source of bleeding. Intravenous fluids are used to help with resuscitation to increase the fluid volume within the blood vessel space, but blood transfusion is not always mandatory. If the bleeding is controlled and the patient becomes more stable, the bone marrow replenishes the lost red blood cells. In cardiogenic shock, treatment is given to restore blood supply and to support blood pressure. Intravenous fluids and medications are given in neruogenic shock to increase the tone in the blood vessel walls. Effective treatment and management of septic and toxic shock is less successful unless the sepsis can be controlled and the source of toxaemia eliminated. Appropriate antibiotic therapy should be given parenterally along with immunotherapy and corticosteroids.

Water Intoxication

When animals are very thirsty particularly after excercise, the ingestion of excessive quantity of water may result in water intoxication under field condition. Calves are most commonly affected, but the disease is also recorded in sheep. The of main clinical signs are 1. heamoglobinuria 2. hypothermia 3. salivation. There is cerebral oedema in post mortem findings. Some nervous signs may also be observed like muscles weakness, tremor, restlessness, ataxia, tonic and clonic conclusion and coma. Water intoxication does not occur commonly and can be avoided by allowing thirsty animal to have only limited access to water. Syndrome will appear to be related to salt poisoning and haemolytic anaemia that can occur in calves drinking cold water.

Treatment

Sedatives and diuretics are used. In severe cases intravenous injection of hypertonic solution is indicated to increase water loss.

Edema

It is the excessive accumulation of fluid in tissue spaces caused by a disturbance in the mechanism of fluid interchange between capillaries, tissue spaces and lymphatic vessel.

Etiology

It results, mainly from an increase in hydrostatic pressure in the capillaries, a fall in osmotic pressure of the blood, obstruction to lymphatic drainage or from damage to capillary wall. Increased hydrostatic pressure is mainly noticed in congestive heart failure and locally in portal hypotension due to hepatic fibrosis causing.

Clinical Findings

Anasarca (swelling of superficial tissue) or ascites (swelling of peritoneal cavity) or hydropericardium (swelling of pericardial sac) are the common clinical. Anasarca in large animal usually confined to the ventral wall of abdomen and thorax, brisket regiontypes of edema In the grazing animal it is usually noticed in intermandibular space. Intermandibular edema may be less evident in animals which do not have to lower their head for grazing. Edematous swelling are soft, painless and pits on pressure. In ascites, there is distension of abdomen and the fluid can be detected by a fluid thrill on tactile percussion.

Diagnosis

- Clinical signs
- Severe hypoalbuminemia.
- Marked protenuria
- Liver function test may be indicated ,when liver disease is the suspected cause of edema.

Treatment

- Congestive heart failure may be treated with digoxin (lancxin)
- Pericarditis –by drainage of sac and feeding of high quality protein
- Restriction of salt in the diet
- Use of diuretics and aspiration of fluid. Fluid aspiration must be carried out very slowly to avoid peripheral circulatory failure.

Pain

Pain is a state of consciousness, a feeling sensation and a mental event, and as such, it can never be observed. Behaviour like writhing, screaming, or drawing the affected part away from pain inducing agent. Thus, pain in other individual or animal cannot be directly experienced by anyoneelse including the clinician. Nearly all the external signs that lead to infer pain in other humans are seen in animal and birds. The behavioural signs include writhing, facial contortions, moaning, yelping or other forms of calling, attempts to avoid the source of the pain, appearance of fear at the prospect of its repetition, and so on. The animals have nervous systems similar to human beings and respond physiologically like human beings do when the animal is in circumstances in which we would feel pain. The impulses, emotions, and feelings nuclei are located in the diencephalon, which is well developed in many other species of animals, especially mammals and birds.

Pain is one of the more difficult manifestations of the disease to conceptualize because it is necessary to describe, quantify, and characterize outward physical responses that have a sensitive, as well as physiologic basis. It is generally stated that free nerve endings of small-diameter serve the function of perception and production of pain. These nerve endings have been identified or found in the superficial layers of the skin, joint surfaces, periosteum, muscle, tooth pulp, and viscera. Stimulation of these receptors results in transmission of pain impulses to the spinal cord, hypothalamus, brainstem and cerebral cortex. The signals are processed in the manner that resembles the processing of information from other types of receptors. When the stimulus is of sufficient intensity to exceed the pain detection threshold, these impulses is centrally processed which permits characterization of the intensity and location of the stimulus. The end result of pain perception is elicitation of multiple motor responses generally indicative of arousal and avoidance.

Classification of Pain

Superficial pain refers to painful responses that is initiated by stimuli applied to the skin or subcutaneous tissues.

Deep pain originates from muscles, joints, bones and connective tissues.

Visceral pain originates from stimulation of nerve endings in the viscera due to localized damage to the visceral organ.

Some common causes of abdominal pain include traumatic reticulo peritonitis (TRP), tympany, abomasal ulcer, gastric ulcers, urolithiasis, spasms, abomasal displacement, peritonitis, abomasal impaction, cystitis, ruminitis, cholelithiasis in ruminants and intestinal volvulus, intestinal torsion, obstruction, intussusceptions, indigestion, colitis, enteritis, ileal impaction, pyelonephritis, meconium impaction, peritonitis. Pleuropneumonia, lung abscess, pleurisy, traumatic reticulo pericarditis pneumonia, choke, fractured ribs, pleuritis, ruptured esophagus are associated with chest pain.

Management of Pain: Proper management of pain and mitigation of suffering speaks about the animal welfare status. Animal in pain should be given immediate attention and should be administered with pain killers. Non-steroidal anti-inflammatory drugs (NSAIDs) primarily are anti-inflammatory due to inhibition of prostaglandin production. So, while prostaglandin production rapidly diminishes, any previously present prostaglandin must be removed to subside inflammation. NSAIDs such as phenylbutazone, flunixin, meloxicam, and carprofen have delayed peak concentrations at the site of inflammation and persist in inflammatory exudates for long periods after plasma concentrations are negligible. This explains the delayed onset and prolonged duration of anti-inflammatory action that does not correlate with plasma pharmacokinetics. In addition, cyclooxygenase inhibition does not explain all of the anti-inflammatory activities of NSAIDs. Some anti-inflammatory action appears to be related to their ability to enter into the lipid bilayer of cell and disrupt normal signals and protein-protein interactions in cell membranes. NSAIDs are more lipophilic at a low pH. In the cell membrane of neutrophils, NSAIDs inhibit neutrophil aggregation, decrease enzyme release and superoxide generation, and inhibit lipoxygenase.

NSAIDs act as analgesics by inhibiting COX and preventing the production of prostaglandins that sensitize the afferent nociceptors at peripheral sites of inflammation. However, there is increasing evidence that some NSAIDs have a central mechanism of action for analgesia and act synergistically with opioids. NSAIDs are likely to be more effective as analgesics when inflammation is a part of the pain process and are more effective as analgesics when given prior to the onset of the inflammatory processes. The time of onset and duration of analgesic properties of NSAIDs does not correlate well with their anti-inflammatory properties—the analgesic effect is likely to have a more rapid onset and shorter duration of action. Therefore, dosage regimens for effective analgesia may need to be different than for anti-inflammatory properties.

Ketoprofen

Ketoprofen (Ketofen®, Anafen®) is a propionic acid derivative available as an injectable formulation and tablets. Typically, the plasma elimination t½ is short, approximately one hour in horses, 1.6 hr in cats, and five hr in dogs. Cats and dogs can be given a dose of 2 mg/kg by injection (IV, IM or SC) the first treatment, followed by 1 mg/kg PO (tablets) q24h. The label dose is for five days of therapy, but 0.25 mg/kg has been recommended for chronic therapy. Adverse effects of ketoprofen are rare. There are reports of hemostasis problems and acute renal failure in animals following anesthesia and surgery when ketoprofen was administered in the perioperative period.

Carprofen

Carprofen, like ketoprofen, is a racemic mixture of "S" and "R" enantiomers. Most of the COX inhibition anti-inflammatory action is attributed to the "S" enantiomer and analgesia is attributed to the "R" enantiomer. Carprofen has greater activity against COX-2 than COX-1, but its overall cyclooxygenase inhibition is weak, so the anti-inflammatory and analgesic activity may be due to central the effects. Carprofen may cause an idiosyncratic hepatopathy in dogs.

Meloxicam

Meloxicam is available as an injectable solution and oral syrup for chronic therapy of osteoarthritis in livestock and pets. Meloxicam has high activity against COX-2. It has no effect on platelet aggregation or renal prostaglandin synthesis, showing a sparing of COX-1. The elimination t½ in the dog is 12–36 hr. Meloxicam is highly efficacious and well tolerated, with few reports of adverse effects. The oral dose in dogs is a one-time loading dose of 0.2 mg/kg followed by 0.1 mg/kg PO q24h. Once a therapeutic effect has been attained, the dose can be titrated to the patient for the lowest possible daily dose. In recent studies injectable, meloxicam given pre-operatively was more efficacious than butorphanol for pain control and did not cause adverse renal or hematological effects.

Dehydration

Dehydration may be defined as disturbance of body water and electrolyte balance in which more fluid is lost from the body than is absorbed resulting in reduction in circulating blood volume and dehydration of the tissues. Dehydration is also defined as the loss of water and salts that are essential for normal body function.

- **Electrolyte imbalances** occur commonly as a result of loss of electrolytes, shifts of certain electrolytes or relative changes in concentrations due to loss of water. Common electrolyte imbalances include hyponatremia (reduced sodioum), hypokalemia (reduced potassium), hypocalcemia (reduced calcium) and hypochloremia (reduced chloride).
- **Acid-base imbalance**, either acidosis or alkalosis, occurs as a result of the addition of acid and depletion of alkali reserve (acidosis), or the loss of acid with a relative increase in bicarbonate (alkalosis).

Etiology

The resons of dehydration can be grouped under two broad categories

1. **Failure of water intake-** Deprivation of water, lack of thirst due to toxemia, and the inability to drink water as in esophageal obstruction etc.
2. **Excessive loss of water-** It is the most common reason of dehydration. It is seen in diarrhoea, vomition, polyurea, loss of fluid from extensive skin wound etc. Severe dehydration also occurs in acute carbohydrate engorgement, acute intestinal obstruction and diffuse peritonitis and in dilatation and volvulus of the abomasum.

Etiology and Pathogenesis of dehydration

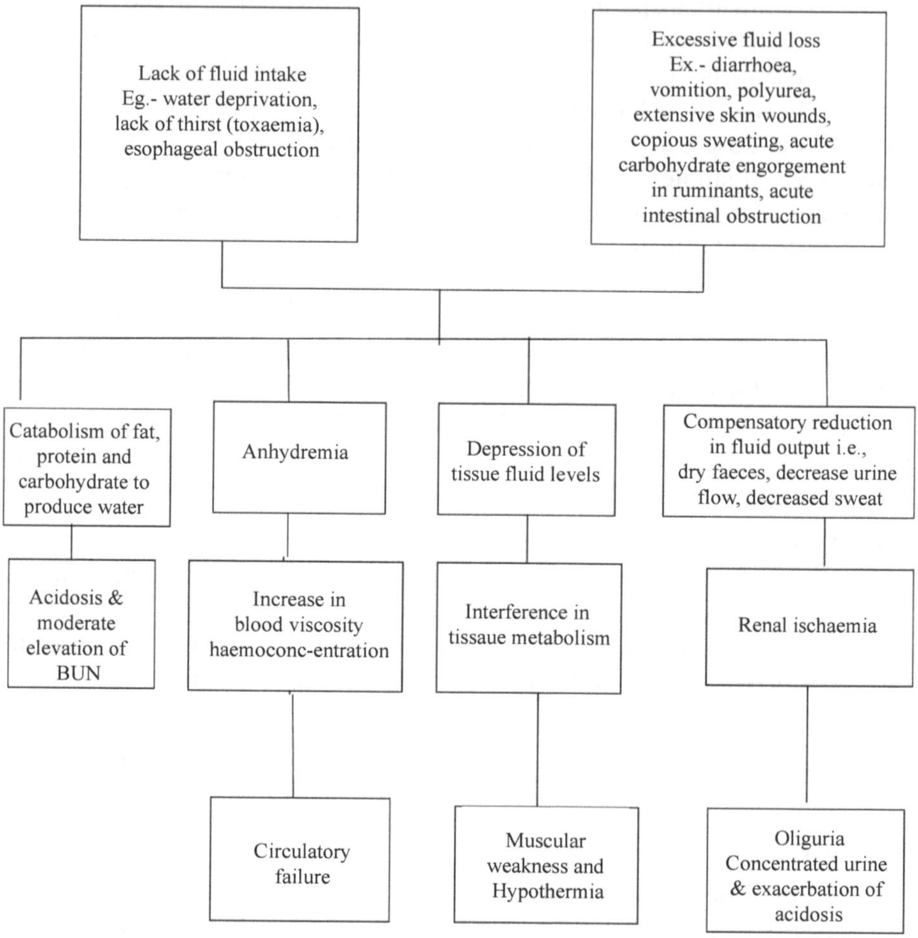

Pathogenesis

- The initial response to negative water balance is the withdrawal of fluid from the tissues in order to maintain the normal blood volume.
- The fluid is drained primarily from the intracellular and interstitial fluid spaces.
- Vital organs including the central nervous system, heart and skeleton contribute a little and the major loss occurs from connective tissue, muscle and skin.
- The loss of fluid from the interstitial and intracellular spaces results in loss of skin elasticity, dryness of the skin and mucosa, and a reduction

and retraction of the eyeball (enophthalmia) due to reduction in the volume of the postorbital fat deposits.

- The secondary response to continued negative water balance is reduction in the fluid content of the blood causing a reduction in circulating blood volume (volume depletion) and an increase in the concentration of the blood (hemoconcentration).
- Hemoconcentration increases the viscosity of the blood, which impedes blood flow and may exacerbate peripheral circulatory failure.
- The loss in circulating blood volume also contributes to the mental depression of dehydrated animals, which is also due to varying degrees of acidosis and toxemia depending on the cause of the dehydration.
- During dehydration, kidneys compensate effectively by decreasing urine output and increasing urine concentration.
- Water is also preserved by reduced faecal output and increased water absorption from gastrointestinal tract which results in dehydration of the contents of the rumen and large intestine and the faeces become dry and scanty.
- Dehydration exerts important effects on tissue metabolism. There is an increase in breakdown of fat, then carbohydrate and finally protein to produce water of metabolism. The increased endogenous metabolism under relatively anaerobic conditions results in the formation of acid metabolites and thus, metabolic acidosis.
- Urine formation decreases because of the restriction of renal blood flow and together with the increased endogenous metabolism, causes a moderate increase in blood levels of non protein nitrogen.
- Dehydration may also cause death, especially in acute intestinal obstruction, vomiting and diarrhoea, but it is mainly a contributory cause of death when combined with other systemic states, such as acidosis, electrolyte imbalances, toxemia and septicemia.

Assessment of dehydration

Body weight loss (%)	Sunken eye & face	Skin fold test persist for (sec)	PCV (%)	Total serum solid (g/l)	Fluid required to replace volume deficit (ml/kg b.wt)
4-6	Barely detectable	-	40-50	70-80	20-25
6-8	+ +	2-4	50	80-90	30-50
8-10	+ + +	6-10	55	90-100	50-80
10-12	+ + + +	20-45	60	120	80-120

Clinical findings

The important clinical findings in dehydration include

- Dryness and wrinkling of the skin
- Shrunken appearance of the eyes. The eyes recede into the sockets
- Skin subsides slowly after being picked up into a fold (skin fold test).
- Rapid loss of body weight
- Muscular weakness
- Inappetence or anorexia
- Decrease in milk yield
- In primary water deprivation, dehydrated animals are very thirsty.
- In dehydration secondary to enteritis, associated with severe inflammation, acidemia and electrolyte imbalance, there may be no desire to drink.
- The best indicator of hydration status in the farm animal is elasticity of the skin of the neck and lateral thorax. This is assessed by pinching the skin between the fingers, rotating the skin fold by 90° and noting the time required after release of the skin fold to disappear (normally < 2 seconds).

Clinical pathology

- Increase in the packed cell volume (PCV)
- Increase in total serum protein which may be modified by the presence of severe enteritis, peritonitis, or proteinuria.

Types of dehydration

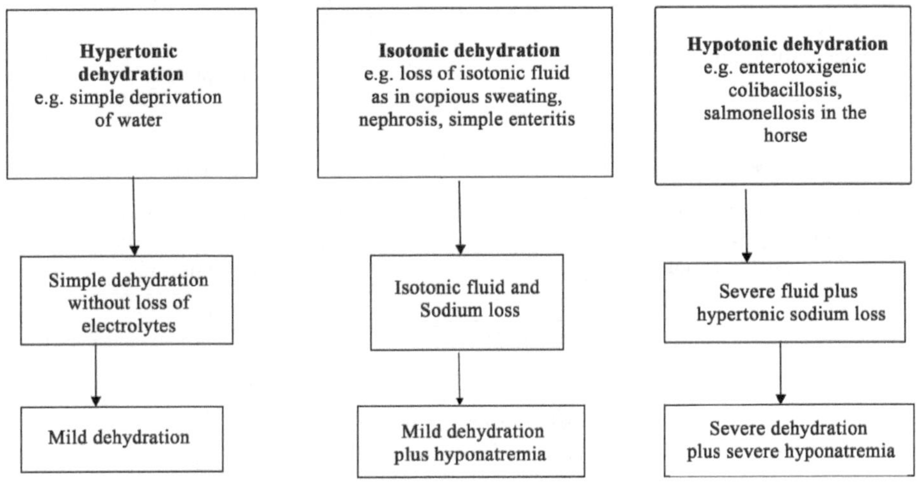

Electrolyte Imbalance

Hyponatremia- abnormally low level of sodium in the blood associated with dehydration

- Sodium is the most abundant ion in the extracellular fluid (E.C.F) and is responsible for the maintenance of osmotic pressure of the extracellular fluid. The most common cause of hyponatremia is increased loss of sodium through the intestinal tract in enteritis, particularly marked in acute diarrhoea.
- In calves with acute diarrhoea due to enterotoxigenic *E. coli* the sodium concentration of the intestinal fluid secreted in response to the enterotoxin is similar to that of plasma, and hyponatremia usually occurs (hypotonic dehydration). Animals affected with diarrhoea for several days continue to loose large quantities of sodium, and the hyponatremia may become severe.

Hyponatremia can become severe when sodium-free water or 5% dextrose used as the only fluid therapy in lready hyponatremic animals. Hyponatremia can also occur in animals with proximal tubular dysfunction.

Etiology and Pathogenesis of Hyponatremia

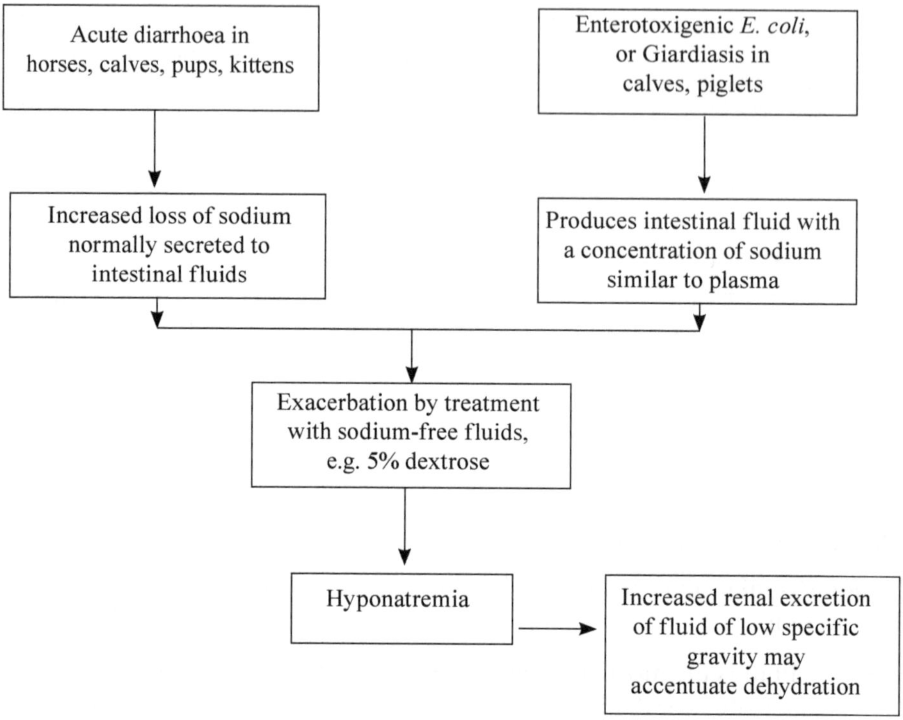

Clinical Findings

- marked dehydration
- hypothermia
- Muscular weakness
- Hyponatremia causes an increase in the renal excretion of water in an attempt to maintain normal osmotic pressure, which results in a decrease in the extra-cellular fluid, leading to a decreased circulating blood volume, hypotension, peripheral circulatory failure and ultimately, renal failure.

Hypochloremia

- Hypochloremia occurs as a result of an increase in the net loss of the chloride electrolyte in the intestinal tract as seem in acute intestinal obstruction, dilatation, enteritis and impaction and volvulus of the abomasum. Normally a large amount of chloride is secreted in the abomasum by the mucosal cells in exchange for bicarbonate, which moves into the plasma.
- The hydrogen, chloride and potassium ions secreted in gastric juice are normally absorbed by the small intestine.
- Failure of abomasal emptying and obstruction of the proximal part of the small intestine will result in the sequestration of large quantities of chloride, hydrogen and potassium ions which leads to a hypochloremic, hypokalemic metabolic alkalosis.
- A severe hypochloremia can be experimentally produced in calves by feeding them a low chloride diet and daily removal of abomasal contents.

Etiology and Pathogenesis of Hypochloremia

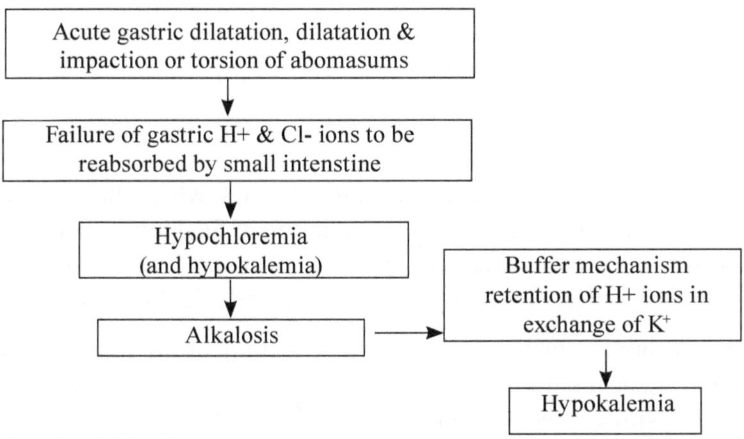

Clinical Findings

- Anorexia
- Weight loss
- Lethargy
- Mild polydipsia
- Polyuria
- A marked metabolic alkalosis with hypokalemia, hyponatremia, azotemia and death.

Etiology & Pathogenesis of hypokalemia

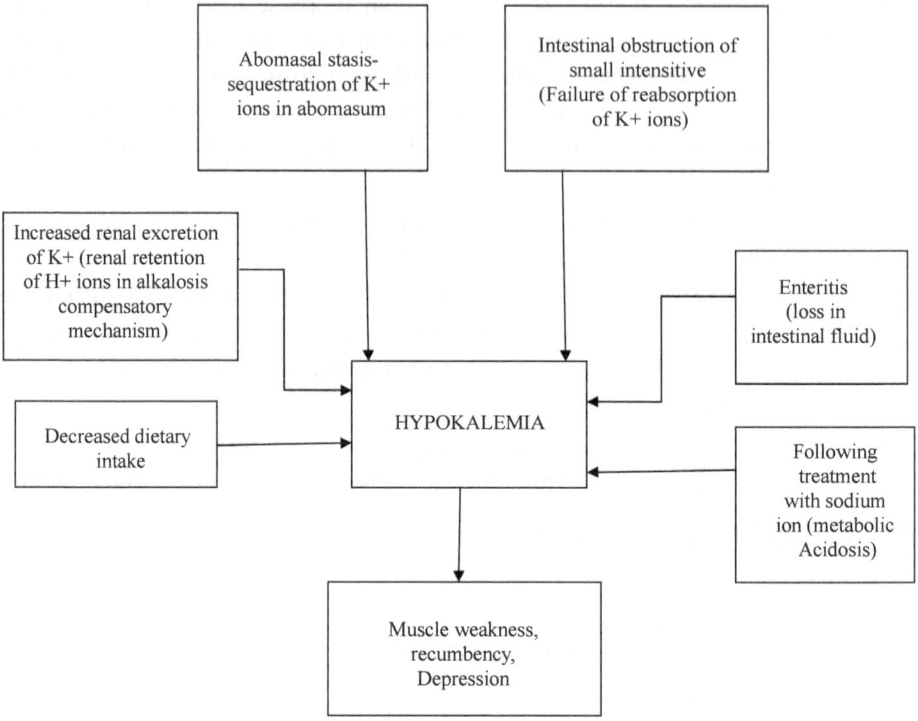

Hypocalcemia- This may occur in recently calved cows which have been anorexic for few days. Also, this can be due to reduction in feed intake because of any illness which may have affected appetite, decreased absorption in diarrhoea it may be the earliest stage of hypocalcemic parturient paresis.

Clinical findings- Anorexia, tachycardia with a reduction in the intensity of the heart sound and occasional arrhythmia, a decrease in the frequency and amplitude of rumen contractions or complete ruminal stasis.

Hypophosphatemia- It also occurs in cattle under conditions similar to those of hypocalcemia. A decrease in feed intake or alimentary tract stasis will result inserum inorganic phosphate cancentration. The condition becomes normal when the feed intake and alimentary tract function are restored to normal.

Acid-Base Imbalance

The pH of the blood is maintained within the normal range of 7.35 – 7.45 by its buffer systems, of which the bicarbonate system is the most important. Any change in the pH may cause alkalosis (increase) or acidosis (decrease).

Acidosis

The general causes of acidosis can be classified into 3 categories on the basis of their pathogenesis.

- Excessive loss of base (bicarbonate)
- Accumulation of endogenous or exogenous acid
- A combination of both processes

Some common specific causes include acute diarrheoa in new born animals, acute enteritis in adult cattle and horses, carbohydrate engorgement in ruminants and horses. Acidosis also occurs where there is retention of carbon dioxide in the blood due to interference with normal respiratory air exchange.

Etiology and Pathogenesis of Acidosis

Alkalosis

It can be caused by an increased absorption of alkali, excessive loss of acid or deficit of carbon dioxide.

Etiology and Pathogenesis of Alkalosis

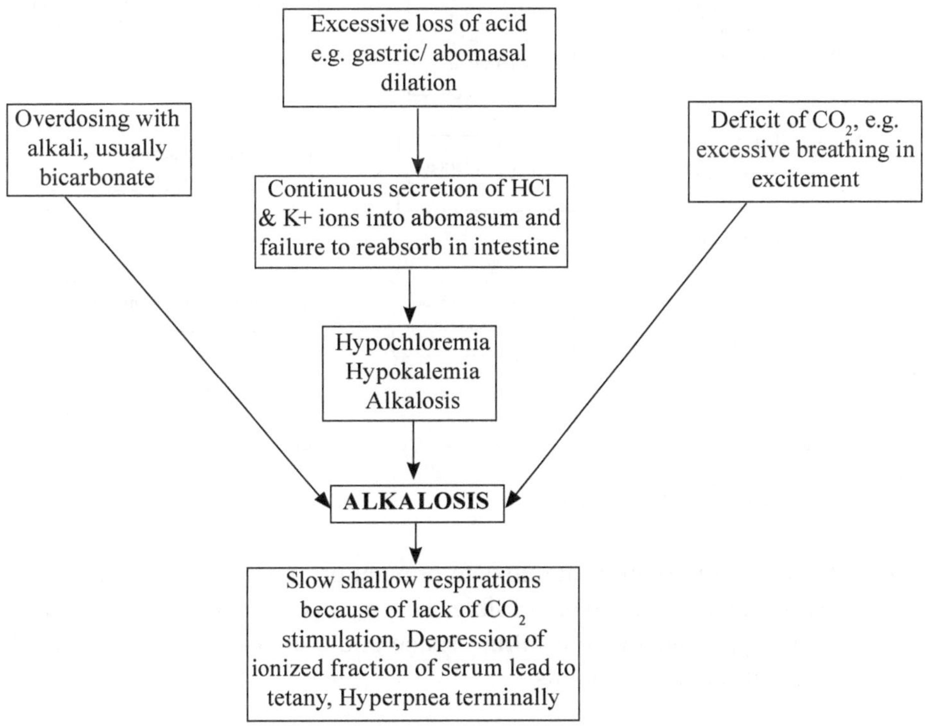

Principles of Fluid and Electrolyte Therapy

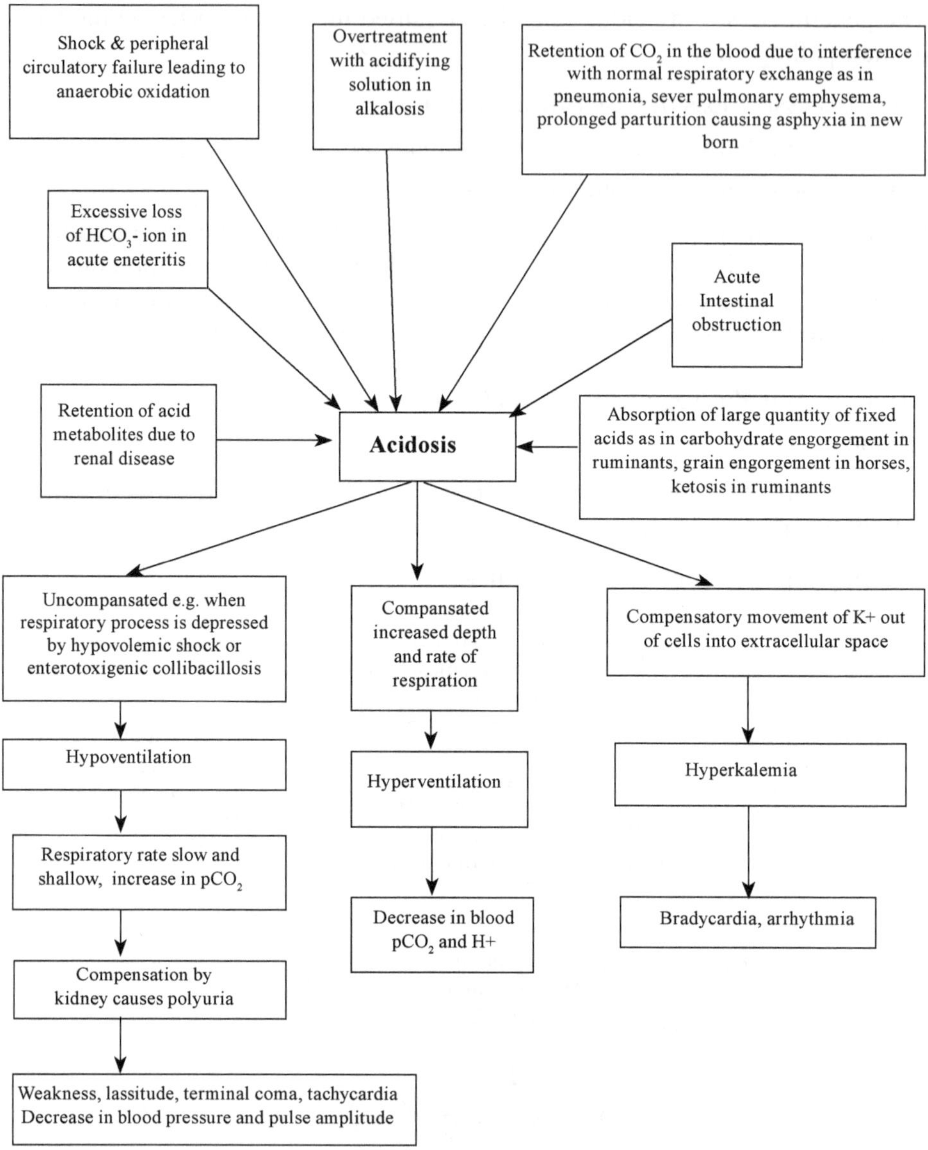

- The most important principle is to prevent or minimize dehydration and electrolyte loss whenever possible. This means the provision of adequate water supply, adequate drinking space and a continuous supply of salt and the necessary minerals.

- The next most important principle is to treat potential losses of fluid and electrolytes as quickly as possible to minimize the degree of dehydration and acid-base imbalance.

Effective Circulating Volume

Effective circulating volume is defined as that part of the extracellular fluid (ECF) that is in the vascular space and effectively perfusing tissues. It varies directly with ECF volume and also with total body sodium, since sodium salts are the primary ECF solute holding water in the extracellular space. Therefore, regulation of sodium balance, by changes in renal sodium ion, and the maintenance of effective circulating volume are closely related.

Plasma Osmolality

Plasma osmolality is a function of the ratio of body solute to body water; it is regulated by changes in water balance. Water intake is derived primarily from three sources: Ingested water, water contained in food, and water produced from oxidation of carbohydrates, proteins, and fats. Water losses occur in the urine and stool, as well as evaporation from the skin and respiratory tract. Alterations in plasma osmolality as little as 1% - 2% are sensed by osmoreceptors in the hypothalamus. These receptors initiate mechanisms that affect water intake (via thirst) and water excretion (via antidiuretic hormone [ADH]) to return plasma osmolality to normal.

Estimation of dehydration percentage based upon physical examination

Estimated Percentage Dehydration	Physical Examination Findings
<5	History of fluid loss but no findings on physical examination
5	Dry oral mucous membranes but no panting or pathological tachycardia
7	Mild to moderate decreased skin turgor, dry oral mucous membranes, slight tachycardia, and normal pulse pressure.
10	Moderate to marked degree of decreased skin turgor, dry oral mucous membranes, tachycardia, and decreased pulse pressure.
12	Marked loss of skin turgor, dry oral mucous membranes, and significant signs of shock.

Calculation of Deficit Volume

Volume of fluid that can be used in replacement therapy of dehydration is calculated taking into consideration the following points

1. Volume for deficit replacement
2. Volume for compensation of counting loss

3. Volume for maintenance requirements
    - The deficit volume is an estimate based on findings from the physical examination or on known changes in body weight.
    - The estimated dehydration is multiplied by the body weight.
    - Also, "Daily maintenance volumes" should also be added to the calculated deficit volume, if the animal is not eating or drinking normally.

Volume of fluid deficit is calculated as = $\frac{\text{Body weight in kg X \% deficit in liters}}{100}$

Normal maintenance requirements in animal is estimated as follows

Small animal : 40ml/kg/day (44-66 ml)

Large animal : 50-100 ml/kg/day

Counting loss is difficult to estimate. Hence a tentative dose shall be = 5ml/kg/hour

Maintenance Volumes for Fluid Therapy

- Maintenance volumes are the normal ongoing losses.
- Ongoing losses are divided into **sensible** and **insensible** losses.
- Sensible losses can be measured and are water losses in the urine and feces.
- Insensible losses are normal but are not easily quantified. Such occur during panting or sweating.
- Generally, one-third of the maintenance volume is made up of the insensible volumes and two-thirds, sensible volumes.

Route of Administration

Route of administration is to be decided depending on the rapidity of loss.

1. In moderate to severe loss, ½ the calculated dose may be given intravenously (first 6 hr) and the remaining givenslowly.
2. In mild loss of fluid, slow rate of administration is followed.
3. If the G.I.T is not affected, oral administration or through stomach tube can check the dehydration.
4. Intraperitonial route is as efficient as intravenous route but hypertonic solution may cause complications (also with subcutaneous route).

Rate of Administration

1. Small animals -90 ml/kg bw/hour intravenously
2. Calves -3-5 lit/hour intravenously
3. Adults 10-12 lit/hour intravenously
4. In severe hypovolumic patients 4 ml./Kg/min for first 20 min and then 20ml/Kg/hr and later 5-10 ml/kg/hr for 24 hrs.

Over hydration- Signs of over hydration are:

- sestlessness
- shivering
- trachycardia
- trachypnoea
- nasal discharge
- vomition
- diarrhoea

5

Body Fluids, Electrolytes and Acid-Base Balance

The two different compartments of the body fluids are extracellular fluid (ECF) and intracellular fluid (ICF) with variation in solute concentrations. The extracellular fluid is the fluid in the cardiovascular system or in between the cells, called interstitial fluid. The fluid present in the gastrointestinal tract or urinary bladder are not included in the either of the fluid compartments. The inter-compartmental distribution of water is maintained by hydrostatic, oncotic, and osmotic forces and the loss of fluid in either of the compartments affects other compartment fluid volume and its composition. The distribution of water in the body and different fluid compartments are given below in a tabular form.

	% of the body weight
Total body water	60
Intracellular water	40
Extracellular water (plasma water + interstitial water)	20
Interstitial water	15
Plasma water	5

Fluid loss: The initial response to negative water balance is withdrawal of fluid from the tissues and the maintenance of normal blood volume. The fluid is drained primarily from the extravascular compartment and the interstitial fluid space. The osmotic pressure of extracellular fluid (ECF) increases with water losses exceeding water intake that activates hypothalamic osmoreceptors and an antidiuretic hormone (ADH) is released from the posterior pituitary gland. Both the increased ECF osmotic pressure and ADH elicit the feeling of thirst. The receptors that elicit thirst have an osmotic threshold higher than the osmoreceptors involved in ADH release. Thus, ADH can act on the kidneys to increase water reabsorption before thirst is elicited. The loss of fluid from these spaces is manifested by loss of skin elasticity, dryness of skin and mucous membranes and reduction and retraction of eyeball (enophthalmia) due to reduction in the volume of postorbital fat deposits. The second outcome of fluid loss is reduced circulating blood volume and an increase in the concentration of blood (hemoconcentration), increased blood osmolarity, sodium, potassium, protein and RBC count, and finally, peripheral circulatory failure. Increased blood level of potassium induces irregularities in heart beat which may lead to death due to heart block.

Electrolyte Imbalance

Most electrolyte imbalances occur due to loss of electrolytes as seen in many disease conditions of digestive system, burns, and excessive salivation and sweating.

Sodium

Serum sodium concentration determines the type of dehydration . Hyponatremia refers to reduced serum sodium level. It is an indication of relatively more loss of sodium than water, whereas hypernatremia is an indication of a relative water deficit. Hypertonic dehydration occurs when water losses exceed the corresponding losses of sodium and potassium. Isotonic dehydration occurs with a balanced loss of water and the electrolytes, and concentration of sodium in ECF remains unchanged.

Hyponatremia is often associated with conditions that cause relatively more sodium depletion. Vomiting, diarrhoea, excessive sweating, blood loss, fluid drainage, gastric reflux and ascites, rupture of urinary bladder, peritonitis, torsion, volvulus of the intestine are associated with hyponatremia. The plasma volume is reduced, and serum sodium concentration decreases due to water retention caused by compensating response of the kidneys. Rupture of the urinary bladder in the neonatal foals is associated with a marked hyponatremia and hypochloremia. Hyponatremia increases the renal excretion of water to maintain the normal osmotic pressure leading to decreased extracellular fluid and circulatory blood volume and manifestation of clinical sings of hypotension, renal failure, peripheral circulatory failure, marked dehydration, polyuria and polydipsia.

Hypernatremia may occur in the initial stages of vomiting, diarrhoea or renal disease when the water loss exceeds the corresponding loss of electrolytes. Food and water deprivation in normal animals is associated with reduced urine and faecal output; but continued cutaneous and respiratory water loss may result in hypernatremia due to only water loss. Hypernatremia also results from administration of hypertonic saline or sodium bicaronate when water intake is restricted. Hypernatremia can also result in case of salt poisoning in cattle.

Chloride

Chloride concentration varies with proportional changes in sodium concentration and inversely with bicarbonate concentration. Acute gastric dilatation, torsion of the abomasum, acute high intestinal obstruction, and failure of reabsorption of H^+ and Cl^- by the intestine are associated with hypochloremia. Hypochloremia alkalosis is a common feature in these digestive troubles and is caused by loss of chloride-rich fluid or its sequestration in the abomasum and rumen. Clinical findings include anorexia, weight loss, lethargy, mild polydipsia and polyuria.

Potassium

Potassium is mainly an intracellular electrolyte and its serum concentration is around 4mEq/l. Altered potassium concentration in serum has a profound muscular effect through change in membrane potential of cell. The decreased serum level, called hypokalemia, results from depletion of the body's potassium stores, redistribution of potassium from the extracellular fluid space into the intracelluler fluid space, or from dietary deficiency. It is mostly seen in vomiting, diarrhoea, vagal indigestion, excessive sweating, and metabolic alkalosis. Administration of insulin or glucose, and rapid administration of sodium bicarbonate in large doses, can result in alkalosis and hypokalaemia.

The metabolic alkalosis and hypokalemia are accompanied by muscular weakness and paradoxic aciduria. Hypokalemia causes excitability of neuromuscular tissues, and resultant muscular weakness. The most prominent signs associated with hypokalemia include muscular weakness, tremors, depression, recumbency, coma and cardiac abnormalities.

Hyperkalemia, increased serum potassium concentration, is a more serious systemic state than hypokalemia. Short-term exercise of horse at high intensity results in marked, but transient hyperkalemia (9-10 mEq/L). It is often associated with a metabolic acidosis, particularly when the acidosis results from volume depletion, and is complicated by renal shutdown. It is usually associated with muscular necrosis,

Acid-Base Homeostasis

The body has excellent homeostatic mechanism to respond to acid-base imbalance as both acids and bases must be regulated to ensure a normal pH. The dynamic regulation of acid-base balance is accomplished through the interaction of the lungs, the kidneys, and the blood buffers. Chemical buffering is almost instantaneous, pulmonary responses occur in minutes, and renal responses are seen in hours to days.

Normal body metabolism tends to result in production of excess acids. Thus, it is important that the body excretes acid at a rate equivalent to its production to maintain pH homeostasis. The lungs and kidneys are responsible for the excretion of excess acids. The lungs excrete volatile acids. The carbonic acid (H_2CO_3) is excreted by the lungs under even ordinary conditions and its concentration is maintained at constant level in the arterial blood. CO_2 is produced continuously in the cells as end-product of aerobic metabolism that diffuses to the systemic circulation where it reacts with water to from carbonic acid. There is a direct, liner relationship between dissolved CO_2 and the concentration of carbonic acid in the blood at normal body temperature. When blood PCO_2 level increases, blood levels of H_2CO_3 increases; thus, PCO_2 can be used as a marker of blood volatile acid level.

Like acids, the bases in the blood stream must also be maintained in a constant balance. The kidney the organ responsible for the regulation of blood bases. The plasma bicarbonate level is the major blood base, which has clinical significance. The HCO_3^- is carefully controlled by the structural and functional unit of kidney, called nephron.

Another important aspect of acid-base homeostasis is the blood buffer system. This important system tends to stabilize the body's pH despite substantial alterations in the concentrations of acids or bases. The buffer may be formed from weak acids and their salts with strong base or from weak bases and their salts with strong acids. The blood has many buffer systems including the bicarbonate buffer system. These buffer systems constitute the first line of defence against abrupt changes in the blood pH. The buffer and its salt are called buffer pair.

Proteins are the most important buffers in the body. They are mainly intracellular and include haemoglobin. The plasma proteins are buffers but the absolute amount is small compared to intracellular protein. Protein molecules possess basic and acidic groups which act as H^+ acceptors or donors, respectively, if H^+ is added or removed. Phosphate buffer ($H_2PO_4^-$: HPO_4^{2-}) is also mainly intracellular. The pK of this system is 6.8, so it is moderately efficient at physiological pH. The concentration of phosphate is low in the extracellular fluid but the phosphate buffer system is an important urinary buffer. H_2CO_3 : HCO_3^- is not an important true buffer system because normal blood pH (7.4) is far from its pK (6.1). H_2CO_3 and HCO_3^- are involved in pH control but they are not acting as a buffer system

Besides metabolic acidosis or alkalosis, ruminants suffer from ruminal acidosis and alkalosis leading to change in the blood pH, subsquent to their absorption. There are alkalizing and acidifying solutions for intravenous administration.

Potassium chloride (1.1%) and sodium bicarbonate (1.3%) solution are used as acidifying and alkalizing solution, respectively in addition to oral drenching of sodium bicarbonate solution or diluted acetic acid to neutralize excess acid or base in the rumen.

Fluid Therapy

Cardiac function, intravascular volume, and vascular tone, integrity, and patency are critical to normal circulation. An abnormality in one or more of these components of circulation leads to compensatory changes to maintain perfusion. The hemodynamic and cellular changes that develop as a result of these abnormalities are called shock. As shock progresses, oxygen and substrate delivery to the tissues becomes insufficient to meet energy requirements for cellular maintenance and repair. If shock progresses and cellular energy demands cannot be met, the ensuing organ failure leads to death. Early recognition of the type and stage of shock is vital to establishing a successful fluid therapy plan.

Shock is typically classified into 3 categories: hypovolemic, cardiogenic, and distributive. Hypovolemic shock develops when there is a blood volume deficit of ≥15%. Cardiogenic shock results when the heart fails as a pump. Common etiologies include pulmonary emboli, cardiac tamponade, valvular insufficiency, cardiomyopathy, and cardiac arrhythmias. Distributive shock is caused by maldistribution of blood flow away from the central circulation as a result of peripheral vasodilation. The different types of shock may have different hemodynamic profiles during the early and middle stages. Frequently, more than one type of shock is present

Changes in fluid and electrolyte balance in response to disease processes may vary widely

- Hypovolemia is common and electrolyte changes are variable. Goal is to correct fluid and electrolyte imbalances before anesthesia, if possible. Many anesthetic agents produce vasodilation and hypotension relative hypovolemia that alterats sympathetic nervous system activity and the endocrine system
- Redistribution of blood flow with changes in vascular resistance
- Reduction in urinary flow rate, renal blood flow, and glomerular filtration rate seen with withholding water (fasting), anesthetic drug effects, and increased ADH levels. These effects can be eliminated or reduced by "filling the tank" with crystalloids.

General Principles of Fluid Administration

Maintenance vs. replacement therapy

- Maintenance fluid therapy is designed to meet the patient's ongoing sensible and insensible fluid losses with normal fluid volume over 1 – 2 days; in the normal animal. This is primarily water loss, with a lesser degree of electrolyte loss.
- Replacement fluid therapy is designed to replenish existing fluid deficits; this usually requires replacement of both water and electrolytes
- The optimal fluid type for each of the above theraptics depends upon serum electrolytes, acid-base status, and concurrent administration of drugs and blood products.

Precautions for rapid fluid administration

- In dogs, maximum fluid administration rate is 90 ml/kg/hr (1 blood volume/hour)
- In cats, maximum fluid administration rate is 60 ml/kg/hr (1 blood volume/hour)
- Cardiopulmonary status should also be monitored carefully during fluid administration.
- Packed cell volume and total plasma protein levels should be monitored to maintain PCV > 20% and TPP > 4 g/dl

Normal fluid administration rates during anesthesia

- Dogs, cats: 10 - 20 ml/kg/hr
- Horses, cattle: 5 - 10 ml/kg/hr

Fluid therapy is used to replenish intravascular volume or interstitial fluid volume, or to correct electrolyte abnormalities. More accuracy is required in formulating the fluid therapy plan for the critically ill than in the usual hospital patients, because the kidneys and cardiovascular system, which can correct most fluid therapy miscalculations, may be in a compromised state. It is important to understand the dynamics between the fluid compartments and the specific components of each fluid to select the best fluid for the individual situation. The volume and rate of administration are guided by pathologic conditions such as cardiac disease, systemic inflammatory response syndrome diseases, fluid loss into the third body fluid space, blood pressure, and pulmonary and cerebral edema.

Fluid Compartment Deficits

Fluid deficit in the intravascular space results in poor perfusion and inadequate tissue oxygenation. This volume deficit results in a lower vessel wall tension and stimulation of the baroreceptors. Physical parameters that reflect perfusion status include heart rate, pulse intensity, capillary refill time, mucous membrane color, and rectal temperature. Fluids administered must remain in the intravascular space, increase the vessel wall tension, and obliterate the need for the baroreceptor compensatory response. Most animals with an intravascular deficit (poor perfusion) also have concurrent extravascular deficits. This warrants the simultaneous administration of crystalloid solutions when colloids are used for correction of the intravascular deficit.

Fluid deficit in the extravascular space (interstitial and intracellular) causes tissue dehydration. This results in tenting of the skin, dry mucous membranes, sunken eyes, and dullness of the cornea. Perfusion parameters should be evaluated simultaneously to determine whether poor perfusion is compounding the dehydration. Crystalloid fluids with the same tonicity as plasma are used to replenish the extravascular spaces. Crystalloids are water-based solutions with low molecular weight molecules that are freely permeable across the capillary membrane. The concentration of these molecules in relation to normal plasma indicates the tonicity of the fluid. The solution is called isotonic if the concentration is similar to normal plasma.

Physical and laboratory parameters are used to quantify the degree of dehydration. Semi-dry oral mucous membranes, normal skin turgor, and eyes maintaining normal moisture indicate 4-5% dehydration. Dry oral mucous membranes, mild loss of skin turgor, and eyes still moist indicate 6-7% dehydration. Dry mucous membranes, considerable loss of skin turgor, and eyes retracted indicate 8-10%. Very dry oral mucous membranes, complete loss of skin turgor, severe retraction of the eyes, dull eyes, and possible alteration of consciousness indicate 12%. dehydration.

The physical guidelines for estimating dehydration are misleading in two common clinical situations. Chronically emaciated animals may have metabolized the fat from around the eyes and the collagen in the skin, resulting in poor skin turgor and sunken eyes despite normal hydration.

Animals with rapid fluid loss into a third body fluid space (a space within the body cavity where fluid from the local interstitial and intravascular spaces leak) have rapid fluid shifts from the intravascular compartments into these spaces before clinical evidence of interstitial fluid loss is seen. Both situations require evaluation of mucous membrane and eye moisture, PCV, and total plasma solids before dehydration can be estimated.

The intravascular space can be replenished using crystalloid solutions alone. However, large quantities of crystalloids may be required to provide volumes sufficient to blunt the baroreceptor response after 1 hr of infusion. The extra interstitial volume for a short period does not cause a problem in most animals, and if renal function is normal, the additional volume is eventually excreted. However, the brain and heart do not have "forgiving" interstitial spaces in disease, and additional interstitial fluid can cause organ failure.

Many conditions can increase capillary permeability and cause systemic inflammation (eg, parvoviral diarrhea, pancreatitis, septic shock, massive trauma, heat stroke, cold exposure, burns, snake bite, and systemic neoplasia). Increased vessel permeability is an additional factor that favors movement of crystalloid fluid from the intravascular space into the interstitial space and complicates maintenance of intravascular volume. A combination of a large molecular weight colloid (to hold the water in the vessels) and crystalloids (to replenish the interstitial spaces) is recommended. In addition, many of these animals have a third body fluid space, most likely due to significant regional inflammation. The end result is massive fluid requirements, which make maintaining fluid balance (especially intravascularly) difficult. It is almost impossible to predict how much fluid will be required to maintain perfusion and hydration in these critical patients. Fluid selection becomes critical, with the rate and volume titrated until the goals of resuscitation have been met (ie, normal heart rate, blood pressure, perfusion parameters).

Three Principles of Fluid Therapy

(1) Replace fluid lost. In practice the problem is usually whether to give saline or dextrose. Most body fluids contain salt but less than plasma.

Features indicating that water (5% dextrose) is needed.

Thirst, Low urine output with high ratio of urine: plasma osmolarity, Dry axilla and groin, raised plasma sodium.

Features indicating that saline is needed:

Fluid lost (excess diuretic, vomit, burns, diarrhoea, sweat), Decrease tissue tugor, postural hypotension, tachycardia, low juglar vein pulse, low urine output, ratio of urine and plasma osmolarity, raised haematocrit.

Features indicating need for another fluid:

If acute blood loss, blood should be trans fuse

If patient is shocked, a 'plasma expander' or 'colloid' is normally given.

(2) Allowance for future abnormal loss. Moderate continuous sweating requires an extra 500 ml of 0.9% saline and 500 ml 5% dextrose per 24 h as does a fever above 39.5 °C.

(3) Maintain normal daily requirements. About 2500 ml fluid containing 100 mmol sodium and 70 mmol potassium per 24 h are required. A good regimen is 2500 ml dextrose-saline with 30 mmol potassium per litre.

Postoperative patients usually need more fluid and more saline.

Patients with heart failure should not be size normal saline. If cntravenous fluids has to be given given 5% dextrose should be adminstered cautiously.

1. Plasma Osmolality

Plasma osmolality is a function of the ratio of plasma solute to water. It is regulated by changes in water balance. Water intake is derived primarily from three sources: Ingested water, water contained in food, and water produced from oxidation of carbohydrates, proteins, and fats. Water losses occur in the urine and stool, as well as evaporation from the skin and respiratory tract. Alterations in plasma osmolality of as little as 1% - 2% are sensed by osmoreceptors in the hypothalamus. These receptors initiate mechanisms that affect water intake (via thirst) and water excretion (via antidiuretic hormone, ADH) to return plasma osmolality to normal.

2. Effective Circulating Volume

Effective circulating volume is defined as that part of the extracellular fluid (ECF) that is in the vascular space and effectively perfusing tissues. It varies directly with ECF volume and also with total body sodium, since sodium salts are the primary ECF solutes holding water in the extracellular space. Therefore, regulation of sodium balance by changes in renal sodium ion, and the maintenance of effective circulating volume, are closely related.

3. Major Effectors of Effective Circulating Volume

Three major effectors altering effective circulating volume: 1) The sympathetic nervous system, 2) angiotensin II, and 3) renal sodium excretion. Volume depletion, sensed by arterial baroreceptors as hypotension, causes an increase in peripheral sympathetic tone. Increased sympathetic tone returns volume to normal by initiating specific compensatory changes. These compensatory changes include the followings:

- Venous constriction: Increased venous return
- Increased myocardial contractibility and heart rate: Increased cardiac output
- Arterial vasoconstriction: Increases systemic vascular resistance and blood pressure

- Increased renin secretion: Increases levels of angiotensin II which is a potent vasoconstrictor
- Increased renal tubular sodium resorption (due to increased levels of angiotensin II and aldosterone)

Sympathetic tone induced changes in effective circulating volume are transient and compensatory; appropriate changes in renal sodium excretion are required to restore normal volume.

4. Body's Main Defense Against Hyperosmolality

The major corrective measures against hyperosmolality (accumulation of excess solute in of body water) is increased thirst. Although the kidney can minimize water losses via the action of ADH, water deficits can be corrected only by increased dietary intake.

5. Hypoosmolality

Hypoosmolality can result from excessive body water retention with subsequent dilution of body solutes or from solute loss in excess of water loss (e.g. diarrhoea). The kidney excretes large volumes of water daily, persistent water retention resulting in hypoosmolality occurs only in the presence of decreased renal water excretion. In patients with normal renal function, hypoosmolality must therefore be due to solute loss in excess of body water loss.

6. Hypovolemia (i.e., dehydration)

Hypovolemia causes an increase in renin secretion. The subsequent increase in angiotensin II causes an increase in blood pressure (as a result of arterial vasoconstriction), as well as renal sodium retention (this is both a direct effect and also the result of increased aldosterone secretion). Water is also retained with sodium retention.

7. Degree of Dehydration in an Animal

Clinical assessment of dehydration is best accomplished by serial body weight monitoring. The physical examination findings often underestimate the degree of dehydration. During the acute phase of volume depletion, these classical physical examination findings are all that are available. The chart below details a general guideline to estimate dehydration percentage.

Table 1: Estimating the percentage dehydration by physical examination findings

Estimated Percentage Dehydration	Physical Examination Findings
<5	History of fluid loss but no findings on physical examination
5	Dry oral mucous membranes but no panting or pathological tachycardia
7	Mild to moderate decreased in skin turgor, dry oral mucous membranes, slight tachycardia, and normal pulse pressure.
10	Moderate to marked degree of decreased skin turgor, dry oral mucous membranes, tachycardia, and decreased pulse pressure.
12	Marked loss of skin turgor, dry oral mucous membranes, and significant signs of **shock**.

8. Fluid Administration Through Subcutaneous route

In mild dehydration, subcutaneous fluids administratin is useful. Isotonic fluids should be used and no more than 5 to 10 ml/lb should be given at each injection site. The rate of subcutaneous fluid flow usually is governed by patient comfort. These fluids are aseptically administered and multiple sites are required to provide adequate fluid volume. Generally, all subcutaneous fluids are resorbed within 6 to 8 hours. The use of intravenous fluids to reestablish peripheral perfusion should be considered if fluids are still noted in subcutaneous after this time.

9. Intraperitoneal Route of Fluid Administration

The intraperitoneal route of fluid administration is quick and easy. The fluids are generally resorbed thus increasing the circulating volume. However, there is potential threat of bacterial peritonitis, perforating viscera, and decreasing ventilation from impeding diaphragmatic excursion. Experience with peritoneal dialysis in dogs has shown that peritoneal fluids often traverse the diaphragm, entering the thoracic space, and further affecting ventilation.

10. Intravenous Fluids Administraton

In general, intravenous fluid administration is indicated in dogs and cats with 7% or greater dehydration. There are numerous potential routes for intravenous fluid administration such on peripheral veins, jugular veins and intraosseous veins.

11. Estimatation of Fluid Volume

The amount of fluid needed for replacement depends on the patient's hydration status and blood volume, restoration of total body water and electrolytes.

12. Phases of Fluid Therapy

- Emergency phase
- Replacement phase
- Maintenance phase

13. Replacement Therapy

The volume of fluid administered during the dehydration phase is based on an assessment of fluid needs for the following:

Returning the patient's status to normal **(deficit volume)**

Replenishing normal ongoing losses (**maintenance volume**)

Replacing continuing abnormal losses **(continuing volume loss)**

14. Deficit Volume Calculation

The deficit volume is an estimate based on findings from the physical examination (Table I) or from known changes in body weight. The estimated dehydration is multiplied by the body weight. It must be remembered that it is difficult to replace all deficits in a 24-hour period. An attempt to do so may result in urinary losses furthering dehydration. Thus, it is recommended that only 75% to 80% of the deficit volume be replaced during the first 24 hours. Also, "daily maintenance volumes" has to be added to your calculated deficit volume if the animal is not eating nor drinking.

Example 1

A 22-lb (10 kg) dog is assessed to have 7% dehydration. What volume of fluid should be given during the first 24 hours?

Total Deficit Replacement Volume = Deficit Volume plus Maintenance Volume

Deficit replacement volume (ml) = % dehydration x body weight (lb) x 454[a] x 0.80

Deficit replacement fluid volume (ml) = 0.07 x 22 lb x 454[a] x 0.80 = 560 ml

a = 454 mls = 1 pound

or

Deficit replacement volume (ml) = % dehydration x body weight (kg) x 1000[b] x 0.80

Deficit replacement fluid volume (ml) = 0.07 x 10 x 1000 x 0.80 = 560ml

b = 1000 ml = 1 kilogram

15. Maintenance volume

Maintenance volume is the amount of fluid required to meet the normal ongoing losses. Ongoing losses are divided into **sensible** and **insensible** losses. Sensible losses can be measured, refers to are water losses in the urine and faeces. Insensible losses are normal but are not easily quantitated. These water losses occur during panting or sweating. One-third of the maintenance volume is made up of the insensibile volumes and two-thirds, sensible volumes.

16. Fluid for Maintenance Volume if the Animal is not Eating nor Drinking?

There is a paucity of data regarding water needs for the dog and cat and many authors recommend dramatically different fluid and energy requirements. Water and energy requirements are numerically the same (1 Kcal of energy = 1 ml of water). Data from recent research has been used to document that energy expenditure or consumption is less than published formulas and recommendations. Estimation of water needs include 50ml/kg/day, 132 kcal X $Kg^{0.75}$, 156 X $Kg^{0.667}$, (30 X kg) + 70, 70 X $Kg^{0.75}$. Indirect calorimetry is being used to estimate energy (and thus water) needs for the dog and cat. These studies reinforce that previously recommended formulae overestimate the energy (water) requirements of the cat and dog.

Example 2

A 22-lb (10 kg) dog is assessed to be 7% dehydrated and has been vomiting. How much fluid should be given during the next 24 hours?

Volume of fluid required = Deficit volume + Maintenance volume

= [0.07 x 22 lb x 454 x 0.80] + [(10 x 30) + 70]

= [560] + [370] = **930 ml**

or = [0.07 x 10 kg x 1000 x 0.80] + [(10 x 30) + 70]

= [560] + [370] = **930 ml**

17. Water Needs in a Sick Animal

The question regarding energy (water) requirements in sick animals continues to elicit controversy. Illnesses, injuries, and surgery results in need for more energy (water). There is mounting evidence in dogs that increased energy requirements are not common in sick or injured dogs. In fact, there are numbers of publications documenting the lower energy (water) requirements for both the normal and sick or traumatized dog. The reserves in injured or sock animals are already minimal and it makes little sense to increase metabolic requirements in order to survive. Sense to conserve available energy and to reduce metabolic (thus energy and water) requirements. Studies on dogs in a critical care unit have documented the presence of significant hypothyroid function. Thus, metabolic requirements are reduced.

18. Continuing Losses

A crude but effective guideline for replacing continuing abnormal losses is to estimate the volume of fluid loss and then double this estimate. The result will be surprisingly close to the actual volume of vomitus, diarrhoea, or urine.

19. Inadequate Fluid Volume

Any acute change in body weight results from losses or gains in water. If the animal is losing body weight while being given crystalloid fluids, the animal is likely receiving inadequate volumes of fluid. If renal function is adequate, a dehydrated animal will have urine specific gravity above 1.025.

20. Overhydration

Classically, pulmonary edema is associated with overhydration. Clinically, pulmonary edema is the terminal event of overhydration. An increased serous nasal discharge, followed by chemosis, and finally pulmonary congestion on ausculation can be noted before plumnaryoedama .

The common parontral crystalloid fluids, their electrolyte composition (m Eq/l), pH, and osmolality

Solution	Na+	K+	Cl-	Ca++	Mg++	Buffer (q/L)	Calories Kcal/L	Osmolality mOsm/L
Dextrose 5% in Water	-	-	-	-	-	-	170	278
Dextrose 2.5% in 0.45% Saline	77	-	77	-	-	-	85	280
Ringer's Lactate Solution	130	4	109	3	-	Lactate 28	9	272
Ringer's Solution	147	4	156	4.5	-	-	-	309
Normosol-R (Multisol-R)	140	5	109	-	3	Acetate 27 Gluconate 23	15	294
Dextrose 5% in Ringer's Lactate	130	4	109	3	-	Lactate 28	179	525
Normal Saline (0.9%)	154	-	154	-	-	-	-	308
Dextrose 50%	-	-	-	-	-	-	1700	2525
Dextrose 5% in Saline (0.9%)	154	-	154	-	-	-	170	-
Potassium Chloride solution	-	2	2	-	-	-	-	-

ii. Colloids

1. General: The term colloids is used to describe fluids that exert oncotic pressure because they contain large particles that cannot leave vascular space. Particle size becomes important if capillaries are leaky as in inflammation or septicemia. If particles leak into interstitium, they take fluid with them that worsen hypovolemia plus cause edema in lungs and peripheral tissues. Synthetic colloids may inhibit coagulation. Hence, it should be used with caution in congestive heart failure and oliguria, where volume expansion may be detrimental.

2. Plasma: Fresh frozen plasma contains all the clotting factors, antithrombin III, a few platelets and alpha-2 macroglobulin as well as albumin. Albumin is the source of oncotic pressure. It is relatively small, 69K Daltons, and can leak from inflamed capillaries.

Plasma transction is a viable choice in inflamation or pancreatitis. It takes 22.5 ml/kg of plasma to raise recipient serum albumin by 5g/L.

3. Hetastarch: Large molecular weight synthetic colloid in 0.9% NaCl

Dose: Cat 5 - 10 ml/kg/day

Dog 20 - 40 ml/kg/day

4. Pentastarch

Dose: Cat 5 – 10 ml/kg/day

Dog 10 – 25 ml/kg/day

Less tissue retention, shorter half-life than HET. More potential for coagulopathy.

5. Dextrans

Dextran 40 MWw - 40K daltons

Dextran 70 MWw - 70K daltons

Dose: Cat 5 – 10 ml/kg/day

Dog 10 – 20 ml/kg/day

21. Hemoglobin Based Solutions

Oxyglobin R: – Long shelf life, typing and cross matching not required. It may improve tissue oxygenation and perfusion (HbO_2 in plasma, dissociates more readily than RBC bound Hb: O_2 at low oxygen tension; low viscosity solution gets to areas of impaired blood flow more readily. Transfeesion many results in discoloration of urine and mucus membranes and alters refractometer reading.

22. Selection of the Parenteral Fluid

In selecting a fluid, it is important to know which electrolytes are lost and the knowledge on the pathophysiology of the disease is essential to institute replacement therapy. The table given below provides an overview of electrolyte changes and replacement recommendations.

	SERUM					
CONDITION	Na^+	Cl^-	K^+	HCO_3^-	Volume	FLUID OF CHOICE
Diarrhoea	D	D	D	D	D	NORMOSOL^R-R + KCl or Lactated Ringer's + KCl
Pyloric obstruction	D	D	D	I	D	0.9% NaCl + KCl
Dehydration	I	I	N	N/D	D	NORMOSOL^R-R + KCl, Lactated Ringer's + KCl, 0.9% NaCl + KCl, 5% dextrose
Congestive heart failure	N/D	N/D	N	N	I	0.45% NaCl + 2.5% dextrose + KCl, 5% dextrose
End-stage liver disease	N/I	N/I	D	D	I	0.45% NaCl + 2.5% dextrose + KCl
Acute renal failure -Oliguria -Polyuria	I D	I D	I N/D	D D	I D	0.9% NaCl, NORMOSOL^R-R + KCl, Lactated Ringer's + KCl,
Chronic renal failure	N/D	N/D	N	D	N/D	NORMOSOL^R-R, Lactated Ringer's solution, 0.9% NaCl
Adrenocortical insufficiency	D	D	I	N/D	D	0.9% NaCl
Diabetic ketoacidosis	D	D	N/D	D	D	0.9% NaCl ($\pm$ KCl)

D-Deficiency / Loss

Intravenous Therapy

Intravenous therapy refers to the administration of liquid substances directly into vein. The word intravenous simply means "within a vein". Therapies administered intravenously are often called specialty pharmaceuticals. It is commonly referred to as a drip because many systems of administration employ a drip chamber, which prevents air entering the blood stream. Compared with other routes of administration, the intravenous route is the fastest way to deliver fluids and medications throughout the body. Some medications, as well as blood transfusions and lethal injections, can only be given intravenously.

Complications

If the cannula is not sited correctly, or the vein is particularly fragile and ruptures, blood may leak into the surrounding tissues. This situation is known as "tissuing" or "blown vein". Using cannula to administer medications cause may extravasation of the drug which can lead to edema, causing pain and tissue damage, and even necrosis depending on the properties medication.

The person attempting to obtain the access must find a new access site proximal to the "blown" area to prevent extravasation of medications through the damaged vein. For this reason it is advisable to place the frost cannula at the most distal at appropriate vein. If a patient needs frequent venous access, the veins may scar and narrow, making any future access extremely difficult or impossible. A peripheral intravenous cannula cannot be left in the vein indefinitely, because of the risk of insertion-site infection leading to phlebitis, cellulitis and sepsis. The US Centers for Disease Control and Prevention updated their guidelines and now advise the cannula need to be replaced every 96 hours. This was based on studies organised to identify causes of Methicillin-resistant *Staphylococcus aureus* (MRSA) infection in hospitals. In the United Kingdom, the UK Department of health published their finding about risk factors associated with increased MRSA infection, now include intravenous cannula, central venous catheters and urinary catheters as the main factors increasing the risk of spreading antibiotic resistant strain bacteria.

Intravenous Drip

An intravenous drip is the continuous infusion of fluids, with or without medications, through an intravenous access device. This may be to correct dehydration or an electrolyte imbalance, to deliver medications, or for blood transfusion.

Intravenous Fluids

There are two types of fluids that are used for intravenous drips; crystalloids and colloids. Crystalloids are aqueous solutions of mineral salts or other water-soluble molecules. Colloids contain larger insoluble molecules, such as gelatin. Blood itself is a colloid. Colloids preserve a high colloid osmotic pressure in the blood. Crystalloids generally are much cheaper than colloids The most commonly used crystalloid fluid is *normal saline*, a solution of sodium chloride at 0.9% concentration, which is close to the concentration in the blood (isotonic). *Ringer's lactate* or *Ringer's acetate* is another isotonic solution often used for large-volume fluid replacement. A solution of 5% dextrose in water, sometimes called D5W, is often used, if the patient is at risk for having low blood sugar or high sodium. The choice of fluids may also depend on the chemical properties of the medications being given. Intravenous fluids must always be sterile.

Composition of common crystalloid solutions

Solution	Other Name	$[Na^+]$ (mmol/L)	$[Cl^-]$ (mmol/L)	[Glucose] (mmol/L)	[Glucose] (mg/dl)
D5W	5% Dextrose	0	0	278	5000
2/3D & 1/3S	3.3% Dextrose / 0.3% saline	51	51	185	3333
Half-normal saline	0.45% NaCl	77	77	0	0
Normal saline	0.9% NaCl	154	154	0	0
Ringer's lactate	Lactated Ringer	130	109	0	0
D5NS	5% Dextrose, Normal Saline	154	154	278	5000

28 mmol/L lactate, 4 mmol/L K^+ and 3 mmol/L Ca^{2+}.

28 mmol/L acetate, 4 mmol/L K^+ and 3 mmol/L Ca^{2+}.

Infusion equipment

A standard intravenous infusion set consists of a pre-filled, sterile container (glass bottle, plastic bottle or plastic bag) of fluids with an attachment that allows the fluid to flow one drop at a time, making it easy to see the flow rate (and also to reduce air bubbles); a long sterile tube with a clamp to regulate or stop the flow; a connector to attach to the access device; and connectors to allow "piggy backing" of another infusion set onto the same line, e.g., adding a dose of antibiotics to a continuous fluid drip.

Oral Fluid Therapy

Whenever possible, the oral route is used to deliver the maintenance requirements. The oral route is preferred for maintenance therapy, provided there are no abnormalities of the digestive tract which interferes with the oral administration or the absorption of fluids. In ruminants such as adult cattle, rumen function must be within normal range for significant absorption of fluids and electrolytes. Oral electrolyte solutions and water should be made available at all times to animals affected with diarrhoea and other diseases in which there are continuous loss of fluid and electrolytes. The provision of water and salt together with glucose and glycine facilitates the absorption of sodium and water in calves with diarrhoea. A wide variety of oral and parental electrolyte replacement solutions are available commercially. Most preparations are made available as powders for mixing with water. They contain sodium, chloride, potassium, glucose and glycine for the correction of dehydration. The glucose and glycine facilitates the absorption of sodium across the mucosa. Oral fluids also contain alkalinizing agents for the correction of acidosis. Bicarbonate is effective immediately but there is speculation that it may interfere with milk clotting in the abomasum which requires an acidic environment for the action of rennin. Some oral electrolyte solutions for diarrheic calves contain citrate, gluconate, acetate or citric acid which when absorbed into the body are metabolized to carbon dioxide and water, and hydrogen ions are consumed in the process. A bicarbonate- rich solution induces the best alkalizing effect and is highly recommended. The use of oral electrolyte solutions without sodium bicarbonate for the treatment of acidosis in diarrhoeic calves may explain the syndrome of acidosis without dehydration. The close relationship between net fluid retention and urine output indicates that urinary excretion may eliminate most of the adminstered fluid and electrolytes in certain circumstances.

6

Diseases of Digestive Systems

The primary function of the digestive system include prehension of food material, its digestion, absorption, excretion of undigested material and maintenance of internal environment. All the these functions are accomplished through the four major functions of the gastrointestinal system.

Motor functions: This function is required for movement of the food material and ingesta and for contraction of the musculature of gastrointestinal tract.

Secretory function: It is responsible for secretion of gastric juice and pancreatic juice

Digestive function: Motor and secretory functions are required to perform the digestive function of alimentary tract.

Absorptive function: Failure of the absorptive function leads to non-absorption of nutrients from the gastrointestinal spinal tract.

Manifestations of Digestive Tract Dysfunction

Abnormality in Prehension, Mastication and Swallowing

Difficulty in prehension is seen in jaw disorder, painful condition of tongue, mal-apposition of teeth and diseases of buccal cavity. Mastication problem is seen in stomatitis, inflammation of mucous membrane. Swallowing disorder is noticed due to foreign body, tumour and inflammation of oesophagus and pharynx, and paralysis of oesophagus.

Drooling of Saliva/ Excessive Salivation

These are seen in cases of salivary gland problem, foot and mouth disease, hyperthermia etc. The drooling of saliva may be local or systemic in origin.

Vomition/ Regurgitation

True vomiting is seen in monogastric animals which is accompanied by retching and coordinated contraction of certain group of muscles. Projectile vomiting occurs due to overloading of stomach with food and water, and the ingesta are ejected out with little effort.

Diarrhoea, Constipation and Scant Faeces

Increased frequency of defecation or fluidity of faeces is called diarrhoea. It is seen in cases of gastrointestinal tract infection, gastroenteritis, and gastrointestinal parasitism. Diarrhoea is generally associated with metabolic acidosis due to loss of bicarbonate. Decreased frequency of defecation and reduced water percentage in the stool is called constipation, and it is associated with difficulty in passage of stool. Scant faeces refer to less quantity of faeces but the consistency is normal.

Paralytic Ileus

Paralysis of gastrointestinal tract is seen in peritonitis, excessive handling during operation, dehydration, acid base imbalance and hypokalemia.

Alimentary Tract Haemorrhage/ Bleeding

Blood in vomitus is called haematemesis, and the presence of digested occult blood in stool is called melena. In melena, the stool colour becomes black. The rupture of blood vessels of GI tract leads to bleeding into the tract and passage of accult (hidden) blood in faeces

Abdominal Pain

In ruminants, abdominal pain is manifested by frequent closing of eye-lid, stamping, looking towards flank, frequent lying down and getting up, frequent bellowing, grinding of teeth. In dogs, abdominal pain is manifested by pressing on ground, frequent lying down and getting up, and animal feels uncomfortable on mild digital pressure.

Tenesmus

Tenesmus refers to persistent straining, may or may not be associated with involvement of gastrointestinal tract. Colitis, coccidiosis, enteritis in calves are the alimentary tract dysfunctions associated with tenesmus.

Shock and Dehydration

Vomtion and diarrhoea are associated with loss of body fluid and electrolyte and imbalance in acid-base equilibrium. The rapid loss of the body fluid may be associated with clinical signs of shrinkage of eye lids, reduced urine output and elasticity of the skin. The loss of fluid to the tune of 10-20% in a short period of time, as seen in acute diarrhoea, may result in hypovolemic shock.

Abdominal distension

This is commonly noticed when there is accumulation of gas, fluid or impacted material in the gastrointestinal tract. Eg. Bloat, impaction of rumen, intestinal tympany.

Complete or partial loss of appetite

Partial loss of appetite (inappetance) or anorexia (complete loss of appetite) is a common sign in many affections of the digestive system. But, this is also seen in fever due to infectious or non-infectious origin.

Diagnosis of GI Tract Disorders

The history of abdominal distension, difficulty in prehension, diarrhoea or constipation, reduced intake of food, pain during mastication, cud drooping etc. give an idea on involvement of gastrointestinal tract disorders. Examination of body parts, particularly mouth, abdomen, per-rectal examination, physical examination such as palpation, percussion and auscultation are then carried out to assess the abnormality. Examination of body fluid such as pH of rumen fluid, biochemical and physical examination of rumen fluid including sediment activity test and cellulose digestion test, medical inaging such as radiography, ultrasonography, and exploratory laparatomy may be conducted to pin-point the disorder.

Diseases of Buccal Cavity

The disease may involve one or more mouth parts such as tongue, palates, gum, teeth, muscles and salivary gland resulting in difficulty in prehension, mastication of the food material and improper buffering of the food with saliva.

Stomatitis

Inflammation of the oral cavity that includes glossitis (tongue), palatitis (palates), gingivitis (gums), is characterized by masking of mouth, painful condition of the oral cavity, difficulty in mastication, and swallowing. Simple inflammation of mouth is frequently met with in horses. Ulcerative or infectious inflammation commonly occurs in young, and occasionally in old, debilitated animals.

Etiology

Non-infectious causes in all species of domestic animals includes

- Trauma caused by physical agents such as injury by sharp objects, chewing and ingesting caustic agents, electrical cords etc.

- Malocclusion of teeth
- Renal failure and associated uremia
- Eating/ drinking of frozen or too hot food/ water
- Chemical agents
- Licking and drinking of irritants, accidental exposure to strong acids and alkali, thallium intoxication in dog and cat
- Immune mediated
- Pemphigus in dogs, lupus erythematosus

Infectious causes of stomatitis

Cattle: FMD, BMC (Bovine malignant catarrhal), BVD (Bovine virus diarrhoea), Actinobacillosis, Actinomycosis, Rhinosporidiosis.

Dogs and cats: Parvo virus Corona virus, leptospirosis, candidiosis, feline viral rhinotracheitis, feline calicivirus, secondary infection to immunosuppression (feline leukemia virus, feline immunodeficiency virus), tooth root abscesses, severe periodontitis, osteomyelitis.

Sheep and Goat: Contagious ecthyma, pox, PPR (Pestes des petit ruminants)

Clinical signs: Stomatitis is associated with partial or complete loss of appetite, painful mastication/ ingestion, empty chewing movements, smacking lips, copious salivation and saliva with blood cells, pus or epithetical tissue, foul and foetid odour from mouth, halitosis, enlargement of local lymphnode, rubbing of mouth against hard objects, frequent movement of jaw, increased desire for water and refusal of animal for examination of the mouth.

Diagnosis: The mouth parts of the animal showing above clinical signs has to be examined for presence of vesicles, ulcers, catarrhal inflammation, erosions and the sings associated with such lesions.

Treatment

Identification of the cause helps in specific treatment of the problem. Non-specific supportive treatment includes avoidance to further exposure to irritant objects, application of antiseptic lotions such as boroglycerine, chlorhexidine, washing with potassium permanganate solution. Systemic antibiotic should be administered in severe cases. Non steroidal anti-inflammatory drugs may be administered to reduce inflammation and pain. Polaprezinc (Chelated form of zinc and L-carnosine) has been found effective in treatment of acetic acid-induced stomatitis and may help in promoting healing of stomatitis in the clinical setting. Animal should be provided with soft palatable diet till recovery.

Diseases of Teeth

Diseases of teeth is characterized by discolouration or deformity of the teeth table, inability to chew, or painful mastication. The causes of teeth disorders may be congenital or acquired as in fluorosis (hydrofluorosis/industrial fluorosis). The teeth colour becomes yellowish and carries, decaying of cement surface appears with chronic exposure to fluoride. Infectious agents like canine distemper in dogs with the enamel formation, and tooth colour becomes dirty yellow. In very young animals, the teeth becomes bluish in colour due to deficiency of calcium.

Teeth disorders are clinically manifested by missing of teeth, presence of damaged, displaced or wearing teeth. There may be malocclusion, presence of foreign body, presence of sharp object between the teeth, discolouration of teeth, and foul smelling from mouth (halitosis).

Diagnosis can be made from history, clinical examination, X-ray examination and clinical pathology. The animal should be treated with the specific drug depending on the cause of the problem. In case of fluorosis in endemic areas, animal should be given chemoprophylactic drug such as aluminium sulphate, calcium carbonate etc. and they should be removed from the affected area after exposure for a certain duration. Antibiotic can be given for 4 to 5 days to check the bacterial growth, and anti-inflammatory should be given to reduce pain.

Diseases of Muzzle

Harelip/ split lip /cleft palate is a hereditary condition, characterized by opening in the hard palate between mouth and nasal cavity, and is associated with difficulty in prehension and mastication of the food material. The disease can be diagnosed by history, clinical signs and physical examination of the patient.

Photosensitization upon exposure to ultraviolet light following ingestion of *Lantana camera* that contain photodynamic substances, is characterized by sever inflammatory changes and the affected area looks reddish purple. The lesions are seen in hairless areas like teat, ear, vulvar region including muzzle. Animal with photosensitized lesions should not be exposed to direct sunlight, and should be treated with antihistamines, liver supporting drugs such as liver tonic, glucose and calcium and antibiotic should be used if the inflamed area has been affected with secondary bacterial infection.

Affections of Gland

Deficiency of vitamin A leads to affection of the salivary gland. Involvement of salivary gland results in the interference with head movement and swallowing process. Affection of glands is treated with antibiotic and anti-inflammatory drug and in case of fistula surgical intervention is required.

Affections of Pharynx

Involvement of pharynx may include inflammation like pharyngitis, pharyngeal obstruction, and pharyngeal paralysis.

Pharyngitis

It is the inflammation of the pharynx caused by infectious agents such as *Actinobacillus* sp. canine distemper, corona virus infection, faulty drenching, ingestion of hot or cold substances, and penetration of the sharp objects. The inflammation of the pharynx is characterized by refusal to take food, painful swallowing, and coughing induction upon external pressure on pharyngeal area, regurgitation of food and water, drooling of saliva, swelling of muscles and lymph nodes. The animal takes a posture with head in an extended position to get relief form pain.

Pharyngeal Obstruction

It may be complete or incomplete depending on the obstructing element. The obstruction may occur due to some fruit, vegetable or bones. Swelling due to actinobacillosis, abscess and chronic growth (polyp) may cause partial or complete obstruction of the pharynx. Appetite remains normal, but it fails to swallow, food comes back to mouth when attempted to swallow. Animal can drink water in case of partial obstruction. Inspiratory noise can be heard on auscultation of pharyngeal region. There may be foul breathe, purulent discharge, laceration of tongue and reduced body condition.

Pharyngeal Paralysis

It may be primary or secondary. Injury to nerve, trauma, encephalitis, central nervous system disorder as seen in rabies may lead to paralysis. The animal has desire to eat but prehension of food and water is not possible and there will be cud dropping. Regurgitation may occur through nostril and there is coughing and aspiration pneumonia and loss of body condition.

Treatment: The underlying cause of pharyngial affections has to be identified for successful treatment. In case of pharyngitis, animal has to be treated with parentral antibiotic along with anti-inflammatory drug. If the cause of pharyngeal paralysis is other than rabies, nervine tonic, a combination vit B1, B6 and B12, should be tried. Pharyngeal obstruction due to food material has to be removed or pushed towards rumen. However, forcible push must not be given as it may result in tearing of the tissue requiring surgical intervention.

Diseases of Oesophagus

Diseases of oesophagus in farm animal practice include oesophagitis, oesophageal diverticulum, oesphagial achalasia and choking. Oesophagitis may result from downward movement of infection from mouth or pharynx. Mechanical causes include drinking of irritant liquid or chemicals. Oesophageal diverticulum is a pocket like structure and an outpouching of mucosa through the muscular layer of the esophagus. It can be asymptomatic or they may cause dysphagia and regurgitation. Diagnosis is made by barium meal contrast radiography. Achalasia is characterised by failure of the smooth muscles of the oesophagus to relax, thus impeding the passage of food from mouth to stomach. Choking is a common accident in cattle and horses. The object may be lodged in pharynx or oesophagus. Greedy eating habits and swallowing foods hastily without proper mixing with saliva result in choke in animals. Cattle frequently become choked on pieces of food as roots and apples that are too large to pass through the oesophagus smoothly. The most common form of choke in horses is seen due to accumulation of dry food in the oesophagus. Animals that have choked should not be given access to feed of any kind to prevent probable aspiration and pneumonia. The administration of drug that stimulates the secretion of saliva such as pilocarpine is a very successful method of relieving the choke in horses and sometimes in cattle.

Simple Indigestion

It is also called mild dietary indigestion, and is mainly seen in adult animals during lactation. Stall fed greedy animals suffer more from such indigestion than animals allowed grazing. It is a minor disturbance in ruminant gastrointestinal function that is seen in cattle, and rarely in sheep and goats.

Etiology: A sudden change in quantity, quality, composition of food or change in feeding time that brings about alteration in ruminal environment can cause simple indigestion. The disease is more common in stall fed animals because of variability in the quality and quantity of their feed. Increase in feed intake especially concentrates beyond the capacity of digestion in dairy animals, and cattle, sheep and goat forced to eat large quantities of poor-quality straw, bedding, or scrub during drought and flood are the common cause of indigestion. Simple indigestion can result from sudden change in the feed, using spoiled or frozen feeds, mouldy feed, introducing urea to a ration, turning cattle on to a lush cereal grain pasture, or introducing feedlot cattle to a high-level grain ration.

The common predisposing factors include supply of less quantity of water for drinking, depraved appetite resulting in intake of inedible things as occurs in phosphorus deficiency, prolonged oral antibiotic administration, ingestion of placenta and allergy. Simple indigestion is primarily ruminal atony. It usually follows a sudden change in pH of the ruminal contents due to excessive fermentation or putrefaction of ingested feed. The simple accumulation of excessive quantities of relatively indigestible feed may physically impair rumen function for 24-48 hr. The primary contraction of the rumen ceases, ruminal flora and fauna are disturbed, and the food does not pass to the next chamber.

Clinical Signs: The signs depend on cause of the disorder. Silage-overfeeding causes anorexia and a moderate drop in production in dairy cattle. There will be cessation of rumination and the left flank may be moderately distended. The rumen is usually full, firm, and doughy on palpation. The primary contractions are almost absent, but secondary contractions may be present. There may be moderate degree of contraction. Temperature, pulse, and respiration are normal. The faeces are normal to firm in consistency but reduced in amount. Recovery is usually spontaneous within 24-48 hr.

Simple indigestion due to excessive feeding of grain results in anorexia and ruminal stasis. The rumen is not necessarily full and may contain excessive fluid. The faeces are usually soft and foul smelling. The affected animal is bright and alert and usually begins to eat within 24 hr. A more severe upset form of ruminal disorder is ruminal acidosis that has been discussed later.

Diagnosis: This is based largely on elimination of other possibilities and a history of a change in the nature or amount of the diet. The disease should be differentiated from following disorders.

Traumatic reticuloperitonitis – There will be systemic reaction and painful responses to deep palpation of the xiphoid. There will be mild temperature, and haematological findings reveal neutrophillia and shift to left. Traumatic pericarditis is manifested by brisket edema and painful walking, particularly on elevated slope.

Ketosis - The history and the absence of ketonuria help to eliminate ketosis, in which case the intake of roughage will be normal.

The possibility of displaced abomasum can be eliminated by auscultation. Vagal indigestion and abomasal torsions become more readily detectable as they progress because they have a longer course, but initial differentiation may be difficult. Grain overload is distinguishable by its greater severity and the pronounced fall in the pH of the rumen contents. In case of bloat, the abdominal swelling will be more intense and there is respiratory distress.

Phytobezoars cause partial or complete anorexia and scant faeces. Per-rectal examination reveals distended loops of intestine and the firm phytobezoar masses are palpable.

Toxaemic diseases: There will be increase in body temperature above the critical limit.

Treatment: Treatment is aimed at correcting the suspected dietary factors. Spontaneous recovery within 24-48 hour is usual. Administration of 20-40 L of warm water or saline via a stomach tube, followed by vigorous kneading of the rumen, may help restore rumen function. Magnesium hydroxide orally seems to be useful when excessive amounts of high-energy feeds have been ingested. If too much urea or protein has been ingested, acetic acid or vinegar may be administered through oral route. If the activity of the ruminal microbes is reduced, administration of 4-8 L of ruminal fluid from a healthy cow will help restoring the rumen function. Besides, other rumenotoric drugs containing probiotic, copper, cobalt, iron, yeast, magnesium oxide and magnesium hydroxide may be administered. The animal should be provided with soft palatable diet

Tympany

It is otherwise known as bloat or hoven. It is classified as primary or secondary, based on its etiology. Continual production of large amount of gas in the rumen through the process of microbial fermentation is a physiological process and they are eructed out. Anything that interferes with eructation leads to over-distension of rumen and reticulum due to accumulation of gas. Such problem is termed as ruminal tympany or bloat. The disorder is perhaps most commonly seen in cattle, but certainly is not uncommon in sheep and goats.

Frothy bloat, otherwise termed as primary tympany, results from failure of eructation mechanism due to trapping of gases of fermentation as stable, persistent foam. As quantities of this foam build up, the rumen becomes progressively distended and bloat occurs. The legumes, such as alfalfa or clover (pasture bloat) are rapidly digested in the rumen, which seems to results in a high concentration of fine particles that trap gas bubbles. Additionally, some of the soluble proteins from such plants may serve as foaming agents that help in trapping of gases inside the bubbles. Also, feeding of a diet with high levels of grain, especially finely grounded (feedlot bloat), undergoes rapid digestion. The abundance of small particles appears to trap gas in bubbles. Some species of rumen bacteria produce an insoluble slime that promotes formation of stable foam.

Free gas bloat, also called secondary tympany, occurs due to failure in eructation process of the free gas produced in the rumen. The obstruction of the esophagus by foreign bodies, abscesses, tumours, or interfere once with rumenoreticular motility as seen in reticular adhesions, damage to motor functioning of the rumen clearly can lead to failure in expulsion of gases. The posture of the ruminant also affects eructation. A ruminant cannot eructate when lying on its back. A cow in a ditch and unable to make itself up right bloats rapidly. Ruminant that has to undergo surgery in dorsal recumbency should be starved for 12 to 24 hours prior to surgery. Otherwise by the time the surgeon is ready to make the incision, the abdomen is already distended.

Regardless of frothy or free gas bloat, distension of the rumen compresses thoracic and abdominal organs. Blood flow in to the abdominal organs is compromised, and pressure on the diaphragm interferes with lung function. The cause of death is usually hypoxia due to respiratory failure.

Clinical Signs: Bloat is an acute disease with a short course in many instance, animals are "found dead". Although it is primarily an acute disorder, chronic, recurrent forms are also seen. The common clinical signs include abdominal distension, and the distension is typically more prominent on left side because of anatomical location of the forestomach. The entire abdomen may become distended with increased in accumulation of gas in the rumen. Animals show reluctance to move and there will be cessation of feeding. Signs of general and respiratory distress such as anxiety, vocalization, rapid breathing, neck extended with protruding tongue are noticed. Respiratory distress and poor oxygenation to tissue may result in staggering. Once an animal with bloat is recumbent, death occurs rapidly due to respiratory failure.

Diagnosis of bloat, irrespective of primary or secondary, is typically straightforward and the clinical picture largely reflects how long the condition has existed. The secondary bloat can be differentiated from the frothy bloat by puncturing a large bore needle or trocar and canula in the paralumbar fossa on the leftside or passing a stomach tube into the rumen through oral cavity,in an attempt to expel the gases from the rumen. Gases come out readily in secondary bloat, whereas lot of froth comes out in primary bloat and expulsion of gases is being hindered by the foams.

Necropsy: The post-mortem examination reveals characteristic lesions, including congestion and haemorrhages in the cranial thorax, neck and head, and compression of the lungs. The pressure from the distended rumen causes congestion and haemorrhage of the esophagus in the neck region, while the esophagus in the thorax remains pale. This demarcation between congestion and pallor seen in the region of the thoracic inlet is called the "bloat line".

Usually, the liver is also pale because of displaced blood and interruption of blood supply. Obvious distension of the rumen is certainly observed in animals that die of bloat. But bloat also occurs rapidly after death from almost any cause in ruminants, and is not a useful diagnostic lesion.

Treatment: Bloat is an emergency problem, and must be relieved with haste. In acute condition, rumen gas should be released immediately by emergency rumenotomy. Insertion of a rumen trocar through the left flank into rumen is sometimes advocated, but usually not very effective unless it has a large bore (i.e. 1 inch), and is often followed by complications such as peritonitis. In less severe cases, a large bore stomach tube should be passed down the esophagus into the rumen. But, passing of stomach tube must not be attempted if rumen is highly inflated and the gas in rumen is seriously compromising the respiration. In such case, an incision should be given in the left flank to relieve pressure immediately. Use of large probang or stomach tube releases the free gas readily, although it may need to be repositioned repeatedly to effectively relieve the pressure. In the case of frothy bloat, antifoaming medications can be delivered directly into the rumen through the tube. The animal should then be closely observed to ensure that the treatment is effective and the animal begins to belch gas, otherwise a rumenotomy may be indicated.

A variety of antifoaming agents have been used to relieve frothy bloat. These include vegetable oils (corn, peanut) or mineral oil (100-300 ml). A number of effective commercial products are available that include agents such as polaxalene (a surfactant) or alcohol ethoxylate (a detergent).

Control

Control of bloat relies on management coupled sometimes with medications, but despite best efforts, it is rarely totally effective. Some of the techniques advocated may be applicable to small herds, but are too labour intensive to use in large herds. Many of the techniques used are based on reducing the rate of fermentation in the rumen. Examples of control strategies include maintaining pastures that have grasses mixed with legumes such as alfalfa, feeding of hay before turning out on bloat-inducing pastures, feeding roughage such as straw or grass hay in addition to concentrate, feeding of cracked or rolled grain rather than finely grounded.

Ruminants allowed grazing in the cities and semi-urban areas ingest polythene bags along with food that chokes the cardiac end of the rumen resulting in chronic secondary tympany. Disposal of polythenes and plastic bags should be proper to avoid ingestion of non-biodegradable materials by the animals. Although not well defined, a genetic component to susceptibility to bloat has been identified, which might be exploited to some extent in reducing herd prevalence of this condition.

Ruminal Acidosis

Ruminal acidosis is caused by ingestion of large quantity of easily fermentable carbohydrate by ruminants, not earlier habituated with such type of diet. The disease is manifested by dehydration, anorexia, diarrhoea, lethargy and neurological signs. It is otherwise termed as D-lactic acidosis, overeating, acute impaction, grain engorgement, grain overload, founder, carbohydrate intoxication and false milk fever etc. The disease is seen both in acute and subacute forms. The subacute form is more common in cows with high level of production as they are to be maintained with high plane of nutrition particularly carbohydrates to meet the energy requirement.

Etiology and pathogenesis: Rumenal acidosis most commonly occus following engorgement of large amounts of starch or other rapidly fermentable carbohydrate. Excessive intake of readily fermentable starch often occurs when animals are first being adapted to a high-concentrate diet, or after accidental ingestion of large quantity of highly fermentable carbohydrate following a period of starvation. The population of Gm +ve bacteria, *Streptococcus bovis* increases following ingestion of large quantity of easily fermentable carbohydrate. This leads to production of more volatile fatty acids (VFA) and lactic acids, thereby reducing the ruminal pH and destruction of cellulolytic bacteria. Finely ground carbohydrate feed exposes large surface area for rapid microbial digestion and acid production leading to fall in rumen pH. Both the acute and chronic forms of the disease are seen depending on kind of food ingested, earlier exposure to that feed, and ruminal environment.

Anaerobic microbes in the rumen and caecum ferment carbohydrates to VFA and lactate. The daily ruminal production of VFA may go above 55 mol. Herbivores absorb these organic acids from the rumen for metabolism by tissues. Abrupt increase in carbohydrate supply following grain engorgement or during adaptation to high-concentrate diets increases the total acid including lactic acid in the rumen. Normally, lactate is present in the digestive tract at only low concentrations, but when carbohydrate supply is increased abruptly, lactate can accumulate, resulting in ruminal lactic acidosis.

Subactue ruminal acidosis is a condition characterised by a rumen pH between 5.0 and 5.5 where the total concentration of short chain fatty acids (SCFA) has been increased, where the ratio between acetic acid, propionic acid and butyric acid has been shifted towards propionic acid and butyric acid, and where accumulated concentrations of lactic acid in the rumen fluid does not exceed

5-10 mmol per litre. The rumen microbial flora is characterised by a dominance of Gram-negative bacteria though the number of Gram-positive bacteria is higher. In contrast, the acute clinical ruminal acidosis is characterised by pH below 5.0, accumulation of lactic acid up to 300 mmol per litre and absence of protozoa (defaunation) in the rumen fluid and the rumen microbial flora is dominated by Gram-positive bacteria.

Rumen fluid osmolality normally ranges from 240 to 265 mOsm/L with roughage diets, and 280 to 300 mOsm/L with concentrate diets. Minerals, VFA, lactate, and glucose are the primary solutes in ruminal fluid those contribute substantially to osmotic pressure. The blood osmotic pressure of 285 to 310 mOsm is maintained by dissolved protein, glucose, BUN and other solutes. Ruminal osmolality may go as high as 515 mOsm in lactic acidosis resulting in water being drawn from the blood vascular system leading to dehydration. Rapid influx of water to neutralize osmotic pressure swells the ruminal papillae and can pull patches of the ruminal epithelium into the rumen by stripping the internal surface layers of the rumen wall from the underlying layers. The damage to the wall of the rumen or small intestine leads to sepsis and liver abscess. Repair of digestive tract leads to thickening of ruminal and reticular wall (hyperkeratosis or parakeratosis) that inhibits rate of VFA absorption for months or years after the damage has occurred. Passage of VFA postruminally for absorption is possible, but abomasal presence of VFA hinders acidification and protein and mineral digestion. Thus, a single bout of non-fatal ruminal acidosis may have prolonged effects.

In reduced ph, fungi such as Mucor, Absidia, Rhizopus etc. multiply and causes mycotic or fungal rumenitis. Acid reaches liver following absorption along with corynebacterium species, Fusobacterium species, and cause hepatic abscess.

As the ruminal pH declines, the amplitude and frequency of rumen contraction decreases and there is ruminal atony at about pH 5. Besides, entry of lactic acid to duodenum exerts a reflex inhibitory action on rumen causing ruminal stasis. Vasoactive substances such as histamine and endotoxins are released during low ruminal pH and alters hemodynamics of peripheral vasculature. These substances cause vasoconstriction and dilation which injures microvasculature. The resultant ischemia causes reduction in oxygen and nutrient supply to the extremities, and physical degradation of junctures between tissues that are structurally critical for locomotion, and animal shows clinical signs of laminitis.

Usually, absorbed lactic acid is buffered by plasma biocarbonate buffering system. The L form of the absorbed lactic acid is being used preferentially, and

D lactic acid accumulates in the body fluid. So the disease is also called D lactic acidosis. The pH of body fluids may or may not be depressed with decreased ruminal pH during acidosis as body fluid pH is buffered by bicarbonate buffering system. Central nervous system function can be disturbed by low bicarbonate concentrations even if blood pH is not depressed. The other clinical signs include anorexia, variable feed intake, diarrhoea, and lethargy.

Type of Acidosis

Depending on the intake of digestible carbohydrate, acidosis is classified in to three different types

i. Acute rumen acidosis (ARA)
ii. Sub – acute rumen acidosis (SARA)
iii. Chronic latent rumen acidosis (CLRA)

Clinical Signs

The affected animals shows signs of anorexia, dullness, ruminal stasis, diarrhoea, nasal discharge, increased heart and respiratory rate, restlessness, lameness, staggering gait, hyperpnoea, abdominal respiration, falling down, grinding of teeth, flank watching, tremor and severe tetanic movement of hind and fore limbs. However, severity of clinical signs starts receding in two days in surviving animals. Subacute ruminal acidosis is manifested by reducing milk production and poor feed digestibility.

Clinical Pathology

Biochemical changes in rumen liquor include decreased pH and increased concentration of lactic acid and TVFA. Changes are most severe between 12 and 72 h after Acceding. The fall in rumen pH is associated with increased production of lactic acid in the rumen due to faster and complete fermentation of starch by amylolytic bacteria in the rumino-reticular compartment. The ruminal pH falls below 5.6 and 5.2, often being used as benchmarks for chronic and acute acidosis, respectively. The blood pH may fall below 7.35. There may be increased liver specific enzymes likes AST, ALT, GGTP and sorbitol dehydrogenase in serum.

Necropsy finding: The visceral organs show congestion. There may be sloughing of epithelial layer from the rumen. Rumenitits and reticulitis are commonly seen and chronic cases of ruminal acidosis are manifested by parakeratosis, liver abscess.

Differential Diagnosis

1. TRP – High rise in temp, leucocytosis, neutrophillia and abducted elbow
2. Milk fever – Hypocalcemia, hotcced mostly withing 72 hours after parturation, starnal or lateral recumbency
3. Nervous form of ketosis, ketone body in urine, sweet smell 4m breathing, mucous coated faeces

Line of Treatment

i. Attempt should be taken to correct ruminal and systemic acidosis. It could be corrected by administration of sodium bicarbonate @ 1-2 gm / kg body weight orally

ii. Systemic acidosis can be rectified by intravenous administration of sodium bicarbonate 7.5% solution, 200-500 ml for adult animal.

iii. Lactic acid production is suppressed by administration of oxytetracycline with equal quantity of distilled water in to rumen.

iv. Antihistaminic drug 10-15 ml forlarge animal and 3-5ml for small animal to be given intramuscularly to suppress elevated histamine level.

v. Corticosteriod like Betamathasone or dexamethasone @ 3-5ml per large animal should be given to prevent shock.

vi. Vitamin B-complex injection should be given to enhance ruminal motility.

vii. Ruminotoric preparation to be given to regain normal micro funna and flora.

viii. Gastric lavage to be performed in acute ruminal acidosis and fresh ruminal cud collected from slaughtered animal may be transplanted to restore ruminal microflora and fauna.

Control: Feeding management can reduce the incidence of acute ruminal acidosis in a dairy farm. The ruminants should not have abrupt change to a concentrate ration to which it does not have prior acquittance.

The goal of producing high milk yields from dairy animals requires feeding of high-energy diets to dairy cattle. The modern dairy cows are able to produce high milk yields, which in turn require an excessively high intake of dry-matter, rich in energy. Therefore, the feeding of rations high in concentrate is necessary. This is, however, predisposes the animals to develop some kind of pathology because of overfeeding. The prevention of SARA can be described by two principles: first, to allow a proper adaptation of the ruminal mucosa in the post-partum period and the microflora in order to absorb and metabolize the high levels of SCFA and secondly, to keep the ruminal pH in physiological ranges in spite of high-energy intake. In other words, the mechanisms applied consist either of prevention of a fermentation disorder or regulation of the fermentation process by direct intervention. The first part can be achieved mainly by management of husbandry practices and feeding, the second is by maintaining fibre-content of the ration within defined borders or adding alkalizing and buffering substances to the ration.

Subacute Ruminal Acidosis

Subacute Ruminal Acidosis (SARA) is a serious common problem in high yielding dairy cows, where the management system has a major focus on higher productivity, and the animals are kept on high plane of nutrition and fed with carbohydrate-rich diet to exploit the production potential of the animals. This a chronic disease and differs from overt cases of ruminal acidosis that occurs following ingestion of highly fermentable and finely grounded carbohydrate ration to which the animal is not earlier accustomed. The later is characterized by signs of anorexia, dullness, nasal discharge, distended abdomen, ruminal stasis, increased respiratory and heart rate, incoordination, blindness, tremor and laminition. Sudden change of feeding to high grain diets in ruminants that are adapted to digest predominantly forage diets, accidental feeding on grain diet in large quantity or overeating following periods of feed deprivation leads to excessive production of lactic acid in rumen, drop in ruminal pH, preferential absorption of D-lactic acidosis and systemic acidosis. Lactic acidosis has severe consequences for the animal is widespread in ruminant production systems and some of the problems associated with lactic acidosis include lameness, polioencephalomalacia, ruminitis, poor immune functions, reduced feed intake, reduced nutrient absorption, liver abscess, grain bloat, clostridial infections, transient diarrhoea, milk fat depression and poor milk production, moderate rumen distension, hemorrhages in lung, and sudden death. In India, 18% cases of anorexia in sheep and goats have been accounted for ruminal acidosis.

Subacute ruminal acidosis (SARA) is a well-recognized digestive disorder in dairy herds with high yielding animals. It is a ruminal fermentation disorder characterized by extended periods of depressed ruminal pH ($\leq$ 5.5). The problem is insidious in nature and more difficult to diagnose. The demand for increased milk production with higher grain and lower fibre diets to maximize energy intake during early lactation leads to drop in ruminal pH. The pH should lie between 6.5 and 6.8 for optimum ruminal fermentation and fibre digestion, and it fluctuates below this level for short periods during the day. The drop in ruminal pH accompanies breakdown of dietary carbohydrates, particularly from cereal grains such as corn and barley. Grains are high in readily fermentable carbohydrates that are rapidly broken down by ruminal bacteria, leading to the production of volatile fatty acids (VFA) and lactic acid. Under normal feeding conditions, VFA are readily absorbed by papillae on the rumen wall. Once absorbed, VFA enter in to the bloodstream and can be used for synthesis of milk constituent. Dairy herds experiencing SARA will have a decreased efficiency of milk production, impaired health and high rates of involuntary culling.

Ruminal pH

The production of acids and inherent buffering capacity of the rumen determines the ruminal pH. In spite of number of complex mechanisms to keep the ruminal pH above the biological threshold of about 5.5 and affected animals' own correcting measure of eating less aftermath of onset of acidosis, the disease continues to be a problem for high yielder on high grain diets. High intake of energy (grain) rich diet in dairy cattle is associated with lowering of ruminal pH. The total daily intake of fermentable carbohydrates depends on total dry matter intake and the density of non-fiber carbohydrates in the diet. This suggests that ruminal acidosis could become an increasing problem with genetic progression aimed at enhancing milk productivity. The better feeding management allows cows to eat more to sustain high level of production.

Ruminal pH varies considerably during the course of a day, and is particularly driven by time and the amount of fermentable carbohydrate meal in each day. As pH drops, lactate-synthesizing bacteria such as *Streptococcus bovis* begin to ferment glucose to lactate instead of VFA. This is a dangerous situation, since lactate has a much lower pK (3.9) than VFA (4.8) and lactate is 5.2 times less dissociated than VFA at pH 5.0. As a result, lactate stays in the rumen longer and contributes to the downward fall in ruminal pH. But, the problem of drop in ruminal pH cannot be solved by frequent feeding of the animals as repeated feedings enhance the total quantity of dry matter intake.

Ruminants possess highly developed mechanisms to maintain ruminal pH within a physiological range from 5.5 to 7. The low ruminal pH that follows intake of large amount of fermentable carbohydrate may be associated with increased osmolarity of the ruminal contents inhibiting the feed intake, the first response after drop in ruminal pH. Ruminants possess a complex system for buffering the organic acids in the rumen, though the buffering is relatively too small. Saliva produces large amount of buffer that contains sodium, potassium, bicarbonates and phosphates and is secreted during the chewing activity. Thus, fiber content of the feed increases saliva secretion as it enhances the chewing activity. However, saliva secretion is not influenced by the lowered ruminal pH. The ability of the rumen to rapidly absorb the organic acids from the rumen contributes greatly to the stability of the ruminal pH. The passive absorption of VFA across the ruminal wall is enhanced by finger-like papillae that provide huge surface area. Ruminal papillae increase in length when cattle are fed high grain diets. This presumably increases the surface area and absorptive capacity that protect the animals from acid accumulation in the rumen. Thus, large dietary changes may not affect the mean ruminal pH but lowest pH level is greatly influenced.

Genesis of SARA

SARA develops when the ruminal pH drops below the physiological threshold of about 5.5 for a protracted period. Lactic acid in the rumen is rarely the cause of depressed pH in the rumen in SARA unlike acute acidosis. It results from excessive VFA production that exceeds the ability of the ruminal papillae to absorb them. Abrupt change from high fibre diets to high concentrate does not allow ruminal bacteria and ruminal papillae adequate time to adjust, thereby leading to the rapid production and accumulation of VFA. Too small particle size of the feed is another cause of SARA as this suppresses rumination and the production of saliva that helps in buffering the rumen pH.

Severe grain-induced SARA is dominated by *Streptococcus bovis* and *Escherichia coli*, whereas mild grain-induced SARA was dominated by *Megasphaera elsdenii,* and alfalfa pellet-induced SARA is dominated by *Pasteurella albensis*. The severity of SARA and degree of inflammation are highly correlated with the abundance of *E. coli* and not with lipopolysaccharide in the rumen. Periodic abundance of available starch allows amylolytic bacteria (e.g., *Ruminobacter amylophilus*, *Streptococcus bovis*, *Lactobacillus* spp.) to proliferate and produce excessive quantities of fermentation acids. Unfortunately, gains in VFA absorption at ruminal pH below 5.5 can be offset by lactate production. As pH drops, *Streptococcus bovis* begins to ferment glucose to lactate instead of VFA. At ruminal pH of 5.0, lactate is 5.2 times less dissociated than VFA, as a result lactate stays in the rumen and contributes to further fall in ruminal pH. This leads to acute ruminal acidosis. Ruminal acidosis is known to be related to diseases such as rumenitis, rumen parakeratosis, liver abscesses (LAs), laminitis and bloat. Laminitis in cattle has been linked to nutrition, specifically in acute acidosis and SARA. Although the exact relationship between SARA and laminitis is not known, one of the theories relates SARA-induced damage to the ruminal epithelium, allowing absorption of histamine and endotoxins. These chemicals and possibly other compounds disrupt normal circulation and cause inflammation within the hoof, leading to the condition commonly referred to as laminitis. A mild episode of SARA does not affect ruminal, epithelial barrier function immediately after the episode but a rapid and more severe acidification (pH 5.2) *in vitro* increases epithelial permeability following the insult.

The periparturient cows are at risk of subacute ruminal acidosis because of the time required for the rumen microflora and papillae to adapt to increased intake of concentrates immediately before parturition and during early lactation when feed intake increases rapidly to meet the energy needs of high-producing dairy cows. The adaptation of the ruminal microflora and papillae from a system appropriate for forage to a system capable of utilizing high-energy lactation rations requires a gradual change over a period of 4-6 wk. Therefore, any increase in energy intake before parturition should take in to account the period of time required for adaptation of the rumen epithelium to dietary changes. Further, cows become more prone to acidosis over time even though intake of grain is decreased to avoid acidosis. The severity of each subsequent bout of acidosis increases, especially for cows fed diets low in physically effective fiber and at high risk of acidosis. Therefore, a bout of acidosis that occurs due to improper feed delivery or poor diet formulation can have long-term consequences on cow health and productivity.

Sings and Diagnosis of SARA

Ruminants suffering from SARA do not exhibit overt clinical signs. However, the consequence of SARA is complex and diverse. The major sign is reduced feed intake. Decreased feed consumption or reduced digestibility of grain also confuse for diagnosis of SARA. On the other hand, interruption in normal consumption pattern also precipitates acidosis. Other signs include lethargy, diarrhoea, appearance of undigested grain in the faeces, foamy faeces containing gas bubbles, excessive salivation, panting, kicking at the belly and general signs of discomfort and stress. The secondary signs in chronic cases of SARA include episodes of laminitis, weight loss, poor body conditions despite adequate energy intake and unexplained abscess. The inflammation and abscess throughout the ruminant's body may occur due to the negative impact of organic acids on the ruminal wall leading to parakeratosis enabling translocation of pathogens in to the blood stream. Thus, SARA should be investigated, if secondary sings are occurring for no apparent reasons. In order to achieve proper diagnosis, SARA has to be considered as herd management problem. Screening of the herd for SARA by rumenocentesis, performed on a sample group, preferably on 12 individuals, may reveal the presence of SARA. The herd screening should include the suspected risk group. Rumenocentesis for diagnosis os SARA may be ethically questionable but the technique remains the most reliable means of diagnosing SARA.

Effects on Production

Milk fat depression is a major sign of SARA and is caused by incomplete saturation of fatty acids within the rumen. Incompletely saturated fatty acids (particularly certain *trans* forms) are potent inhibitors of milk fat synthesis in mammary gland. Feeding high levels of unsaturated fatty acids increases the *trans* fatty acid uptake from the rumen. Ruminal acidosis may also facilitate *trans* fatty acid uptake from the rumen, perhaps by inhibiting certain bacteria, which are normally responsible for biohydrogenation in the rumen.

Consequences of SARA include depression in feed intake, reduced fiber digestion, milk fat depression, diarrhoea, laminitis, liver abscesses, increased production of bacterial endotoxin and inflammation, characterized by increases in acute phase proteins. Presumably, heightened volatile fatty acid production stimulates satiety receptors in cattle, which in turn results in the commonly observed "off-feed" or low intake syndrome. Rumen digestion of neutral detergent fibre (NDF) from grass hay, legume hay and corn silage decreases in animals suffering from SARA. In addendum, dietary neutral detergent fibre (NDF) content higher than 33.8% of DM had lower ($P < 0.01$) fecal endotoxin than those with a dietary NDF content lower than 33.8% of DM. Poor feed digestibility and absorption also lead to reduced production. The associated secondary problems are also responsible for poor production performance of the animals.

Public Health Concern

Ruminal acidosis can have direct public health concern. Low ruminal and intestinal pH due to high grain diet have been reported to increase the risk of shedding enterohemorrhagic *E. coli*. It has been established that switching cattle to a high forage diet just prior to slaughter decreases such shedding.

Management of SARA

Monensin either as controlled release capsule or premix was tried for attenuation of SARA in Holstein cows. Neither of them had effect on ruminal VFA concentration but reduces the acetate and propionate ratio. Monensin-premix treated cows produce more milk as a result of higher dry-matter intake but with reduced milk fat content. Similarly, supplementing the diet with direct-fed microbials that enhance lactate utilizers in the rumen may reduce the risk of SARA. Yeasts, Propionobacteria, Lactobacilli and Enterococci have been used for enhancing lactate utilization.

The risk of developing SARA can be reduced by adopting a feeding regime, which balances ruminal buffering with the production of volatile fatty acids from fermentation of carbohydrates. This can be accomplished by feedstuff selection and/or by the addition of dietary buffers such as sodium bicarbonate or potassium carbonate. Cows do not prefer voluntary intake sodium bicarbonate to attenuate SARA. Therefore, adjustments of suboptimal feeding and management routines are believed to be essential prophylactic steps. It is recommended to avoid the following events to minimize the risk of SARA, 1) a daily mean ruminal pH lower than 6.16, and 2) a time period in which ruminal pH is <5.8 for more than 5.24 hr/day. Thus, the key aspect of SARA prevention is careful control of the intake of rapidly fermentable carbohydrates. This is accomplished by providing adequate chemical fibre, processing grains properly, including high fibre concentrates as needed and offering feed to cows in a manner that allows them to consume small, frequent meals on a regular basis. Feed additives and supplements can provide an additional margin of safety for preventing SARA.

Cows receiving the MFC (medium concentrate: forage) treatment have lower daily mean ruminal pH (below 6·0) for a longer duration compared with the HFC (high forage: concentrate) diet. Additionally, cows receiving the MFC diet have a greater reduction in milk fat concentration (g/100 g FA) of FA C16 (17 vs. 9%), trans-10 18:1 (159 vs. 21%) and trans-9, cis-11 conjugated linoleic acid compared with cows receiving the HFC diet.

Increasing dietary cation and anion difference (DCAD) increases urine pH and modifies the urinary excretion of minerals. With low DCAD, 70% of Cl and only 16% of Na are excreted in urine whereas with high DCAD, 33% of Cl and 53% of Na are excreted. Increasing DCAD allows cows to increase dry matter intake because of the ability of positive DCAD to maintain blood acid-base status. A localized rumen buffering effect could not be excluded and could be linked with a higher amount of HCO_3 recycled into the rumen. Main mechanisms involved in regulating blood pH might be renal excretion of protons and strong ions and renal HCO_3 reabsorption. Dietary supplementation with acarbose in dairy cattle fed high-production rations may be effective in reducing the time for which rumen pH is suboptimal, with no negative effects on ruminal fermentation and blood metabolites.

Supplementing feed of the dairy cows with active dry yeast increases the mean, minimum and maximum ruminal pH; decreases time spent in subacute rumen acidosis, and decreases total VFA concentration in the rumen.

Conclusion

SARA is a major production limiting health problem in dairy cattle, expected to produce more with feeding of larger quantity of highly fermentable carbohydrates. Milk production may increase temporarily by over-feeding of grain. However, the long-term health effects due to development of SARA and its economic consequences may become quiet frustrating. The prevention of SARA includes the establishment of feeding and management guidelines designed to minimize rumen acid load. Limiting the intake of rapidly fermentable carbohydrates, providing adequate ruminal buffering and allowing the ruminal adoption to high grain diet are the basic principles of preventing SARA. Regular monitoring may facilitate early recognition of the condition and limit economic losses. Some degree of SARA may be inevitable, and presents a challenge to the dairy industry as consumers become increasingly concerned about the welfare of production animals.

Vagus Indigestion

The lesion on the vagal nerve, possibly due to traumatic reticuloperitonitis, leads to distension of rumen, reticulum and abomasums, and is characterized by diminished appetite, decreased ruminal contraction, gradual reduction in milk production, and scanty and sticky faeces, and papple shaped abdomen. However, vagal nerve lesions are not noticed in all cases in post-mortem examination. Affection of dorsal part of the vagal nerve hinders passage of food from rumen and reticulum; whereas affection of ventral part does not allow food to pass beyond abomasum.

Etiology and Pathogenesis

Injury, inflammation, or pressure on the vagal nerve or mechanical obstruction of the cardia or reticulo-omasal orifice (eg, papillomas or ingested placenta) results in ruminoreticular distention syndrome leading to distension of the rumen, reticulum and abomasum. There are 4 types of vagal indigestion based on the site of the functional obstruction. Type I vagal indigestion, or failure of eructation, results in free-gas bloat, and occurs most commonly due to inflammatory lesions in the vicinity of the vagus nerve, such as localized peritonitis, adhesions (a sequelae of traumatic reticuloperitonitis), or chronic pneumonia. Less common causes include pharyngeal trauma, which affects a more proximal part of the vagus nerve, and esophageal compression by abscesses or neoplasia, such as lymphosarcoma. Type II vagal indigestion, or failure of omasal transport, develops as a result of any condition that prevents ingesta from passing through the omasal canal into the abomasum. Adhesions and abscesses (reticular or single liver abscesses) are the most common causes.

They are usually seen on the right or medial wall of the reticulum near the route of the vagus nerve. Reticular abscesses and adhesions are almost invariably due to traumatic reticuloperitonitis. Mechanical obstruction of the omasal canal by ingested material (eg, placenta) or masses (eg, lymphosarcoma, squamous cell carcinoma, granulomas, or papillomas) can also cause chronic ruminoreticular distention due to failure of omasal transport. Type III vagal indigestion is abomasal impaction that develops due to feeding of dry, coarse roughage, such as straw, in a chopped or ground form with restricted access to water, usually during extremely cold environmental temperature. Vagal indigestion can develop in cattle after abomasal volvulus without abomasal impaction. Type IV vagal indigestion, or partial forestomach obstruction, is poorly defined, and develops in cattle during gestation. It may be related to the enlarging uterus shifting the abomasum to a more cranial position, which inhibits normal motility.

Clinical signs

There is a gradual development of ruminoreticular and abdominal distension over a period of days to weeks. Distention of the dorsal and ventral sacs of the rumen results in an "L-shaped" rumen on per rectal examination. Left dorsal and left and right ventral distention of the abdomen causes a "papple" (pear plus apple) shape of the rumen. There will be reduced appetite, gradual loss of milk production, fecal output is reduced, faeces becomes scant and sticky, and often contains long hay particles.

The strength of rumen contractions is decreased, but the motility may be increased. Ruminal contraction sounds are not audible as contents become frothy due to the prolonged contractions and failure of the rumen to empty. Temperature and respiration rate are usually normal. In some cases, there will be decreased heart rate. Tachycardia develops as the disease progresses. In chronic cases, the animal develops a rough hair coat, loses condition, and becomes weak, dehydrated and recumbent.

Per rectal examination reveals distended rumen filled with gas or froth.

Clinical Pathology

Hematologic examination may reveal increased PCV suggesting dehydration, or decreased PCV because of bone marrow depression. Lymphocytosis can be seen in vagal indigestion due to lymphosarcoma. Leukopenia may be present with diffuse peritonitis. Increased serum globulin and total protein can be seen with abscesses.

Vagal ingestion causes hypochloric, hypokalemic metabolic alkalosis. Low chloride indicates reflux of chloride from the abomasum into the rumen and obstruction at the level of the abomasum. The chloride levels of the rumen fluid may be increased. Metabolic alkalosis is typically present if serum chloride is decreased. The chloride is usually normal if the lesion is cranial to the abomasum. Potassium is usually low due to decreased potassium intake in the feed.

Diagnosis

The subacute to chronic ruminoreticular and abdominal distension creates suspicion for vagal indigestion. This is associated with change in abdominal Silhousette and L-shaped rumen on per rectal examination. Vagal indigestion is a subacute to chronic disease and must not be confused with acute ruminal tympany. Other causes of abdominal distention, such as ascites and uterine enlargement can almost invariably be ruled out by rectal palpation due to the absence of ruminoreticular distension. Occasional cases of longstanding obstruction of the cecum or small intestine can cause severe ruminoreticular and abdominal distension and can be differentiated by per-rectal examination of palpable enlarged caecum or small intestine. Diagnosing the specific cause of vagal indigestion is more difficult but is important because of differences in treatment and prognosis. Physical examination, rectal examination, blood cell count, blood acid-base determination, and serum chemistry values are often useful. Peritoneal fluid analysis can support the diagnosis of peritonitis if total protein or nucleated cells are increased. Radiographs of the reticulum should be taken to identify a radiopaque linear foreign body (eg, wire) or reticular abscess. Definitive diagnosis often requires exploratory surgery. The prognosis of the disease is unfavourable or unpredictable.

Treatment

Medical management alone is almost ineffective. A left paralumbar fossa laparotomy and rumenotomy provides the opportunity for definitive treatment in some cases. Emptying the rumen at the time of surgery may help restore normal rumen motility. Stimulation of low-threshold tension receptors in the reticulum occurs under normal circumstances and causes reflex reticulo-ruminal contractions. However, severe distension causes stimulation of high-threshold receptors that have the opposite effect and inhibit contractions. Ruminal lavage may help in removal of the rumen content, thus reducing abdominal distension, thus reducing abdominal distension.

Supportive or symptomatic therapy should be provided in all cases, which typically involves correcting dehydration as well as calcium and electrolyte deficits, commonly with oral fluids and electrolytes. The affected ruminant may be treated with 20L of Dextrose saline for three days. Laxative may be given for 5 days in cases of impaction. Prokinetic drugs such as metaclopromide injection may be administered.

Control

The most common cause of vagal indigestion is traumatic reticuloperitonitis, which causes adhesions and abscesses that interfere with vagal nerve function. Therefore, prevention of traumatic reticuloperitonitis is important. Good management practices will prevent some cases of vagal indigestion resulting from chronic pneumonia. Early diagnosis of right-sided abomasal displacements and abomasal volvulus, and prompt surgical correction may prevent some cases. Prompt removal of the placenta from the cow's enclosure after parturition will prevent the ingestion of placente by the animal and there by poeventing the obstruction of cardia, reticulo-omasal orifice, or pylorus.

Traumatic Reticuloperitonitis

This is the inflammatory condition of the reticulum and peritoneum due to piercing of the sharp foreign body into the reticular wall. Such clinical condition may result without complete perforation of the reticular wall. The common sequelae of traumatic reticuloperitonitis (TRP) include acute local peritonitis, acute diffuse peritonitis, or acute pericarditis. Either of these results following perforation of the reticular wall by the sharp foreign objects such as needle, nail etc, allocoing the reticular contents to come out and infect the surrounding. Chronic local peritonitis may result in vagus indigestion or diaphragmatic hernia. Acute pericarditis may lead to chronic pericarditis or death due to congestive heart failure. Uncommon sequelae include rupture of left gastroepiploic artery or rupture of coronary artery causing internal bleeding, cardiac temponade and death.

Clinical Signs

Acute local peritonitis is manifested by grunting while walking down hill, rigidity of back muscles called tucked up, recumbency and inability to rise, and acute abdominal pain. In case of chronic local peritonitis, the pain is not evident although gait is slow and careful. Chronic or moderate bloat may be present. Acute diffuse peritonitis is associated with cessation of alimentary tract movement, and increased pulse rate.

Clinical Pathology

Traumatic retiucloperitonitis is associated with leucocytosis and neutrophilia with shift to left. The neutrophil count may go as high as 95%. The chronic diffuse peritonitis is associated with leukopenia due to associated toxaemia.

Diagnosis: The sudden onset of grunting pain, ruminal stasis, complete anorexia, severe pain on palpation of ventral abdomen, moderate degree of fever, leukocytosis and fall in milk yield arouse suspicion for traumatic reticuloperitonitis. Bamboo test, sharp lifiting of bamboo on either side just behind xploid cartilage elicits sharp pain, is used to diagnose of traumatic retiucloperitonitis.

Treatment: The animal should be allowed to stand on an elevated floor so that the sharp foreign body does not pierce further and perforate the reticular wall. Anti-inflammatory and antibiotic or sulfonamide should be administered for healing of the inflammed area. Magnet feeding should be practised in order to restrict the sheep foreign object within the reticulum & preventing from penetration into the reticular wall, these reducing the incidences of TRP.

Traumatic Pericarditis

Perforation of pericardial sac by sharp material coming from the reticulum through the reticular wall causes inflammatory condition of the pericardium. The problem is mostly seen during advance pregnancy during last trimester of pregnancy or at parturition, due to pressure on pericardium.

Clinical Signs

Engorment of jugular vein, swollen ventral abdomen, easily palpable jugular pulse, pericardial friction rubs that increases or decreases with respect to respiratory sound are the commonly seen clinical signs in affected animal. Heart sound is muffled i.e. not clearly audible, and there will be dyspnoea, depression, diarrhoea, and anorexia. In some cases, acute condition may turn to chronic.

Diagnosis can be made from the clinical signs and the history of traumatic reticuloperitonitis. Metal detector test can diagnose the problem if the foreign body is metallic. Differential count shows increased neutrophil with shift to left with increased total leukocyte count. Bamboo test/ Fist test elicit pain reflexes. The prognosis is generally unfavourable.

Treatment

Antibiotic should be administered for 5 to 7 days. Anti-inflammatory preferably non-steroidal drug should be administered in non-pregnant animals. Diuretics should be given to reduce oedema. Vitamin B complex should be administered to improve general health condition of the animal. Dextrose (40ml/Kg body weight), around 12L in adult animal may be administered. Avoiding ingestion of metals can reduce the incidence of the problem.

Diaphragmatic Hernia

Diaphragmatic hernia is the protrusion of reticulum and rumen through a rupture of diaphragm and is characterised by clinical signs of chronic ruminal tympany, anorexia and displacement of heart. Hernination of reticulum and sometimes abomasum through the diaphragm has been recorded in unusually high proportion in buffaloes in India, particularly in Punjab state.

The lesion due to traumatic reticuloperitonitis makes the diaphragm weak, and become susceptible to rupture, through which abdominal organs particularly reticulum, sometimes abomasum enters in to the thoracic cavity. The food can get into the rumen but cannot pass from rumen to abomasums. The over-distension of rumen leads to hypermotility and frothy bloat. There will be capricious appetite, loss of body condition, chronic tympany, grinding of teeth, pasty and scanty faces, displacement of heart (to its normal position), normal temperature, bradycardia, no rumination and regurgitation.

Diaphargmatic hernia should be differentiated from chronic bloat, presence of non metals like polythene or leather in rumen with occlusion of the cardiac opening, amphistomiasis, secondary tympany and ruminal acidosis.

Treatment: Medical treatment is not recommended and surgical treatment is mostly unsuccessful. The clinical signs could be partly relieved by keeping the animal confined with forequarters at an elevated floor.

Peritonitis

Inflammation of the peritoneum is accompanied by abdominal pain, fever, toxemia and reduction in the amount of feces.

Etiology

- Traumatic reticuloperitonitis
- Perforation or leakage of abomasal ulcer
- Secondary to ruminal trocarization
- Concurrent abomasal displacement and perforating ulcer
- Necrosis and rupture of abomasal wall after abomasal volvulus
- Rumenitis of cattle subsequent to acute carbohydrate engorgement
- Complication of caesarean section
- Rupture of vagina in young heifers during violent coitus with a young male
- Intraperitoneal injection of nonsterile solutions

- Spontaneous uterine rupture during parturition, or during manual correction of dystocia

Pathogenesis

Six factors associated with peritonitis account for the clinical findings.

1. Toxemia and septicaemia

Toxins produced by bacteria and by the breakdown of tissue are absorbed readily through the peritoneum. With rupture of the alimentary tract wall and the spillage of a large quantity of gut contents into' the peritoneal cavity, an acute peritonitis does develop, but death is usually too sudden, within 2-3 hours in horses. These animals die of endotoxic shock due to absorption of toxins from the gut contents.

2. Shock and hemorrhage

The shock caused by sudden deposition of gut contents, or infected uterine contents, into the peritoneal cavity, plus the hemorrhage resulting from the rupture, may be significant contributors to the common fatal outcome when an infected viscus ruptures.

3. Abdominal pain

In acute, diffuse peritonitis, the toxemia may be sufficiently severe to depress the response of the animal to pain stimuli, but in less severe cases the animal usually adopts an arched-back posture and shows evidence of pain on palpation of the abdominal wall.

4. Paralytic ileus

Paralytic ileus occurs as a result of reflex inhibition of alimentary tract tone and movement in acute peritonitis. The end result is a complete absence of defecation, often a large amount of mucus without any faces is present in the rectum.

5. Accumulation of fluid exudate

Accumulation of large quantities of inflammatory exudate in the peritoneal cavity may cause visible abdominal distension and, if severe enough, interfere with respiration by obstructing of diaphragmatic movement.

6. Adhesions

Trauma to the peritoneum results in a serosanguineous exudate, which contains two closely bound proteins: fibrinogen and plasminogen. Cattle have a high capacity to respond to trauma with fibrin deposition and adhesion formation is the most important factor in localizing peritonitis after peritoneal trauma from penetrating foreign bodies or abomasal ulcers. However, these adhesions can cause mechanical or functional intestinal obstruction.

Clinical Findings

- Inappetence and anorexia
- Toxemia and fever
- Disinclination to move,
- Disinclination to lie down,
- Lying down with great care and grunting with pain.
- The posture includes a characteristically arched back,
- The gait is shuffling and cautious, with the back held rigid and arched.
- Grunting at each step of walking and during defecation and carination.
- When urine is eventually passed it is usually in a very large volume.

Clinical Pathology

- **Hematology:** leukopenia, neutropenia and a marked increase in immature neutrophils (a degenerative left shift).
- **Abdominocentesis :** The ease of collection of the sample as a guide to the amount of fluid present
  - Whether it is bloodstained, indicating damage to a wall of the viscus
  - The presence of feed or fecal material, indicating intestinal ischemic necrosis or rupture
  - Presence of clots and high protein content of peritoneal fluid indicates inflammation
  - The number and kinds of leukocytes present are an indication of the presence of inflammation, and also its duration
  - Microbiological examination revealing presence of bacteria

Necropsy Findings

- In acute diffuse peritonitis, the entire peritoneum is involved but the most severe lesions are usually in the ventral abdomen. Gross hemorrhage into the subserosa, exudation and fibrin deposits in the peritoneal cavity and fresh adhesions that are easily broken down are present.
- In less acute cases, the exudate is purulent and may be less fluid, often forming a thick, cheesy covering over most of the viscera.

Diagnosis

- The diagnosis of peritonitis can be difficult because the predominant clinical findings are often common to other diseases.
- The clinical features that are the most reliable indicators of peritonitis are:

1. Abnormal feces -in amount and composition
2. Alimentary tract stasis based on auscultation and evaluation of the passage of ingesta or feces
3. Abdominal pain is evinced as a groan with each respiration or on light or deep percussion of the abdomen
4. Abnormality of intestines on per rectal palpation fibrinous or fibrous adhesions on rectal palpation
5. Abnormal peritoneal fluid with an increased leukocyte count collected by paracentesis
6. A normal or low blood leukocyte count with a degenerative left shift

Treatment

- Broad-spectrum antimicrobials
- Fluid and electrolytes adminstration
- Nonsteroidal anti-inflammatory drugs : Flunixin meglumine is recommended at 0.25-1.1 mg/kg body weight intravenously every 8-12 hours when the peritonitis is accompanied by shock.
- **Lavage :** Peritoneal lavage with large volumes of fluid containing antimicrobials

Enteritis

Inflammation of the small or large intestines is caused by many infectious and non-infectious agents and is characterized by symptoms of diarrhoea and abdominal discomfort. In many cases, enteritis is accompanied with inflammation of stomach; such condition is termed as gastroenteritis.

Etiology

Non-infectious diseases associated with enteritis include cardiac failure, lymphosarcoma, toxins and poisons, spoiled silage etc. Overfeeding or intolerance to particular food type may result in inflammation of the gastrointestinal tract. Chemicals such as arsenic, fluorine, copper, lead, molybdenum, mercury and nitrate may cause intestinal and gastric inflammation and resultant clinical signs of diarrhoea or vomition

Infectious agents responsible for causing gastroenteritis are given below

Bacterial enteritis: Colibacillosis, salmonellosis, pasteurellosis and enterotoxaemia (caused by *Clostridium perfringes* types B and C), shigellosis in foals, *Mycobaterium paratubeculosis* and anthrax.

Viral enteritis: Rinderpest, mucosal disease, bovine malignant catarrh (BMC), rota virus, corona virus, parvovirus

Fungal enteritis: Candidiosis, following anti-bacterial therapy, opportunist fungal growth may occur leading to diarrhoea

Protozoal enteritis: Coccidiosis, intestinal trichomoniasis

Parasitic enteritis: Abomasal worm (*Ostertagia ostertagi)* in cattle, stomach flukes (*Paramphistomum* spp.), *Trichostrogylus* spp., *Cooperia* spp., *Chabertia* spp. and *Nematodirus* spp. Hookworms in cattle (*Bunostomum* spp.), heavy tapeworm (*Monezia* spp.) infestation in sheep, *Strongylus* spp., *Trichonema* spp. and Ascaris in horses

Pathogenesis

Inflammation caused by infectious and non-infectious agents provides an ideal breeding ground for infectious agents normally present in intestinal tract. Parasitic gastro-enteritis refers to the infection of the abomasum (the true stomach) and intestine with nematode worms. *Ostertagia ostertagi*, called abomasal worm, is the most significant parasite, particularly in young calves during the summer and early autumn. The worms larvae are ingested by the cattle while grazing, enter the abomasum and become adults in about three weeks. During this time they cause severe damage to the lining of the abomasum, leading to digestive disturbances. Apart from existing and known causes of enteritis, nowadays one of the most frequent causes of enteritis in small animals particularly in dogs and cats, is intolerance to one or more foods. If intestine is the target organ for intolerance to food, relapses of the disease occurs after the pharmacological treatment of the gastroenteritis. Besides, necrotic enteritis, a disease of unknown etiology, is seen in spring-born suckling calves usually of 6 to 16 weeks of age.

The inflammation of the intestinal mucosa is associated with increased motility of the gut, decreased sojourn time of the ingesta, decreased absorption with increased secretion, loss of fluid and electrolytes, acid-base imbalance.

Osmotic diarrhoea is associated with increased osmotic pressure due to presence of food materials and indigestible feeds, and results in accumulation of fluid inside the lumen of the intestine. This accumulation occurs due to osmotic transfer of fluid from the body fluid compartments to the lumen of the intestinal tract and result in tissue dehydration. The best example of osmotic diarrhoea is lactose intolerance in horses and D-lactic acidosis in ruminants.

Exudative diarrhoea occurs in acute or chronic gastroenteritis when there is necrosis of mucosal epithelial cells and increased fluid production.

Secretory diarrhoea is seen in cases of infection with *E. coli* resulting from imbalance in secretory-absorptive mechanism and intestinal hypersecretion. The increased secretion is due to increase in cyclic AMP stimulated by prostaglandin. In this case, the mucosal integrity is maintained and secretory fluid is isotonic resulting in isotonic dehydration.

Denudation of epithelium and vessels in facilitates prompt absorption of toxic products and may result in shock, In chronic enteritis, the intestinal wall becomes thickened, and there is stimualated mucus secretion leading to decreased absorption. The faeces becomes thin, watery and contains much mucus.

Clinical Signs

Acute enteritis is manifested by diarrhoea and abdominal pain. If gastritis accompanies enteritis, vomition may be one of the prominent clinical signs. Diarrhoea is the characteristic sign of acute enteritis with soft or fluid consistency faeces and unpleasant odour. Faeces may become pale yellow due to dilution of bile pigments. It may contain blood, shreds of mucosa and mucus especially in chronic type. However, abdominal pain or colic is seldom present or indistinct in chronic enteritis. Soiling around the anus or the hind portion of the animal suggests presence of diarrhoea in animals. Straining may occur especially in calves and intussusceptions or rectal prolapse may accompany severe straining particularly in young animals. The pattern of the feacal output may suggest the disease; smudge and pasty faeces in coccidiosis to projectile fluid discharge in cases of rinderpest and Johne's disease. In helminthes infestation, there is little smearing on the pin bones but the tail and inside of the hocks are largely coated. Feces may be tarry coloured in dogs suffering from infestation due to release of blood in to the intestinal lumen at the site of attachment of the worm and subsequent formation of acid hematin. There may be complete anorexia in acute enteritis to normal appetite in chronic cases. Thirst is usually increased.

Auscultation of the abdomen reveals fluid gurgling sound due to increased motility of the intestinal tract and fluidity of lumen content. The heart rate may be increased in some cases and signs of dehydration are common in enteritis associated with diarrhoea or vomition. The specific signs of the primary disease such as fever and other specific lesions are common due to systemic involvement accompanied with septicemia or toxemia.

Clinical Pathology

Examination of the faeces reveals the fluidity. Microscopic and cultural examination of faeces reveals the causative bacteria, helminthes, protozoa etc. The level of dehydration should be monitored by skin tenting test and examination of blood protein level and packed cell volume. Fluid, acid-base and electrolyte balance should be monitored for assessing the severity and institution of therapy. Haematology and serum biochemistry including test for differential count, total leukocyte count, hemoconcentration is of clinical importance for the prognosis of the disease.

Diagnosis

Acute enteritis is easy to diagnose because of the presence of fluid faeces and abdominal pain. Diarrhoea may occur in other forms of hypermotility, but abnormal odour of the faeces, excessive mucous or systemic reaction is not present. Chronic enteritis due to John's disease and parasitic infestation can be differentiated by laboratory examination of faecal content for the presence of mycobacterium and parasitic ova, respectively.

Treatment

The treatment of enteritis associated with diarrhoea is aimed at replenishing fluid, electrolyte and acid-base imbalance, reducing hypermotility and diarrhoea through administration of astringent, spasmolytic, anticholinergic durgs and opiates, and specific treatment against the causative agents involved in enteritis. Hypermotility can be reduced with the use of spasmolytic drugs and astringent and protective preparations are prescribed to reduce fluid loss. However, purgatives are being used in few cases, to remove toxic material from the bowel and thereby reducing further absorption into the body. Antibiotics are given to check the multiplication of the bacterial infectious agents or to check the secondary bacterial infection in viral diseases associated with diarrhoea.

In cases of toxic gastroenteritis, the stomach should be washed with normal saline or magnesium sulphate solution by means of a stomach tube, and animal should be treated with specific antidotes for each toxicant or poison. The sulfa drug preparations available for oral administration in ruminants include slowly absorbed sulphonamides, short-acting sulphonamides, long-acting, sulphonamides, and sulphonamide-trimethoprim combination.

The initial dose in the case of slowly absorbed sulphonamides and short-acting sulphonamides should be 60-100 mg/kg body weight. A dosage of 20-30 mg/kg body weight is considered sufficient for the newer long-acting sulphonamides and the sulphonamide-trimethoprim combination. Follow-up doses of 1/2 to 2/3rd of the initial quantity are required at 12 to 36 hour intervals. Therapy should be continued for 3-5 days. Dewormers should be given in cases of helminth infestations and coccidiocidals for coccidia infection.

Anti-secretory drugs such as loperamide hydrocholoride, chlorpromazine and progstagladin inhibitors may be administered to reduce hypermotility and excess fluid secretion. Fluid therapy should be undertaken irrespective the cause of diarrhoea or vomition in cases of enteritis to replenish fluid, and electrolyte and to correct acid base imbalance. Vomtion is generally associated with alkalosis and diarrhoea with acidosis. The systemic acidosis and hyponatreamia associated with diarrhoea can be corrected with intravenous administration of hypertonic sodium biocarbonate solution (5%) isotonic solution (1.3%). Normal saline solution or Dextrose saline solution may be given to check dehydration and compensate fluid loss to avoid hypovolemic shock.

7

Diseases of Liver and Pancreas

Affections of Liver

Liver is the largest exocrine gland located in right side of the abdominal cavity obliquely from lumbocostal angle downward and forward to intercostal space, about 3-4" (10 cm) above the abdominal floor.

Manifestation of hepatic dysfunction

1. Icterus or jaundice
2. Gastrointestinal abnormalities
3. Intermittent pyrexia
4. Ascites
5. Abdominal pain
6. Alternation in liver size
7. Edema of body parts due to hypoproteinemia and emaciation
8. Photosensitization
9. Haemorrhagic diathesis
10. Hepato-encephalopathy.

(A) Jaundice / Icterus

Yellowish dircolouration of skin and visible mucous membrane (sclera and vaginal mucosa) due to hyperbilirubinemia.

Types of Icterus

1. Haemolytic jaundice- without impairment of bile flow
2. Obstructive jaundice- impairment of bile flow

Metabolism of bilirubin:

Production:

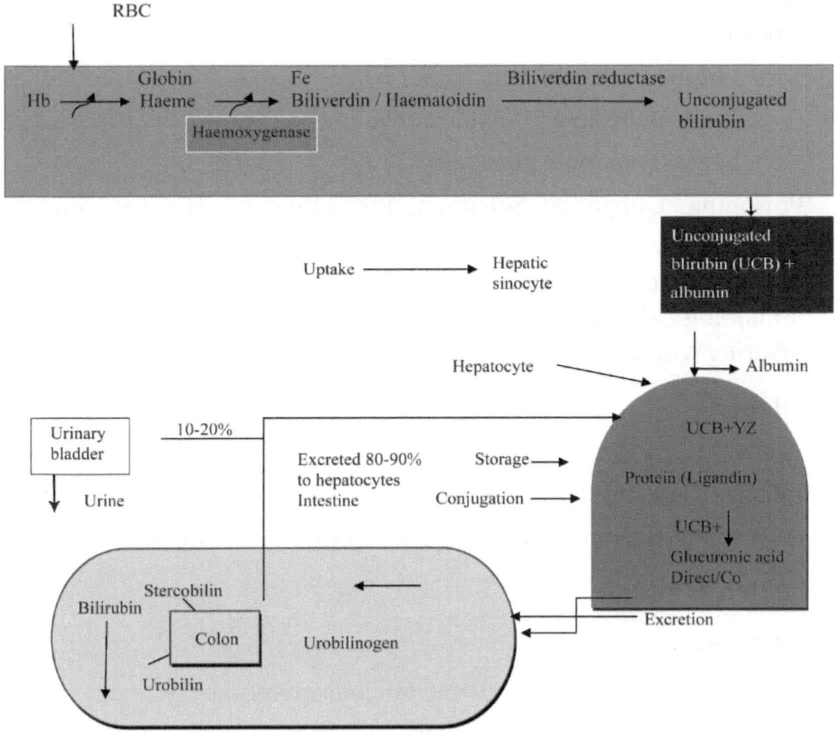

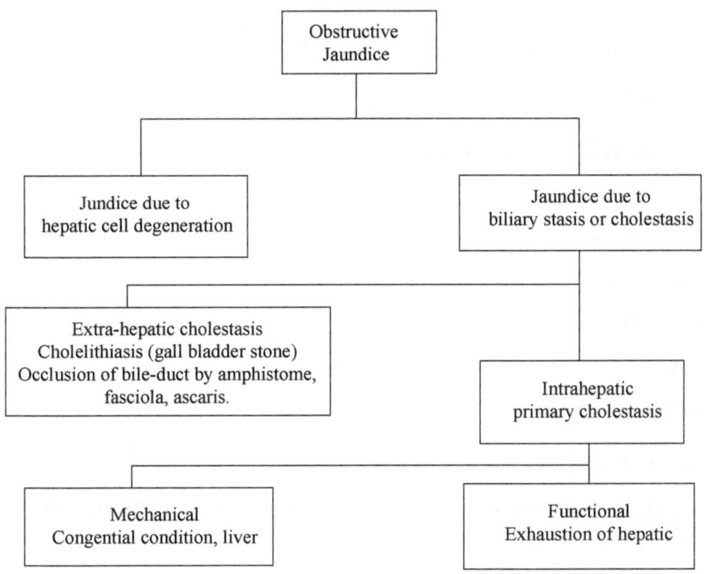

Causes of Hemolytic Jaundice

- Bacteria: Bacillary hemoglobiuria caused by *Clostridium haemolyticum*, leptospirosis.
- Virus: Equine infectious anaemia, HIV.
- Protozoan: Babesiosis, Anaplasmosis
- Deficiency: Hypophosphatemia
- Poisoning: Copper & Selenium, Phenothiazine, Bracken fern, Snake venom
- Immunological causes Neonatal isoerythrolysis isoerythrolysis: (In immnological jaundice there is reaction of sensitized erythrocytes of ofspring with immunoglobulins in colostrums of dam causing hemolysis)

Clinical Signs

- Anaemia
- Increased unconjugated bilirubin (indirect bilirubin) in serum.
- Absence of unconjugated bilirubin in urine (as it is insoluble in urine)

Obstructive Jaundice

Clinical Signs

- Yellow discolouration of visible mucous membrane.
- Intense yellow urine due to more bilirubin in urine (conjugated and soluble).
- Pale and whitish faeces (clay coloured facaes).
- Increased bilirubin in serum.

Bile has got the following functions

- Laxative.
- Emulsification.
- Fat digestion.
- Disinfectant.
- Fluidity.
- Peristaltic movement.

(B) Gastrointestinal abnormalities

- Constipation followed by diarrhoea, nausea, vomition and regurgitation and distension of GI tract due to gas accumulation.

- Stretching of nerve ending of distended part leading to reflex nerve spasm resulting in colic or abdominal pain.
- Distension causes drawing of more fluid to the part, hence further distension. When it crosses critical limits, there is no distension, pain and colic disappears and it causes paralytic ileus.
- When more fluid are drawn to a part then dehydration occurs resulting in hypovolemia, arrhythmia and lastly shock.

(C) Intermittent pyrexia

- Infection is associated with liberation of toxin. These toxin causes stimulation of immune response and there is release of cytokines and interleukins, which cause pyrexia.
- When detoxifying capacity of liver is reduced, there is accumulation of toxic substances which causes toxaemia and increases in temperature.

(D) Ascites

- Portal hypertension occurs due to dysfunction of liver. It leads to increase in hydrostatic pressure of plasma as it draws fluid from the system.
- When there is disruption to protein metabolism, there is hypoproteinemia or hypoalbuminemia which reduces osmotic pressure of plasma and more fluid is drawn from vascular system resulting in ascites.

(E) Alteration in liver size and shape

- Infection of liver leads to hepatomagaly. In terminal stage , liver fibrosis leads to decrease in size of liver.

(F) Emaciation

- Liver dysfunction impairs protein metabolism. Hence, anabolism of aminoacids in liver is hampered leading to emaciation.

(G) Photosensitization

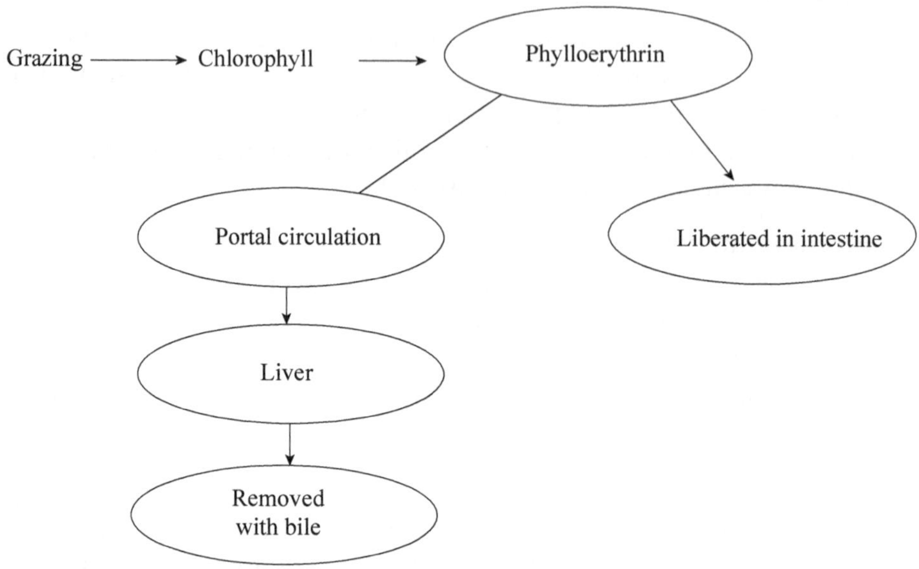

In liver diseases, phylloerythrin cannot be removed out and get accumulated in skin throughout the body (photo-dynamic substances). It reacts with radiant energy of U.V ray and there is peroxidation of cellular lipid and formation of free radicals. These radicals cause cell injury at whitish non-hairy part and there is dermatitis and sloughing of skin.

(H) Haemorrhagic Diathesis

Liver disease ⟶ decrease vitamin-K absorption ⟶ increase in blood clotting time ⟶ continuous haemorrhage by leakage of erythroytes.

(I) Hepato-encephalopathy/Hepaticencephalopathy

Liver disease ⟶ accumulation of amines, NH_3 and phenols ⟶ affects brain and CNS ⟶ Nervous disorder.

Diagnosis of Liver Diseases

1. Palpation at abdominal area immediately next to last costal arch only possible in dog and cat.
2. Liver biopsy- cumbersome and highly invasive procedure.
3. Ultrasonography.
4. Liver function test- sulpho-bromophthaline test, indole cyanine green excretion test, urea tolerance test, takatara test.

5. Enzyme test: ALT, AST, SDH and LDH.
6. Bile acid estimation mostly cholic acid, lithocholic acid and deoxycholic acid.

Treatment

1. Glucose solution intravenously to counter hypoglycaemia.
2. Amino-acid mixture containing methionine to counter hypo-proteinemia.
3. Provision of diet rich in carbohydrate, protein and calcium.
4. Choline citrate to repair hepatocyte.
5. Liver extract injections.
6. Anthelmintics to reduce parasitism.
7. Operative surgery.

Affections of Pancreas

Pancreatitis

It refers to inflammation of pancreas. It is important in case of small animals like dog and cat. It may occur in two forms:

1. **Acute pancreatitis**- No irreversible damage to pancreas and can be recovered.
2. **Chronic pancreatitis**- damage to pancreas and persist for long periods.

Etiology

1. **Infectious agents** like bacteria, viral and mycoplasmal agents. It starts with generalized systemic infection, later on causing pancreatitis.
2. **Dietary origin:** Diet containing more fat and less protein causes hyperlipidemia. Triglyceride concentration in pancreatic capillaries increases leading to increased breakdown of triglyceride by lipase which increases the production of toxic fatty acids eventually causing pancreatitis.
3. **Drugs:** Diuretic like thiazide and frusemide and long term use of sulfonamide and tetracycline cause pancreatitis.
4. **Duodenal reflux:** The obstruction or intestinal overload, leads to fluid distension and highly acidic duodenal fluid returnes to pancreas causing pancreatitis.
5. **Hypercalcemia:** Increased calcium level in blood stimulates pancreatic activity and may lead to pancreatitis.

6. **Scorpion venom:** Experimentally, scorpion venom causes pancreatitis by stimulation.
7. **Obstruction of pancreatic duct** due to neoplasm, surgical wound, hyperplasia and parasites may cause pancreatitis.

Pathogenesis

The most important way in which pancreatitis occurs is auto-digestion due to failure of excretory, process of pancreas by any means. Excretory failure causes unwanted effect on lysosomes and zymogen granules. Lysosomes present in cytoplasm causes lysis of bacteria. But when fusion occurs, zymogen enters into lysosomes and acts as trypsin inhibitors. There will be activation of trypsinogen which digests the same cells. This phenomenon is called auto-digestion.

Clinical Signs

1. Anorexia, depression, dullness and weakness.
2. Nausea and vomition are regular features.
3. Sometimes diarrhoea.
4. Vomition and diarrhoea leads to dehydration.
5. Congestion of visible mucous membranes.
6. Abdominal pain and softening of abdomen.
7. Peculiar position of dog (Prayer position).
8. Mild rise in body temperature.
9. Secondary symptoms like jaundice, respiratory distress and cardiac arrhythmia may be seen.

Clinical Pathology

1. Blood

- Leucocytosis.
- Hb and PCV % increases
- Hyperglycaemia due to lack of insulin.
- Hyperglucagonemia.
- Azotemia.
- Increased concentration of pancreatic enzymes in serum.

Treatment

1. Feeding should be withheld for 3-5 days in suspected cases and fluid therapy should be given with electrolytes and plasma expanders.
2. Antiemetic like metoclopramide and ondansetron may be given to counteract vomition.
3. Insulin treatment subcutaneously.
4. Start with proteinaceous diet or carbohydrate diet.
5. Hepatotonic and digestive enzymes are recommended
7. Vitamin-K injection is given if there is bleeding.

8

Cardiovascular Systems

The primary function of cardiovascular system is to maintain blood circulation so that normal exchange of fluid, electrolyte, oxygen, carbon dioxide, nutrient and excretory and secretory end products can take place between tissue and blood. Failure of circulation to any degree interferes with the transport and exchange mechanism.

Compensatory Mechanism

The body compensatory mechanism is activated to maintain the homeostasis. The failure of the compensatory mechanism leads to reduced body function. Heart and peripheral blood vessels are either affected at the same time or independently resulting in heart failure or peripheral circulatory failure. A failing heart utilizes the cardiac reserve and compensatory mechanism including involvement of peripheral circulation. Similarly, the problem in peripheral circulation also leads to altered functioning of the heart. Involvement of heart alone is called heart failure and that of peripheral blood vessels is called peripheral circulatory failure. Circulatory failure also occurs when there is reduced circulatory blood volume.

Pericardiatis

Inflammation of pericardium or pericardial sac is known as pericarditis. It causes an audible friction sound initially followed by muffling of heart sound and congestive heart failure with fluid accumulatim in the pericardial sac.

According to nature of pericarditis, it is divided into

- Acute
- Chronic

According to inflammation -

- Fibrous type
- Adhesive type

Aetiology

- Bacteria like *Pasturalla multocida*, Streptococcus, Salmonella, Leptospira
- Viral infection like glasser disease in pig, canine distemper in dog
- Fungal diseases like Coccidiomycosis
- Trauma & surgical injury may lead to pericarditis
- Pulmonary tuberculosis, pneumonia, pleurisy, myocarditis, endocarditis may lead to pericarditis.

Pathogenesis

Early stage- Infective pericarditis produces bacterimia or viremia along with toxemia. Hyperemic changes over the pericardium, lead to deposition of exudates in pericardial sac which is fibrinous in nature. Fibrinous deposit roughen the pericardial surface, resulting in friction between two pericardial layers during cardiac movement, which is audible on auscultation. Due to heavy deposition of the exudate, there may be detachment of pericardial surface, as a result heart sound is audible as murmur heart sound. Due to intense pressure of exudates there is incomplete filling of ventricle of heart and there will be interference with the function of heart. Hence, passive venous congestion and chronic heart failure develops.

Clinical Finding

- Pain over the pericardium
- Restricted movement, disinclination to lie-down
- Extension of head and neck
- Well marked jugular pulse
- Edema of brisket region.
- Arching back due to pain
- Deflection of elbow in outward direction (Abducted elbow)
- Pulse is quick and feeble, later on small and unsteady
- Temperature is high but may remains normal or sub normal
- Increased area of cardiac dullness - Auscultation reveals feeble, muffled heart sound, with some adventitious sound like frictional rub, humming, splashing, gurgling sound.

Diagnosis

- Based on clinical finding

- Echo-cardiography is the most valuable diagnostic procedure that shows the presence of fluid in the pericardial sac.
- Lateral thoracic radiography at $6^{th}/7^{th}$ inter costal space on standing position may be of diagnostic value.
- Electrocardiographig it can add to diagnosis. Electrocardiographic changes include sinus tachycardia in animal with right sided heart failure & hydro thorax and diminished QRS amplitude
- Examination of pericardial fluid - The smell is sufficiently diagnostic in cattle with traumatic pericarditis. However, cytological examination can be carried out for confirmation.

Treatment

- A broad spectrum antibiotic should be used. A combination of penicillin and gentamycin is commonly used and provides the cover against organisms associated with the infection
- Pericardiocentesis with 0.9% NCl solution and drainage should be conducted as required to release the fluid present in the pericardial sac
- Corticosteroid may be given
- Enzymatic therapy is advisable for fibrinolysis
- Salt free diet should be given

Myocarditis

Inflammation of the myocardium is known as myocarditis. Pericarditis and endocarditis lead to myocarditis. The causes of myocarditis are as follows

Aetiology

- Non-infective agents, include mercury, calcium, selenium, uremia, auto immune conditions
- Infective agents

  Virus- FMD, Canine distemper, canine parvo virus

  Bacteria- BQ, strangles, Staphylococcus

  Fungus- *Cryptococcus neoformans*

  Parasite- Trypanosoma, Toxoplasma, Strongyle spp.
- Nutrional deficiency – Vit.E, Selenium, chronic copper deficiency (falling disease), Co deficiency
- Venom – snake venom
- Embolic infarction- emboli from vegetative endocardiatis

- Braken fern poisoning in cattle
- Drugs including succinyl chloride, catecholamine, xylazine, monensin, overdosing of doxycycline

Pathogenesis

Most commonly myocardial diseases result in arrhythmia and conduction disturbances. There may be minimal evidence of cardiac disease when the animal is at rest. Myocardial weakness affects the cardiac output leading to passive venous congestion and chronic heart failure resulting in death.

Clinical Finding

- Early exhaustion and collapse
- Temperature is elevated in infective process
- Cardiac enlargement and dyspnoea
- Chronic venous congestion and chronic heart failure
- Animal may die without any sign

Clinical Pathology

- Electrocardiography and echocardiography are used as special examination
- Serum biochemical examination reveals elevated level of AST, ALT and lactate dehydrogenase (LDH), creatine kinase

Diagnosis

It is difficult to differentiate myocarditis from endocarditis and pericarditis except cardiac murmur. Electrocardiography is necessary for pinpoint diagnosis.

Treatment

- Correction of primary cause with proper therapeutic measure
- Symptomatic treatment
- Digitalization may be helpful
- Medical treatment does not become helpful in large animals

Tiger Heart Disease- Grossly, the ventricular wall appear streaked with patches of yellow tissue interspersed with apparently normal myocardium. Calves infected with FMD virus, may die suddenly due to myocarditis and typically evidenced tiger hert disease during post-mortem examination.

Endocardiatis

It denotes inflammation of the endocardium. It affects the inner lining of the heart as well as valves within it. It may be two type; acute and chronic

Etiology

- Bacteria are the most important cause of endocarditis such as infection with Streptococcus, *Corynobacterium pyogenes*, *Actinobacillus equi*, Black Quarter (*Clostridium septicum*)
- Influenza virus is considered as one of the etiological factors

Pathogenesis

Some infections of oral cavity or upper respiratory tract may help the organism to settle in some areas of the heart. The organism settles in healthy valves and set up the process of infection and on inflammation.

- **Stage of bacteremia-** Following infection by bacteria in other system, infectious agents get dislodged, enter the blood and circulate in blood stream.
- **Stage of implantation-** The exact site of implantation is governed by mechanical factor. Bacteria can settle and start producing pathological changes
- **Formation of vegetation-** Vegetations are formed in the endocardial surface of the valve. It can be produced by fibrin, platelet, bacteria and inflammatory cells. Then vegetation may get dislodged causing embolism in the coronary artery
- **Extension of infection to myocardium** - Small area of myocardial infarction due to occlusion of small branches results in small area of necrosis surrounded by inflammatory cells.
- **Extension of infection to pericardium-** Occasionally, pericarditis may develop due to extension of infection.
- **Disruption of cardiac rhythm** Takes place due to toxemia and septicemia

Clinical Finding

- Prolonged low grade pyrexia
- Pain in the joint and limb
- Weakness, progressive loss body weight
- Loss of appetite

- Anaemia
- Progressively increasing pallor of the mucosa due to toxic depression of bone marrow
- Change in cardiac function

Clinical Pathology

- Examination of blood- anaemia and leucocytosis
- Culture of blood sample to isolate the bacteria, and *in vitro* antibiotic sensitive test to screen out the specific antibacterial agent.

Diagnosis

- Based on clinical and clinico-pathological finding
- **Electrocardiography**- Findings suggestive of endocarditis are sinus tachycardia and decreased QRS amplitude in a base apex lead. Ectopic foci may be present
- **Echocardiography**- Findings suggestive of endocarditis are hypo echoic and ecogenic masses, irregular thickening of valves and rupture of chordae tendinae

Treatment

- Antibiotic therapy of higher doses through parental route. In travenous route is preferraed, Crystalline penicillin up to 20 times each, IU indicated 4-6 hr interval against hemolytic streptococcus and other gram positive organism. Supportive therapy is given to correct anemia. High protein diet, vit.C, folic acid, iron preparations may be given

Congestive Heart Failure

Congestion in venous circulation due to inability of heart to maintain circulatory equilibrium at rest because of intrinsic defects is termed as congestive heart failure (CHF). It is associated with dilation of vessels, edema of lungs, enlargement of heart and increased heart rate.

Etiology

Endocarditis, congenital valvular defect, rupture of valve, myocarditis, myocardial depression, pericarditis, pulmonary hypertension, congenital defect of atrial and ventricular septum, vascular abnormality

Pathogenesis: The generalized congestion of the veins associated with increased hydrostatic pressure results in passage of more fluid from the peripheral circulation particularly at the capillary bed with passage of protein into the tissues. Accumulation of protein along with fluid results in tissue edema. There is improper filling of the ventricles due to accumulation of blood in the peripheral circulation and sufficient ejection of blood during ventricular systole is not attained leading to reduced glomerular filtration rate and decreased urinary output. Increased pulmonary congestion results in decreased compliance in rate in terms of exchange of oxygen and carbon dioxide that results in increased rate and depth of respiration as compensatory mechanism, and exercise intolerance.

Clinical Finding

In general, the CHF is manifested by respiratory distress, cardiac enlargement, moderately increased resting heart rate, increase in rate and depth of respiration, dyspnoea, coughing with moist rales and crackling sounds, cyanosis and exercise intolerance.

In right sided CHF, there is congestion of the anterior and posterior vena cava and the vein draining blood from the systemic circulation to these large veins. The increased hydrostatic pressure due to accumulation of the blood results in edema of the dependent body parts and cavities. On the contrary, the left sided heart failure is associated with accumulation of the blood in the pulmonary vein resulting in edema of the lungs. However, the either sides of heart failure leads to affection of the other side. There is increased heart rate, edema, anasarca, ascites, hydrothorax and hydro-pericardium. Anasarca is characteristically limited to ventral surface of body, neck (brisket edema) and jaws. The respiration is deep and rate may be increased. There may be passage of low amount of concentrated urine. Hepatic congestion results in enlargement of liver and impaired digestion. Faeces are usually normal, but in later stage profuse diarrhoea, loss of body condition, loss of appetite and dilatation of jugular vein may be noticed. Prognosis varies to a certain extent with the cause but in most cases it is unfavourable in large animal.

Diagnosis

1. Clinical symptoms
3. Edema of brisket region may be noticed at the end of pregnancy particularly in cows.
4. Clinicopathological findings of proteinuria

Treatment

1. Cardiac glycoside- Digoxin should be given with diuretic agent. Digoxin should be given intravenously as it is destroyed in rumen, but

not intramuscularly as it causes muscle necrosis. It can be given @ 2.2 mg/100 kg body weight, in cattle, and @ 1-1.5 mg/ 100 kg body weight in horses.

2. If treated animals are not taking food, the daily oral administration of KCl is recommended to restore potassium concentration in blood.
3. Diuretic like frusemide, acetazolamide, spironolactone can be used to mobilize and eliminate excess body fluid. Frusemide in given @0.25-1 mg/kg body weight in horse and 2.5-5mg / kg in cattle
4. Salt feeding should be stopped. Stall rest and avoidance of violent exercise should be practised.

Acute Heart Failure

Acute heart failure can occur when there is severe defect in filling and failure of heart as a pump, caused by severe tachycardia, bradycardia or arrhythmia; and where there is sudden increase in workload. It is sudden and characterized by loss of consciousness, falling with or without convulsion, severe pallor of mucosa. Either death or complete recovery may occur. It is a major consideration as a cause of sudden death in large animals especially when death is associated with exhaustion and excitement.

Etiology

Organisms are associated with acute heart failure are as follows

Cattle; Streptococci, *Corynebacterium pyogenes, Clostridium chauvoei.*

Horse; Actinobacillus, Streptococcus, Migrating *Strongylus* spp. larvae

Pig/Sheep; Erysipelothrix, Escherechia, Actinomyces, Strepto cocus

- Atrial and ventricular rupture
- Aortic and pulmonary artery rupture
- Myocarditis
- Severe copper and selenium deficiency
- Certain plant poisoning
- Electric shock and lightening stroke
- Bradycardia due to intravenous calcium therapy, xylazine administration
- Concentrated solution of potassium chloride
- Heavy work load due to rupture of aortic valve and
- Acute anaphylaxis.

Clinical Signs

- It may occur at rest but commonly during excitement and heavy exercise
- Dyspnoea, staggering and falling down leading to immediate death
- Marked pallor of mucosa
- Clonic convulsion
- Deep asphyxia, gasping
- Physical examination reveals absence of pulse rate, tachycardia or absence of heart sound.
- Hydrothorax and mild ascites may develop in the animals surviving for some days.
- The major presenting sign is respiratory distress and it is the main cause of sudden death in horses during racing
- In cattle, a frequent history of ill thrift with periodic and temporary fall in milk production having loss of body condition along with intermittent lameness.
- Cardiac murmur on auscultation or a thrill on palpation of cardiac area.
- Poor exercise tolerance
- Moderate fluctuating fever is common.
- Peripheral lymphadenitis, embolic pneumonia, nephritis, arthiritis, myocarditis, pallor of mucosa and increased heart rate.
- Course of endocarditis may be as long as several weeks or months or death may occur without showing any premonitory clinical signs.

Sows

It is common for agalactiae to develop in 1st two to three weeks after farrowing followed by a loss of body weight, exercise intolerance, dyspnoea at rest etc.

Endocarditis is also a cause of acute heart failure and sudden death in sows.

Diagnosis

1. Presence of cardiac murmur or persistent tachycardia in conjunction with clinical and laboratory evidence of chronic bacteraemia.
2. Echocardiography is a major aid for diagnosis. Endocarditis without cardiac murmur is the bottleneck for diagnoses. Such cases are suspected where there is chronic recurring bacteremia.

Treatment

Not usually practicable in large animals due to sudden onset. Culture of blood and antibiotic therapy like penicillin, cefotaxime, ceftriaxone for a long period may be provided. The prognosis is poor, if signs of congestive heart failure is present.

Congenital Cardiac Defects

The cause of congenital cardiac defects is unknown, but it is assumed that these defects results from prenatal insults during developments or from single recessive genes or polygenic sets that have location specific effects on cardiac development.

1. **Ectopic heart:** Abnormal position of heart outside the thoracic cavity is the most common congenital defect in cattle where the displacement is usually near the lower cervical region. The heart is easily noticed and palpated. Affected animal may survive for years but those with a displacement through the defective sternum or ribs, rarely survive for few days.
2. **Patent foramen ovale (PFO):** It is seen in 30 % of congenital cardiac defect cases. This defect of atrial septum is common in cattle, but usually causes no clinical signs, when it is present as an isolated defect and is detected only at necropsy. The foramen ovale may be patent, but normally a flap like opening allows a shunt from right to left atrium. Atrial septal defects are more significant when they are present with other cardiac defects. If these results in severe right ventricular hypertrophy, the shunt may reverse and cyanosis may occur.
3. **Ventricular septal defect (VSD):** This is one of the most common cardiac defects in sheep, cattle and horse and has high prevalence in calves and lambs. In absence of other defects, their presence results in shunting of blood from left to right ventricle. The fate of the animal is determined by the size of the defect and the degree of resistance to flow from right ventricle. The shunt of the blood can be considerable amount and animal may die at birth or show clinical signs for few weeks to few months of age. The major sign during this period is lassitude, failure to grow well, dyspnoea with moderate exercise. If the shunt is less severe, it allows an apparently normal existence until maturity or causes no apparent problem in life. On auscultation, cardiac murmur is audible, which is loudest and most obvious.
4. **Tetralogy of fallot**: This is almost always a lethal defect in farm animals. The tetralogy consists of VSD, pulmonary stenosis, dextral position of

aorta, so that it overrides both ventricles and secondary right ventricular hypertrophy. The condition is associated with clinical signs very early in life, frequently results in death, and has been reported in calves and foals. Affected animals show dyspnoea after minor exhaustion during milk suckling. Cyanosis may or may not be present depending on pulmonary stenosis. On auscultation, a murmur and sometimes a thrill may be noticed.

5. **Patent ductus arteriosus (PDA):** This results from failure of closure of ductus arteriosus following birth which is a common defect in horses. Clinically, murmur associated with a patent ductus arteriosus which are frequently heard during first day after birth and may persist up to 5th day.
6. **Constriction of aorta**: Constriction of aorta at the site of entrance of ductus arteriosus causes a syndrome similar to that of stenosis of the aortic semilunar valve with systolic murmur and a slow rising pulse of small amplitude.
7. **Persistence of right aortic arch:** It causes constriction of oesophagus with dysphagia and regurgitation. Aorta is situated to the right side of oesophagus and trachea. Clinical signs are evident soon after birth with regurgitation of milk through mouth and nostrils after suckling of milk.
8. **Persistent truncus atreriosus:** It has been recorded in animals in low percentages.
9. **Fibroelastosis:** It has been observed in calves and pigs. The endocardium is converted into a thick fibroelastic coat. Although the wall of left ventricle is hypertrophied, the capacity of ventricle is reduced. The defect may cause no clinical abnormality until the animal is mature.
10. **Subvalvular aortic stenosis**: stenosis of aorta at or just below the point of attachment of aortic semilunar valve has been recorded in pigs. Clinically, affected animals may die suddenly with asphyxia and dyspnoea.

9

Diseases of Blood and Blood Forming Organs

The blood is considered as the connective tissue, and consists of fluid component called plasma, and cellular component. Cellular component consists of erythrocytes, leikocytes and thrombocytes. Blood cells produced during different stages of life (prenatal and postnotal) differ in morphology and function. The primitive erythrocytes (Red blood cell) are produced on yolk sac, and later from liver, spleen and bone marrow. Thus, hematopoiesis of erythroid cells occurs at multiple sites within the embryo and extra embryonic tissue, other haematopoietic cell lineages are generated in the yolk soc during primitive stage of haematopoitic development. The circulating blood cell numbers in young animals differs from that of adults. The circulating leukocytes count (WBC) at birth is approximately 20% of counts in adults. Platelets counts in neonates are approximately one-third of that in adults. Bone marrow is the major haematopoietic organ in adults and a primary lymphoid organ.

The important function of the blood is to carry the oxygen and carbon dioxide nutrients and waste products of the metabolism for excretion. Haemoglobin inside the erythrocytes transports oxygen. Leukocytes are comprised of granulocytes and agranulocytes (monocycte and lympocytes) act as body defense system and protect the animal from invading pathogen. Neutrophil number increases as manifold following inflammation. Megakaryocytes in the blood play important role in production of platelets that help in clotting mechanism.

The process of formation of erythrocytes is known as erythropoiesis. The stages of erythropoiesis, include pleuripotential stem cell, erythroblastic cells, rubriblasts, prorubricytes, rubricytes, meta-rubricytes, reticulocytes and finally erythrocytes. As erythroid precursors mature, the cells become smallers, the nuclear-cytoplasmic ratio decreases, and the nuclear chromatin condense. In mammals, the neucleus is extruded before maturation of erythrocytes. This process of erythropoiesis takes place in distinct erythroblastic islands in the bone marrow. The pleuri potential stem cells are a population of unspecialized precursor cells with capacity for self renewal and differentiation.

Anaemia

It is defined as a deficiency of circulating erythrocyte, and may be caused by (1) haemorrhages or by (2) increased destruction or (3) inefficient production of erythrocytes Anaemia can be classified as haemorragic, hemolytic or due to decreased production of RBC.

Types of Anaemia

Haemorrhagic anemia: Anaemia associated with blood loss due to bleeding or blood sucking parasites is termed as haemorrhagic anaemia

Haemolytic anemia: The causes of this type of aneamia include blood protozoa, parasitic infection, babesiosis, theileriosis, trypanosomiasis, anaplasmosis.

- Bacillary hemoglobinuria, caused by Clostridium haemolyticum
- Leptospirosis, caused *Leptospira ictero haemorrhagica leptospira pomona, Leptospira hardjo*
- Post-parturient hemoglobinuria .
- Excess feeding of potatoes or onions.
- Weed poisoning.
- Phenothiazine and chronic copper poisoning
- Treatment with long acting oxytetracycline
- Heavy infestation with tick, lice and endoparasites
- Calves drinking large quantity of water following excercise
- Blood transfusion reaction
- Snake bite
- Iso erythro haemolysis
- Autoimmune hemolytic anaemia recorded under 6 months old claves.

Aplastic Anemia

- Nutritional deficiency of cobalt, copper and iron
- Folic acid, pyridoxine deficiency
- Radiation injury
- Poisoning by bracken fern, furazolidone, and phenyl butazone
- Chronic intestinal parasitism
- Temporarily for several weeks after sudden movement to high altitude.

Pathogenesis

Irrespective of causes of anemia, the primary abnormality in function is anaemic anoxia. There is loss of circulating blood volume and plasma protein. Hemolytic anaemia causes hemoglobinuria and may result in hemoglobinuric nephrosis and depression of renal function. Aplastic anemia is caused by toxins. Anaemia due to nutritional deficiency is reversible. In a situation where erythrolysis occurs after drinking large volume of cold water, hemolysis occur in the capillary of intestinal wall. Plasma osmotic pressure decreases as a result of fluid intake and hemolysis takes place due to influx of fluid into the erythrocytes. The primary response to tissue anoxia caused by anaemia is an increased cardiac output through increased stroke volume, heart rate and decrease in circulation time. In terminal stages when tissue anoxia is sufficiently severe there may be moderate increase in respiratory activity lowering tissue oxygen tension.

Clinical Signs

1. Pallor of mucosa
2. Muscular weakness
3. Depression
4. Hypoxia or anoxia
5. Increased heart rate leading to tachycardia and decrease in intensity of heart sound and weak pulse
6. In terminal cases, there is laboured breathing, oedema, jaundice and hemoglobinuria.

Treatment

Treatment of primary cause is essential to stop further bood loss.

Non specific treatment includes

1. Blood transfusion in acute haemorrhage.
2. Haematinics preparations are used in less severe cases as supportive to transfusion like imferon, jectofer plus, belamyl parenterally and hepatoglobin, sharkoferrol, cadisol –DC orally, iron tonic administration orally or parenterally is a common practice in horses which is much superior treatmnent to other expensive drugs.
3. Vitamin B_{12} is widely used as a non specific hematinics in anaemia
4. Nutritionally balanced food should be provided.
5. Cases of hemolytic anaemia respond well to corticosteroid therapy.

Haemorrhages

The rapid loss of whole blood from the vascular system causes peripheral circulatory failure and anaemia leading to shock and death.

Etiology

1. Spontaneous rupture /traumatic injury to large blood vessels
2. Minor surgical wounds like castration or dehorning .
3. Severe ecto and endoparasitic infestation.
4. Nasal bleeding .
5. Rupture of uterine artery during prolapse following parturition.
6. Abomasal ulcer and some bacterial and viral diseases

Pathogenesis: The major defects of haemorrhages are loss of blood volume, loss of plasma protein and loss of RBCs. If the rate of blood loss is rapid, the loss of circulating blood volume results in peripheral circulation failure. Anaemic anoxia results from loss of erythrocyte leading to death.

Clinical signs: The major clinical signs include pallor of mucosa, weakness, staggering, recumbency, rapid heart rate, cold extremities, subnormal temperature, restlessness, dullness. In fatal cases, animal dies in coma in lateral recumbency.

Clinical pathology: Examination of haemoglobin/ blood and heamatocrit level and erythrocyte count provides an index to the progress of the disease. The packed cell volume (PCV) and total protein concentration falls to lower level in 12-24 hour following hemorrhages.

Treatment

1. The source of haemorrhage should be determined and the cause should be rectified.
2. A decision for blood transfusion should not be taken very early as the procedure is time consuming, costly and has some risk. In the period immediately following hemorrhages, PCV should be monitored over the next 24-48 hr. If there is a fall to less than 12%, a transfusion of blood is indicated, but a stable PCV between 12-20% is not usually an indication for blood transfusion.
3. Treatment of hypovolemic shock- Fluid may be given with electrolyte like Na+. Plasma expander (hacmacil-dextran) may be useful. Blood transfusion replaces all elements of blood and in case of severe haemorrhages, blood transfusion is the most satisfactory treatment.

4. Apart from this, liver extract, Fe, Vit-B complex therapy should be given to compensate stress to the animal.
5. To check haemorrhages. Anti haemorrhage drugs like Stryptovet, Dicynene, Vit-k (kapisin), Butropase injection should be givev.

Abnormality in Cellular Constituents

The cellular constituents of the blood include erythrocytes, reticulocytes (immature erythrocytes), leukocytes, and platelets. The major function of the erythrocytes (Red blood cells) is to carry oxygen and carbon dioxide. Decrease in erythrocyte population as noticed in anaemia is associated with poor oxygenation of the blood, called anaemia anoxia, and is manifested by laboured and deep breathing and poor exercise tolerance. The leukocytic series include granulocytes such as neutrophil, eoisonophil and basophil and agranulocytic cells such as monocyte and lymphocyte. The platelet population in blood are responsible for clotting of the blood in case of trauma. Decreased platelet count is clinically manifested by bleeding from the blood vessels and the blood clotting time is prolonged.

Leukocytosis

Physiologic Leukocytosis

Leukocytosis may occur as a result of exercise or excitement; this response is mediated by increased epinephrine. Epinephrine centralizes the marginal pool; thus, the effect of excitement may double the total WBC count within minutes. In addition, splenic contraction releases WBC and RBC into the peripheral circulation. The leukocytosis is usually due to a mature neutrophilia without a left shift. A lymphocytosis also may be present, especially in young horses or cats.

Corticosteroid-induced or Stress Leukogram

Treatment with exogenous corticosteroids or endogenous release results in a typical leukogram with lymphopenia as a consistent feature and invariably accompanied by neutrophilia. The net effect on the total WBC count is a function of the species and its normal differential WBC count. In dog, neutrophils are the predominant circulating WBC. In cattle, in which lymphocytes predominate, the WBC count is variable depending on the degree of neutrophilia and lymphopenia. There is usually a reversal of the neutrophil to lymphocyte ratio. Stress leukograms have a characteristic WBC differential count consisting of mature neutrophilia, lymphopenia, and eosinopenia. Neutrophilia is due to decreased adherence to the vascular endothelium, which prolongs circulating time and shifts the marginating cells to the circulating pool, and increased marrow release of neutrophils. Lymphopenia is due to redistribution or lysis of lymphocytes. Monocyte numbers are variable; however, a monocytosis often occurs in steroid or stress reactions in dogs and horses.

Other Leukogram Alterations

Although the specific features of leukocytosis and leukopenia vary with species, there are some generalities. Radiation and radiomimetic drugs (eg, many antineoplastic drugs) produce leukopenia. Lymphocytes are extremely sensitive to radiation, but mature granulocytes—unlike their precursors in the bone marrow—are not particularly radiosensitive. Pancytopenia, which includes leukopenia, may result from drug toxicities (eg, estrogen toxicity in dogs, bracken fern toxicity in cattle), nutritional deficiencies, stem-cell alterations (possibly immune-mediated), and space-occupying lesions in bone marrow (myelophthisis). Generally, viral infections, particularly acute infections are not associated with extensive tissue necrosis, produce leukopenia and neutropenia and may have mild lymphocytosis or lymphopenia. In viral infections of longer duration (2-3 week) with secondary bacterial complications, the total WBC count may be increased or within normal limits due to concurrent neutrophilia and lymphopenia. Ehrlichiosis in dogs is associated with thrombocytopenia, but persistent leukopenia may be seen, especially in chronic cases.

The four major types of leukocytoses are inflammatory, glucocorticoid-associated, catecholamine-associated, and neoplastic. These leukocytoses are distinguished by leukocyte concentrations and microscopic features of leukocytes. All laboratory findings need to be interpreted within the context of the case information, including signalment, history, and physical examination findings. Newer assays are being used to differentiate the different forms of leukocyte neoplasia and to distinguish between hyperplastic and neoplastic proliferations.

Leukocytosis, or elevated WBC count, is a commonly encountered laboratory finding. Distinguishing malignant from benign leukocytosis is a critical step in the care of a patient, which initiates a vastly different decision tree. Confirmation of the complete blood cell count and the WBC differential is the first step. Examination of the blood smear is essential to confirm the automated blood cell differential count or affirming the manual differential performed on the blood smear. Next is separation of the leukocytosis into a myeloid versus a lymphoid process. Distinguishing a reactive lymphoid proliferation from a lymphoproliferative disorder requires examination of lymphocyte morphology for pleomorphic lymphocytes versus a monomorphic population, with the latter favoring a lymphoproliferative neoplasm. Samples suspicious for lymphoproliferative disorders can be confirmed and characterized by flow cytometry, with molecular studies initiated in selected cases; precursor lymphoid neoplasms (lymphoblasts) should trigger a blood smear microscopic examination. Myeloid leukocytosis triggers a differential diagnosis of myeloid leukemoid reactions verses myeloid malignancies. The manual differential is the key, along with correct enumeration of blasts and blast equivalents, immature granulocytes, basophils, and eosinophils and identifying dysplasia to identify myeloid malignancies. Confirmation and characterization of myeloid malignancies should be performed with a blood smear microscopic. examination and the appropriate ancillary studies. Myeloid leukemoid reactions commonly result from infections and show activated neutrophil changes on morphology.

Automated hematology analyzers rapidly analyze the whole blood samples for the complete blood cell count and differential count, including WBC count, RBC count, platelet count, hemoglobin concentration, hematocrit, RBC indices, and the leukocyte differential count. The newer generation of hematology analyzers can examine thousands of leukocytes using flow cytometry–based methodology, some in combination with cytochemistry or fluorescence or conductivity, to elucidate different types of WBCs, including neutrophils, lymphocytes, monocytes, basophils, and eosinophils (ie, the 5-part differential). Nucleated RBCs are also detected routinely, and some analyzers also quantitate immature granulocytes. Based on proprietary algorithms, hematology analyzers will flag high or low numbers of specific cell types and possibly abnormal populations of leukocytes, including immature granulocytes, blasts, and variant/atypical lymphocytes. The automated hematology analyzers used in laboratories within physicians' office may use older methodologies for cell analysis, such as impedance technology, which generates a 3-part leukocyte differential that includes lymphoid cells/basophils, neutrophils/eosinophils, and monocytes/other mononuclear cells. Whereas these smaller instruments may work well for screening a normal, healthy population, the presence of abnormal cells may cause error flags and inaccurate counts, resulting in a high review rate when used in a hospital-based population. Spurious elevations of the WBC count can also be seen, including platelet clumps, nucleated RBCs, incomplete lysis of RBCs, cryoglobulins, and cryofibrinogen.[5] Regardless of the instrument used, a flagged blood sample triggers action before the CBC and WBC differential can be released; most commonly, this is a review of a peripheral blood (PB) smear.

Neutrophilia

The increase in absolute number of neutrophil in the circulation may result from movement of neutrophil between circulating and marginal blood pools, change in movement of cells from storage pool to blood pool or alteration in the rate of movement of the cells out of the blood pool. Increase in immature neutrophil in the circulation is termed as shift to left and occurs as a compensatory mechanism with release of more of immature cells to the circulation to meet the immediate body demand. A regenerative left shift is characterized by an absolute increase in neutrophils accompanied by appearance of immature neutrophil where as a degenerative left shift is associated with normal, low or falling total leukocyte count. Degenerative left shift indicates inability of the bone marrow to produce mature cells in response to infections. Neutrophillia is recorded in the following conditions

- Localized infections, particularly those produced by pyogenic bacteria are associated with significant increase in neutrophil population. Localized traumatic peritonitis or traumatic reticuloperitonitis (TRP) is manifested by 90-95% neutrophils in the circulation and large number of immature neutrophil.
- Systemic infections also results in neutrophilia. However, it is frequently preceeded by leukopenia.
- Non-infectious diseases stimulating stress reaction such as metabolic disturbances and toxic chemicals
- Tissue destruction irrespective of the cause including both physiological and pathological causes. Eg. Prolonged surgical invervention
- Haemmorhages including bleeding to serous cavities such as peritoneum, pleura, joint and subdural space
- Exogenous or endogenous increase in glucocorticoids

Monocytosis

Absolute number of circulating monocytes greater than the reference range is called monocytosis

Species

1. Absolute count in dogs: $1.3 \times 10^9/l$ or >1300/μl or mm^3;

2. cats: $0.9 \times 10^9/l$ or 900/μl or mm^3

Monocytes are formed in the bone marrow and play an important role in normal immune system functioning. Inflammatory disorders, infection and certain forms of cancer are the most common causes of monocytosis. Symptoms commonly include fatigue, weakness, fever or an overall feeling of being ill. Managing this condition involves diagnosing and treating the underlying cause of the blood cell elevation

Inflammatory conditions such as infection or autoimmune disturbances are primary causes of monocytosis. Some of the common types of infection that might lead to this condition include tuberculosis, syphilis and Rocky Mountain spotted fever. Autoimmune disorders such as lupus or rheumatoid arthritis may also lead to monocytosis. Some blood disorders lead to a high number of monocytes as well. The use of medications including antibiotics or steroid can sometimes return the blood cell counts to normal, although the condition may become chronic in some patients.

Leukemia or a form of lymphoma known as Hodgkin's disease are types of cancer that are known to cause monocytosis. These cancers affect the blood or the bone marrow and restrict the body's natural disease-fighting abilities. The immune system is compromised as a result of these cancers, placing the patient at an increased risk of developing serious complications, even from ordinarily mild types of infection.

There are no specific symptoms associated with the development of monocytosis. Most find the condition only through the routine examinations.

Monocytosis is actually a symptom of some other disease process and not a medical condition of its own, so treatment options vary widely. The primary goal of treatment is to accurately diagnose the underlying cause of the abnormal monocyte count.

Pathophysiology

- Monocytes are derived from hematopoietic stem cells named colony-forming unit granulocyte, monocyte (CFU-GM). The CFU-GM is responsible for neutrophil and monocyte production, with the appropriate stimulus. The cells from this unit differentiate into monoblasts (or myeloblasts) and then into monocytes.
- The production, differentiation, and release of monocytes is regulated by variety of chemicals, including colony stimulating factor, antichalones, PGE_2, and various interleukins. Production to release of monocytes takes approximately 6 hours, and thus cells in circulation are relatively young.
- Monocytes exit the circulation to reside in various tissues, begin another phase of differentiation, and then become part of the mononuclear phagocyte system and are referred as macrophages and histiocytes. They reside in lymph nodes, bone marrow, spleen, liver (Kupffer cells), lungs (alveolar macrophages), bone (osteoclasts), pleural and peritoneal cavities, and central nervous system (microglial cells).

- Several macrophages may fuse to form multinucleated giant cells. This is a common response to fungi, mycobacterium, syncytial virus, and foreign material.
- The ratio of macrophages to circulating monocytes is approximately 400:1. The accumulation of monocytes in an area of acute or chronic inflammation is caused by chemotactic factors that attract monocytes to these specific foci. Most macrophages in a region are migrating circulating monocytes but under specific microenvironmental stimuli, they can be derived from local production.
- The functions of the mononuclear phagocyte system include phagocytosis, microbiocidal activity, tumor cytolysis, regulation of the immune system, coagulation, fibrinolysis, and bone repair. The mononuclear phagocyte system is vital in controlling certain pathogens, including intracellular bacteria (e.g., Mycobacteria, Listeria, and Brucella), mycotic agents, protozoa, and viruses.

Nomenclature of Monocytes in Various Systems

- Respiratory system alveolar macrophages
- Hemic/lymph/immune system lymph nodes (histiocyte proliferation), spleen (proliferation of red pulp and mononuclear phagocyte system proliferation), and bone marrow
- Hepatobiliary system Kupffer cells
- Musculoskeletal system osteoclasts
- Central Nervous system microglial cells
- Thoracic and abdominal cavities-macrophage and mesothelial proliferation

Signalment

- Breed predisposition: Irish setter--chronic granulocytopathy syndrome
- Young animals have higher monocyte counts than adults.
- Geriatric dogs have monocytosis.

Causes of monocytosis

- General: Any process that stimulates neutrophilia, as monocytes and neutrophils share the same stem cell precursor (CFU-GM)
- Glucocorticoids: Corticosteroids stimulate absolute monocytosis in dogs and less frequently in cats. Monocytosis develops within hours of steroid exposure and resolves within 24 hours after removing the corticosteroid stimulus. Causes include glucocorticoid treatment, stress of a disease, and hyperadrenocorticism.

- Inflammation (infectious): mycotic (e.g., Aspergillus and Blastomycosis), protozoal (e.g., Toxoplasma), viral (e.g., Fline infectious penito), bacterial (e.g., Mycobacteria, Brucella) infections.
- Inflammation (non-infectious): Foreign material, necrotic tissue, malignant tumor, hemolytic anemia, trauma, neutropenia with compensatory monocytosis, and immune mediated disease
- Monocytic or myelomonocytic leukemia: Neoplastic proliferation of the monocyte cell line or a combined myeloid and monocyte cell line produces monocytosis. Immature, bizarre cells are present in the circulation. Careful examination of the feathered edge of the blood smear should permit identification of these cells.
- Granulocytopathy syndrome in dogs: Cellular defect in monocytes, a familial disease in Irish setters dogs
- Cyelichematopoiesis (silver-gray collies): The cyclic neutropenia at 11-14 day intervals is usually followed by high numbers of other cell lines, including monocytes, thrombocytes, and neutrophils
- Older dogs: Absolute monocytosis, lymphopenia, and eosinopenia can be seen.

Diagnosis

- Severely stressed or ill dogs may have monocytosis due to production of endogenous glucocorticoids
- Concurrent alopecia, "pot belly," thin skin, and muscle atrophy may be due to hyperadrenocorticism
- Fever of undetermined origin may be due to endocarditis and immune-mediated disease
- Mycotic infection and foreign body associated with draining cutaneous wound
- Spleenomegaly, hepatomegaly, or lymphadenopathy may be associated with leukemia

Laboratory Findings

Certain techniques for counting monocytes can yield errors. Mechanical blood-spreading devices shift larger cells (monocytes) into the "counting area," with resultant absolute, artifactual monocytosis. Incorrect identification of metamyelocytes and other immature neutrophils in a left shift also can result in erroneous monocytosis.

CBC/Biochemistry/Urinalysis

- Severe monocytosis (i.e., > 20,000 monocytes/µl) may be due to leukemia or rebound phase of cyclic hematopoiesis
- Immature, bizarre, and abnormal cells in circulation is due to monocytic leukemia and myelomonocytic leukemia
- Mature neutrophilia, lymphopenia, and eosinopenia is observed in stress and hyperadrenocorticism
- Neutrophilia along with monocytosis may be due to pyogranulomatous diseases
- Anemia along with monocytosis may be due to immune mediated hemolytic anemia

Treatment

Treatment is directed at the underlying cause of the monocytosis. Levamisole increases the rate of migration of monocytes, enhances chemotaxis, and increases phagocytosis

Other diseases that affect the mononuclear phagocyte system but do not cause consistent monocytosis:

- Malignant and systemic histiocytosis of Bernese mountain dogs
- Lysosomal storage diseases
- Recovery from leukopenia and neutropenia can cause monocytosis (> 20,000/µl). The rapid induction of monocytes with their uniquely short marrow transit time causes monocytosis that precedes the rebound neutrophilia.

EOSINOPHILIA

Eosinophils are produced in bone marrow, circulate in blood for a few hours, and migrate into tissues where they survive for several days. Increased production of eosinophils is mediated by factors produced by some activated T lymphocytes. Corticosteroids decrease blood eosinophil numbers but increase the marrow pool of eosinophils.

Increased numbers of circulating eosinophils may be seen in hypersensitivity reactions, as with certain forms of parasitism and allergic conditions. The presence of mast cell tumors in an animal may also be associated with eosinophilia. Basophilia sometimes occurs concurrently with eosinophilia. Idiopathic "hypereosinophilic" syndromes are seen infrequently in cats.

Eosinophilia refers to increased number of eosinophils in circulation. It is most commonly associated with parasitism (especially those parasites with a tissue migration phase) and hypersensitivity reactions.

Eosinophil count rises in parasitic worm infections (roundworm, hookworm) in the body and inflammations occurring in the body like rheumatoid arthritis, inflammatory bowel disease, autoimmune diseases, and inflammations in the respiratory tract like asthma.

Cancerous Conditions and Allergy

Eosinophils may increase due to some form of cancers like Hodgkin lymphoma, lung and stomach cancer. Certain neoplasms can also promote production and release of eosinophils. This is most commonly seen with mast cells tumors, but has also been described with lymphoma, squamous cell carcinoma, and some other tumor types. The mechanism of this paraneoplastic eosinophilia is not always known, but can be due to release of cytokines by the neoplastic cells that promote eosinophil production (e.g. IL-5). Another potential cause for eosinophilia is Addison's disease.

Allergies like seasonal allergies, hay fever, asthma can increase eosinophils count. Lung disease and certain medications can cause an increase in eosinophil count. Drug interactions or allergic response to a particular drug can also lead to eosinophilia.

Eosinopenia

Eosinopenia refers to decreased number of eosinophils. It may be difficult to document because the eosinophil normal range may go down to zero. Eosinopenia is most commonly attributed to increased corticosteroids (stress leukogram).

Basophilia

Basophils are granulated leukocytic series cells and are produced in the bone marrow. The neucleus is multi-lobed and almost similar in size to that of neutrophils with purple cytoplasmic granules. These granules contains histamine, heparin, chondroitin sulfate, and other substances. Basophils constitute only 0-2% of the total blood leukocytes and are rarely noticed during routine differential counting of the blood cells in thin blood smears. An increase in the absolute number of basophils is also rare. However, basophilic granulocytic leukemia, respiratory and skin diseases, heart worm infections in dogs and hyperlipoproteinemia are associated with basophilia. Immune reaction to ticks in cattle and guinea pigs also reveals basophilia during blood smear examination.

Basophils are normally similar in size to neutrophils, or may be slightly larger. The nucleus is multilobed, but with less distinct indentations than neutrophils. The distinctive feature of basophils is their lavender to purple cytoplasmic granules (containing histamine, heparin, chondroitin sulfate, and other substances) and their long "ribbon-like" nuclei. The morphology of these granules varies slightly with species. There may be a few purple granules but not enough to fill the cytoplasm in dogs, and the remainder of the cytoplasm is light purple. Cat basophils have oval light lavender granules that fill the cytoplasm, and only occasionally may have a few large purple granules. Horses and cattle have a more classic appearance of basophils, with cytoplasm that is completely filled with dark purple granules.

The basophil number in blood is very small in all species normally, but a few can usually be found in smears from healthy horses and ruminants.

Increased number of basophils (basophilia) is a relatively rare finding, which usually occurs in association with eosinophilia. Since most healthy animals have no basophils in blood, the reference interval usually includes zero basophils, therefore basopenia is not a relevant finding.

Leukopenia

It does not occur as a specific disease, but is a common manifestation of a number of diseases. Viral diseases particulary, Hog cholera, is frequently accompanied by panleukopenia in early stages. Leukopenia has also been observed in leptospirosis in cattle although bacterial infection is usually accompanied by leukocytosis. Acute local inflammation may cause a transient fall in the leukocyte count, Leucopenia reduces the resistance of animal to bacterial infection that may lead to septicemia and death.

Treatment of the leukopenia should include administration of broad spectrum antibiotic to prevent bacterial infection.

Leukemia

It is manifested by abnormal proliferation of myeloid or lymphoid tissue causing a marked increase in number of circulating leucocytes accompanied by enlargement of spleen and lymphnodes. Bovine viral leucosis is a common example associated with increased leukocytic count. Bone marrow samples are examined for confirmation, and are easily obtained from sterum in animal in standing position. In farm animals, only common form of leukemia is enzootic bovine leucosis.

10

Diseases of Respiratory Systems

The functional efficiency of the respiratory system depends on the ability to oxygenate the blood and to remove CO_2 as it passes in the respiratory circulation resultant. Interference with this function can occur in a number of ways but the resultant defect in all cases is lack of adequate oxygen supply to the tissues. The respiratory insufficiency like anoxia or hypoxia is responsible for most of the clinical signs of respiratory diseases leading to respiratory failure and finally death.

Anoxia

It is defined as inadequate supply of Oxygen to tissue or reduced tissue oxygenation. It occurs in a number of ways.

1. **Anoxic anoxia:** It occurs when there is defective oxygenation of blood in pulmonary circulation which is usually caused by primary diseases of respiratory tract.
2. **Anemic anoxia:** It occurs when there is deficiency of hemoglobin per unit volume of blood for which oxygen carrying capacity of blood is reduced. For example, hemoglobin is converted to methemoglobin in nitrate and nitrite poisoning and in excess of carbon monoxide to carboxy hemoglobin thus, reducing oxygen carrying capacity of haemoglobin leading to anemic anoxia.
3. **Stagnant anoxia:** It is the state in which the rate or velocity of blood flow to the capillary is reduced. Stagnant anoxia is the basic defect in congestive heart failure, peripheral circulatory failure and venous obstruction. Arterial hypoxia occurs in adult cattle which are restrained in dorsal recumbency for abdominal surgery.
4. **Histotoxic anoxia:** It occurs when there is adequate oxygenation of blood but ther is failure of tissue oxygenation. The cyanide poisoning is the only common cause for this type anoxia.

Anoxic anoxia may occur when oxygen tension in the inspired air is too low to oxygenate the pulmonary blood efficiently, but the common causes are lesions or dysfunction of the respiratory tract reducing the supply of alveolar air. Abnormality of alveolar epithelium occurs in pneumonia, pulmonary atelectasis, pneumothorax, pulmonary edema and congestion. Decreased amplitude of chest movement due to pain in chest wall also reduces the oxygen tension of blood. Obstruction of air passage by accumulation of exudates and depression of respiratory centre by drugs or toxin has the same effect.

Anoxic anoxia is the basic defect in congenital heart diseases associated with mixing of arterial and venous blood. Anoxic anoxia also occurs when there is paralysis of respiratory muscles as in tick paralysis, botulism, tetanus, and strychnine poisoning. Several compensatory mechanisms operate if development of anoxia is slow. There is an increase in depth of respiratory movement (hyperpnoea) as a result of anoxia and it is mediated by the chemoreceptor of the carotid and aortic arteries. Stimulation of spleenic contraction and erythropoesis in bone marrow are produced by anoxia resulting in polycythemia. There is also increase in heart rate and stroke volume. The signs of dysfunction of respiratory system start appearing in various organs, if these compensatory mechanism are insufficient to maintain an adequate supply of oxygen to the tissue. Central nervous system is more susceptible to anoxia showing symptoms of cerebral anoxia along with myocardial asthenia, renal and hepatic dysfunction and increase in motility and secretory activity of alimentary tract. Respiratory inefficiency also results in faulty elimination of $CO_2$and it's accumulation in blood and tissue.

Respiratory Failure

Respiratory movements are involuntary, and are stimulated and modified by respiratory centre in medulla. The activity of this center is regulated by pH and O_2 as well as CO_2 tension in the cranial blood supply. Stimulation of all afferent nerves may cause reflex change in respiration and stimulation of pain fibres. Respiratory failure is the terminal stage of respiratory insufficiency in which the activities of respiratory centre diminishes to the point where movement of respiratory muscles ceases. Respiratory failure can be paralytic, dyspnoeic, asphyxial or tachypnoeic depending on primary disease. In asphyxial failure there is hypercapnea and anoxia. Hypercapnea stimulates the respiratory centre resulting dyspnoeic respiratory movement followed by alternating periods of gasping and apnea just before death. Paralytic respiratory failure is caused by poisoning with respiratory centre depressants or by nervous shocks. Acute heart failure or haemorrhages may cause paralytic respiratory failure, but there is usually a variable degree of dyspnoea and gasping which is not as severe as in typical asphyxial failure. In typical paralytic failure the respiratory centre are paralysed so that respiration become shallow, rapid and less frequent and ceases without appearance of dyspnoea or gasping. Tachypneoic respiratory failure is a least common form and arises when pulmonary ventilation is increased, as in hyperthermia, so that there is hypoxia but no CO_2 tension is observed. Because of lack of CO_2 to stimulate respiratory movements, they are shallow and rapid which is termed as tachypnoeia. The differentiation of these types of failure is of some importance in determining the line of treatment. In paralytic form O_2 is the rational treatment and in taachypnoeic form, both O_2 and CO_2 should be provided.

Manifestation of Respiratory Insufficiency

Hyperpnoea and Dyspnoea: Hyperpnoea is defined as increased pulmonary ventilation. It includes increased respiratory movements which appear to cause distress to the animals. Hyperpnoea becomes dyspnoea at an arbitrary dyspnoeic point. Dyspnoea is a physiological occurrence after vigorous exercise and is abnormal when it occurs at rest or other little exercise. It is usually caused by anoxia and hypercapnea arising most commonly from diseases of respiratory tract. In pulmonary dyspnoea, one other factor may be of contributory importance that is there may be an abnormally sensitive reflex. This is most likely to occur when there is inflammation or congestion of lungs and pleura resulting shallow and rapid breathing. Dyspnoea of pulmonary emphysema is characteristically expiratory in nature i.e. expiratory dyspnoea and is caused by anoxic anoxia and the need for forced expiration to achieve successful expulsion of tidal air. Cardiac dyspnoea results from backward failure of left ventricle with congestion and edema of the lungs. Stagnant anoxia plays some part in production of this form of dyspnoea. Dyspnoea is never marked in anaemic anoxia when patient is at rest because there is absence of hypercapnoea. In acidosis, release of CO_2 stimulates respiratory centre and dyspnoea may occur and in some cases like encephalitis, stimulation of the centre may cause neurogenic dyspnoea. Dyspnoea and hyperpnea are the clinical signs most likely to attract attention to the possible presence of disease in respiratory tract.

Disease Causing Dyspnoea at Rest or Lack of Exercise Tolerance

1. Respiratory tract diseases: These diseases cause interference with supply of O_2 and CO_2 discharge from alveolar epithelium like
   (a) filled alveoli in pneumonia and pulmonary edema,
   (b) compressed alveoli in pneumothorax, hydrothorax, haemothorax, emphysema, diaphragmatic hernia and
   (c) blocked air passage in nasal obstruction, pharyngeal, laryngeal, tracheal and bronchial obstruction.

2. Cardiovascular diseases: Those cause inadequate perfusion of lung lobes.
   (a) Cardiac diseases such as congestive heart failure and acute heart failure
   (b) Peripheral circulatory failure in shock and dehydration
   (c) Increased blood viscosity in haemoconcentration
3. Diseases of blood: Those cause inadequate supply of O_2 to tissue and CO_2 discharge from tissue resulting from inadequate haemoglobin in circulation.
   (a) Anaemia due to insufficient HB
   (b) Altered haemoglobin level due to met–haemoglobinemia or carboxy-haemoglobinemia
4. Nervous system diseases: The movement of respiratory muscles are affected by impairment of their nerve supply including
   (a) Paralysis of respiratory muscles in tetanus, tick paralysis and botulism
   (b) Paralysis of respiratory centre in poisoning by nicotine sulphate
   (c) Stimulation of respiratory centre in encephalitis
5. General systemic states: Pain, hyperthermia, acidosis
6. Environmental cause: Lack of O_2 in high altitude disease, lack of O_2 in fire place or exposure to toxic gases
7. Miscellaneous poisons: Number of poisons cause dyspnoea as a prominent sign such as
   (a) Farm chemicals (Methaldehyde, dinitrophenols)
   (b) Organophosphates, carbamate, urea etc.

Coughing

Cough is an explosive expiration of air from lung. It is initiated by reflex stimulation of cough centre in medulla oblongata by irritation of sensory receptor in respiratory tract. The stimulus may originate in pharynx, larynx, trachea and bronchi. Coughing may also be initiated by irritation of the oesophagus particularly in choking. The purpose of coughing is to remove the excess mucous, inflammatory products or foreign material from the respiratory tract. Coughing indicates presence of primary or secondary respiratory disease. Coughing can be assessed according to several characteristics. Generally, it is infrequent in early stages of respiratory tract disease, but may become frequent as the degree of inflammation of larynx, trachea and bronchi become more severe. A simple cough of short duration indicates mild inflammation. Coughing is usually painless and indicates widespread inflammation of larynx trachea and bronchi. A cough is productive if there is expulsion of mucous and inflamed debris through nasal or oral cavity. A productive cough indicates presence of exudative lesions resulting in large quantities of inflamed debris and mucous. A non productive cough is usually called as dry cough indicating inflammation with minimal exudation. When cough is infrequent and does not spontaneously arise during clinical examination, it may be necessary to induce coughing. External manipulation and slight compression of larynx or trachea will induce a cough in presence of laryngitis and bronchitis. Occlusion of nostrils with towel for 30-60 seconds will also result in coughing as a result of hypoxia which causes an immediate deep inspiration following removal of obstruction. An undesirable consequence of coughing is the spread of exudates and mucous of low viscosity distally into bronchial lumen leading to spread of infection further into lungs.

Respiratory Noises

Respiration may be accompanied by audible abnormal respiratory sounds or noises like sneezing, snoring, wheezing, roaring and expiratory grunting.

Sneezing is a sudden noisy expiration through nasal cavities caused reflexly by irritation of nasal mucosa. Sneezing occurs in rhinitis and obstruction of nasal cavities and by digital manipulation or examination of nasal mucosa.

Wheezing is a high pitched sound produced by air coming through a narrow lumen such as inflameed nasal cavity.

A **snore** or **stertor** is a deep guttural sound on inspiration originating from vibration of pharyngeal mucosa. It is often intermittent depending on animal posture. A fatty young bull will often snore when he is dozing half asleep with his head long down but snore will disappear when he is alert and his head is held in a normal position.

Stridor is an inspiratory stenotic sound originating from a reduction in the caliber of larynx as occurs in laryngeal edema and abscess.

Expiratory grunt is a clearly audible noise synchronous with expiration. It is most common in cattle with diffuse pulmonary disease. A painful grunt may occur in diseases of thorax such as fibrinous pleuritis and is not associated with inspiration or expiration.

Roaring may occur during exercise and is produced by air passing through larynx of reduced lumen or paralysed larynx as seen in rabies.

Snuffling, bubbling or rattling sounds may be audible over trachea or base of the lungs when there is accumulation of secretion or exudates in nasal cavities, larynx or trachea which are most clearly audible on inspiration.

Cyanosis

It is the bluish discoloration of the skin, conjunctiva and visible mucosa caused by an increase in the absolute amount of the reduced haemoglobin in blood. It can also occur when there is incomplete oxygenation of the Hb in the blood even if the Hb concentration in blood is normal. It can occur in all type of anoxic anoxia and stagnant anoxia, but not in anaemic anoxia because of insufficient amount of Hb. On the other hand, polycythemia (increased PCV) predisposes to cyanosis. Methemoglobin is accompanied by discoloration of skin and mucosa, but colour is browner than blue and can't be accurately called as cyanosis. The most marked cyanosis occurs in congenital cardiac defects and is never marked in acquired heart diseases. It is not usually marked in pulmonary diseases unless degree of pulmonary collapse is severe. It is also a common and a life threatening sign in severe cases of laryngeal obstruction as occurs in sever laryngitis .

Nasal Discharge

Excess of abnormal nasal discharge is usually an indication of respiratory tract disease. It is common in all farm animals. Cattle may remove some or all of nasal discharge by licking with their tongue. Horses donot remove any nasal discharge. The discharge may be copius, serous, mucoid, purulent, caseous, streak as with blood (ozena), foul smelling or contain feed particles. The discharge may originate from lesions in nasal cavity, congenital defect of hard palate like cleft palate in new born animals, para nasal sinuses, guttural pouch in horses, pharynx, larynx, trachea and lungs. Disease of esophagus and stomach which cause dysphagia and regurgitation or vomition can also cause nasal discharges. Copious bilateral serous discharge is characteristic of early infllammation of nasal cavities in viral rhinitis. Bilateral mucous discharge suggests infllammation of few days duration. A bilateral purulent discharge indicates infllammation with concurrent infection with pyogenic bacteria of upper or lower respiratory tract. A copius bilateral caseous discharge suggests an allergic or bacterial rhinitis. Foul smelling discharge is usually associated with necrosis of tissues anywhere in nasal cavity, guttural pouch in horse or severe necrotic and gangrenous pneumonia. A bilateral foul smelling discharge containing feed particles suggests dysphagia, regurgitation or vomition. In most cases a chronic unilateral nasal discharge suggest lesion of one nasal cavity or paeranasal sinuses. A bilateral discharge suggests lesion posterior to the nasal passage. In animals with evidence of an infectious disease of respiratory tract accompanies bilateral serous to muco-purulent discharge. It is usually assumed that the discharge is usually primary or secondary. Nasal swab may be collected aseptically and given for microbial examination if suspected for infectious disease. However transtracheal fluid examination or pharyngeal swabs are most reliable for cytological examination. Physical examination of paranasal sinus for evidence of pain and facial deformity will assist in diagnosis of sinusitis. Examination of pharynx and larynx in cattle can be done simply through oral cavity. The use of a flexible fiber optic endoscope is necessary for detailed examination of the upper and lower respiratory tract of horse along with radiographic examination of the head.

Epistaxis and Haemoptysis

Epitaxis or nose bleeding in most instances is a disease of the upper respiratory tract. However in pulmonary haemorrhage in horses, epistaxis is manifested by severe nose bleeding. It is commonly noticed in anthrax in cattle and guttural pouch mycosis in horse. It is usual presenting sign in exercise induced pulmonary haemorrhage particularly in race horses. Such blood is coughed off from lungs which are termed as haemoptysis and appears at the nostrils. Coughed off pulmonary blood coming from nose is also a feature of thrombosis of posterior vena cava in cattle. Haemoptysis is spitting or coughing off blood from lungs or airways, seen in pulmonary or bronchial haemorrhage which may result from injury, infectious diseases, neoplasm or warfarin poisoning.

Thoracic Pain

It is a spontaneous pain evidenced by grunting with each respiratory cycle called as pleural pain from a fractured rib, traumatic injury including haematoma of pleura. The following points are carefully studied before arising at diagnosis.

1. History

- Age, sex and breed- Most viral diseases causing respiratory problem in dogs are commonly noticed in young age group whereas pulmonary neoplasm is seen in old animals. Small toy breed dogs suffer from tracheal collapse.
- Main complaints by animal attendant includes neezing, coughing, nasal discharge, breathing difficulty, panting etc
- Duration of present illness, which differentiates acute from chronic form of the disease
- History of previous illness with clinical signs
- Nature of work assigned to animals
- History of housing (indoor/ outdoor, kept outside the room under tree etc).
- History of drenching, confinement in water logged area, high environmental temperature, strong cold wave and season etc.

- History of geographical distribution: Animals of some regions commonly suffer from hemorrhagic septicemia. Similarly, heart worm infection is common in certain belt, where intermediate host (anopheles, culex and aedes) are prevalent
- Details of treatment done previously.
- History of immunization, colour and consistency of stool.

2. Physical examination

(a) Nasal discharge –unilateral or bilateral

(b) Odour- foul, rusty etc

(c) Nature of discharge – serous, mucoid, serosanguineous, mucopurulent, haemoptysis, epitaxis etc.

(d) Nasal passage-visualization, inspection of epiglottis by pulling tongue.

(e) Abnormal swelling- Any growth, enlarged lymphnodes in neck and thoracic region, edema of chest wall, localized swelling of thorax etc.

(f) Rate of respiration either increased or decreased, rhythm of respiration altered, if any

(g) Any abnormality of the type of respiration

(h) Palpation for fracture of nasal bone, enlargement of any respiratory organ etc.

(i) Percussion for audible sounds from various organ on auscultation

3. Others Methods of Diagnosis

(a) Rhinoscopy- visualization of any abnormalities within nasal passage and nasopharynx.

(b) Laryngoscopy- visualization of any abnormalities within larynx.

(c) Bronchoscopy- visualization of any abnormalities within bronchial mucous membrane which is done by flexible bronchoscope.

(d) Plain or contrast radiography reveals lungs parenchyma exudation, fibrosis, calcification, fluid shadow, abscess, presence of any foreign body, tuberculosis nodules etc.

(e) Blood- Total WBC and differential count, erythrocyte sedimentation rate, blood urea nitrogen, glucose, serum enzymes and bloods smear examination for occult heart worms

(f) Sputum for microbial population

(g) Aspiration of tracheal or bronchial fluid done by a thin plastic tube inserted by a tracheal canula for cytological, bacteriological and parasitological examination.

(h) Thoracocentesis: Aspiration of fluid from thoracic cavity or pleural cavity is called thoracocentesis for pleural fluid can be collected by this method. The site for insertion of needle is $6^{th}/7^{th}$ intercostal space. Presence of blood denotes heamothorax or fluid denotes hydrothorax and air denotes pneumothorax.

(i) Faecal sample examination to find-out presence of egg/ larva of lungworm and other worms of respiratory tract.

(j) Tuberculin test- Single intradermal test SID and double intradermal test is performed to detect tuberculosis in cattle.

(k) Exercise tolerance test: Time taken to return to normal respiration rate after exercise is recorded to test excercise tolerance. In case of pulmonary emphysema, animal takes longer time to restore to normal respiration rate.

(l) Lung tissue bioposy: This is taken using trocar and canula at the place of 8th and 9th intercostal space through suction by attaching a syringe to the end of canula. Tissue is processed for histo-pathological and cytological examination.

(m) Test for vital capacity of lungs: Spirography is used to measure respiratory volume and residual air. CO_2 content of expired air can be estimated capnography.

Diseases of Upper Respiratory Tract

Rhinitis/Coryza

It is the inflammation of the nasal mucous membrane characterized by serous, mucoid or purulent nasal discharge. It may be acute or chronic and may be associated with inflammation of all the upper airways.

Acute Rhinitis

It is an acute inflammation of the nasal mucosa which often spreads to all the air passage, producing serous or mucoid nasal discharge.

Etiology

- Exposure of animal to cold and humid weather
- Ill ventilated shed
- Inhalation of dust, smoke and other factory fumes.
- Inhalation of chemical vapours like ammonia, chloride, sulphur etc.
- Sudden change of environmental temperature from too hot to too cold and vice versa

- Individual susceptibility and malnutrition
- Under stress and strain like hard work
- Viral diseases: Parainfluenza, canine distemper, mucosal disease and rinderpest in cattle, infectious bovine rhinotracheitis, adenovirus, blue tongue virus in sheep, equine rhinovirus, sheep pox, feline viral rhinotracheitis infection.
- Bacterial infection: Streptococcus, Staphylococcus, strangles, glanders, haemorrhagic septicemia etc.
- Fungal infection: Aspergillosis, rhinosporidiosis, mucor and rhizopus in dog.
- Parasitic infection: *Schistosoma nasalis* in cattle, *Linguatula serrata* in dogs, *Verminous pneumonia* in cattle.
- Allergic origin - dust fumes, pollen grains, dusty stables produce chronic rhinitis in horses.
- Rhinitis may be caused by tumour or infection of the sinus or teeth.
- Traumatic injury is one of the significant causes leading to epistaxis followed by rhinitis.

Pathogenesis

Irritation of nasal mucous membrane by above causes leads to swelling and congestion of mucous membrane. There is hydropic degeneration of epithelial cells which causes excessive nasal secretion. The nasal secretions remain serous initially, but soon becomes mucoid to mucopurulent due to bacterial invasion. These changes are due to presence of inflammatory cells and tissue degeneration.

Clinical Findings

- Unilateral or bilateral nasal discharge which may vary from serous, mucoid, mucopurulent, haemorrhagic to caseous.
- Copius or scanty and orange to yellow colour or greenish nasal discharge.
- Continuous or intermittent discharge and may have foetid odour.
- Nasal mucosa shows erosion, erythema or ulceration.
- There may be elevation of temperature due to bacteremia or viremia.
- Sneezing is evident in allergic rhinitis and conjunctivitis in severe cases.
- There is enlargement of sub maxillary lymphnode.
- There is shaking of head and rubbing of muzzle, nose on ground due to irritation, which induces bleeding.

- Difficulty in respiration due to presence of edema of nasal mucosa.
- There may be blockage of nasal passage causing dyspnoea and snoring in case of nasal granuloma.
- Thickening of mucoid discharge especially in horse blocks the nose resulting in open mouth breathing.

Clinical Pathology

Nasal swab may be examined for microbial load or any fungus. Examination of nasal mucous scraping is carried out for inclusion bodies. Cytological study is performed for nasal eosinophilia. Nasal discharge is examined for Schistosoma egg and nasal washing for cytological examination and presence of any parasitic ova.

Treatment

Flushing with physiological normal saline removes exudates from the nostrils. In order to remove nasal exudates, antiseptic inhalant vapour may be used like eucalyptus oil, tincture benzoin, tincture Camphor etc. Nasal decongestants may be used in small animals. A course of antihistaminics should be given in allergic rhinitis. Penicillin @10,000- 40,000 units for 4-5 days i/m., tetracycline or oxytetracycline @5-20 mg/kg wt. intravenous or i/m, sulfamethaxine or sulfadimidine @7.5 mg/kg body weight is mostly used in large animals in order to check secondary bacterial infection. Ampicillin and cloxacillin, cefotaxim, ceftriaxone may be tried in acute rhinitis. In fungal infection, thiabendazole @10 mg/kg body weight suspension in 10-20 ml of water should be given twice daily through nasal tubes. Oral thiabendazole can be given @20 mg/kg body weight daily for 6 days to overcome the parasite infection.

Chronic Rhinitis

It is the chronic inflammation of the nasal mucous membrane characterised by mucopurulent nasal discharge.

Etiology

- As a sequale to acute rhinitis, if untreated
- Some adenocarcinoma or nasal tumour not responding to conventional therapy
- Pus in teeth or air sinus
- Glander in horse and *Schistosoma nasalis* in cattle
- Rhinosporidiosis caused by Rhinosporidium producing nasal polyps

- Infestation of nasal cavities with Pasteur mites may be possible causes.
- Fungus like Maduromycosis and Helminthosporium have been reported as a cause of bovine atopic rhinitis.

Clinical Signs

- Mucopurulent nasal discharge which may be serosanguineous in case of nasal granuloma.
- Ulceration of the nasal mucosa and congested and thickened mucous membrane.
- Large amount of mucopurulent discharge may be expelled.
- Snoring sound due to granulomatous lesions and difficulty in respiration
- Open mouth breathing is noticed in chronic cases.
- Enlargement of submaxillary lymph gland
- Extension of head and neck with head shaking

Treatment

1. Nasal granuloma - Anthiomaline @ 20 ml I/M followed by 15 ml in two occasions at 3 days interval.
2. Rhinosporidiosis - Surgical intervention is required. Systemic antibiotics like sulfonamide may be given along with antiseptic inhalants. Vitamin B complex, liver extracts, arsenical preparation may be given. Acetyl arsan @ 2 ml in small animal and 5-10 ml in large animals on alternate days intramuscularly.

Laryngitis

It is an acute or chronic inflammation of the laryngeal mucosa or sub-mucosa and may be associated with catarrhal inflammation of pharynx, trachea and bronchi.

Eticology

1. Exposure to cold, faulty drenching, smoke, fumes etc.
2. Presence of foreign bodies
3. Excessive barking in case of dog
4. Passing of stomach tube or probing in large animal
5. Viral disease like canine distemper, hepatitis, rabies, parainfluenza, equine viral rhinopneumonitis
6. Bacterial infection like *Haemorrhagic septicemia Streptococcus, Corynebacterium pyogenes, Spherophorus necrophorus*

7. Non specific bronchitis, rhinitis and pharyngitis may precipitate the disease condition
8. Chronic laryngitis may be produced by irritation due to chronic lung infection, actinobaccilosis and tuberculosis.

Clinical Signs

Acute Laryngitis

- Short, harsh, dry, painful cough that becomes more prolonged and moist.
- Cough is induced by dust, drinking cold water and pulling of head with collar.
- Coughing on external palpation of larynx.
- Elevation of body temperature ($\geq$105^{0}F), snoring sound, scanty, serous, mucoid or mucopurulent nasal discharge
- Abducted elbow with lowering of head and open mouth breathing while standing.
- Swelling of sub-maxillary lymphodes, if not treated properly. Severe dyspnoea and death due to asphyxia

Chronic Laryngitis

- Commonly seen in dogs dry, harsh and hacking type of cough, which is aggravated on exposure to cold, excitement, dust and exercise
- Stall-fed cattle which are exclusively confined develop persistent cough due to chronic laryngitis unless they are allowed to graze on pasture.
- Pharyngitis may augment chronic laryngitis in equines in which inspiratory stertorous type of laryngeal breathing is observed.
- Excessive hot, humid or chilled atmosphere may aggravate the symptoms resulting in collapse due to hypoxia.

Diagnosis is made from history and symptoms. Differential diagnosis is made from other respiratory diseases like bronchitis, pneumonia, tracheitis etc. Confirmation of laryngitis is made by laryngoscopy.

Treatment

- Provision of well ventilated warm room
- Cold and damp surrounding should be avoided
- A course of antibiotic like ampicillin, cloxacillin, penicillin, amoxicillin, cefotaxime is given intramuscularly for 5-7 days.
- Cortisone given to reduce swelling along with sedative expectorant.

- Intravenous administration of Sodium iodide @2-3 gm/150 kg slowly for 5-7 days in horses.
- Inhalation of steam added with few drops of tincture benzoin may be useful.
- In case of severe dyspnoea, epinephrine @1:1000 spray may be useful.
- Generalized malaise and fever may be checked by giving acetyl salicyl group of drugs.
- Persistent cough can be treated with expectorant drugs like codein sulfate.
- Drenching of liquid medicine should be avoided and it should be given in form of electuary.

Bronchitis

It is the inflammation of the epithelium of the bronchi and bronchiole, which extends in various depth of mucosa of bronchial tubes. Inflammation of trachea and bronchi occur frequently together, called trachea-bronchitis, which extends to lungs parenchyma causing bronchopneumonia. Bronchitis is manifested by production of mucoid and muco-purulent type of nasal discharge with productive husky cough. Bronchitis is classified as acute or chronic bronchitis.

Causes

- Inhalation of irritants, dusts, industrial gases, toxic fumes, chemical, smokes etc
- Sudden change in environmental temperature
- Exposure to cold weather
- Overcrowding of animals during long distance travel, and housing in poor ventilated shed
- Too much bathing of animal with cold water
- Malnutrition and exhaustion during transport
- Drinking of cold water after exercise
- Bacteria like *Bordetella bronchoseptica* infection in dogs, *Streptococcus, Staphylococcus, Pastuerella, Klebsiella* etc
- Virus like influenza, distemper, canine adenovirus type-II, infectious bovine rhinotracheitis
- Parasites like ascaris larva, lungworm infection, filaroids infection
- Disease of other organs like cardiac diseases, enteritis, dermatitis may be secondary attributable causes

Pathogenesis

Mucosa of bronchi and bronchiole becomes inflammed, thickened and congested with infiltration of inflammatory cells, mainly neutrophils. There is secretion of mucous due to increased activity of mucous secreting cells and goblet cells. In severe cases, the epithelium of the mucosa may be destroyed and covered by exudates, which is catarrhal, fibrinous or purulent in nature. Irritation of mucosa causes increased elasticity of bronchial epithelium and swelling which causes partial obstruction of the air passage resulting in inspiratory dyspnoea, and coughing causes expulsion of the exudates. In case of chronic bronchitis, there is edema and swelling of the bronchial mucosa due to exudation. Goblet cells are hypertrophied, and secrete excess mucous. Cellular infiltration and edema cause narrowing of bronchial lumen. There is spasm of bronchial muscle and ulceration leading to formation of granulation tissue and fibrosis. Narrowing of lumen is responsible for ronchi (dry rales) and presence of exudates is responsible for moist sound. There may be spread of infection from bronchi to surrounding lung parenchyma.

Clinical Signs

Production of dry and harsh type of cough is noticed, which is spasmodic in nature. Cough is noticed in the morning hours. Animal may expel large volume of mucous with coughing. There is elevation of body temperature and respiration rate. Mucoid nasal discharge initially leads to mucopurulent at later stage, extension of head and neck. In severe cases, there is dyspnoea and mouth breathing. Auscultation reveals moist rales in early cases with dry and crepitant rales leading to emphysema at later stage.

Clinical Pathology

Haematological examination reveals increased leucocytes due to bacterial infection or eosinophilia due to irritation and allergic reaction.

Examination of bronchial fluid is performed for cytological investigation and presence of any parasite. Bronchitis should be differentiated from the followings:

- **Chronic pulmonary tuberculosis** - Diurnal variation in temperature, sputum for acid fast organism, X-ray, tuberculin test, consolidation of lung.
- **Bronchiectasis**- It can be diagnosed by radiography and honey comb appearance of lungs field.
- **Bronchogenic carcinoma-** Cytological examinations of sputum, pleural fluid, bronchial wash etc.

- **Pneumonia-** High rise of body temperature, severe dyspnoea, moist rales, vesicular murmur, toxaemia, isolation of causative factors are important in diagnosis of disease.
- **Cardiac disease-** Cardiac murmur, no rale sound, cardiac arrhythmia, ECG findings.

Treatment

A course of antibiotics like amoxicillin and cloxacillin, ampicillin and cloxacillin should be given along with a course of antihistaminics like chlorpheniramine maleate, cetrizine, levocetrizine. Expectorant should be given to depress cough. Antiseptic inhalation like Tincture Benzoin, Tincture Camphor and eucalyptus oil may be used. Parasitic infestation should be treated with anthelmintics along with rest and proper hygienic condition.

Pneumonia

It is the inflammation of the lung parenchyma usually accompanied by inflammation of bronchioles (bronchopneumonia) or with pleura known as pleuropneumonia, clinically manifested by rapid shallow breathing, coughing, and fever with vesicular rale sound. Bacterial pneumonia may produce signs of toxaemia. All species of animal irrespective of age may suffer from pneumonia.

Etiology

1. Predisposing factors: Exposure of animals to damp and cold condition, ill-ventilated shed, exhaustion of workload, long transportation by truck or ship, severe hunger and malnutrition, exposure to cold wave during winter, sudden change in weather, cardiac weakness, inhalation of dust and other irritating vapour.

2. Immediate factors:

I. Bacterial agents

- Cattle - *Streptococcus, Staphylococcus, Corynebacterium, Klebsiella, Mycoplasma, Pseudomonas*
- Horse - *Streptococcus, Staphylococcus, Salmonella, Corynebacterium, Escherichia coli, Pasteurella, Pseudomonas*
- Sheep/ goat - *Streptococcus, Staphylococcus, Pastuerella, Mycoplasma, Acinobacillus lignierresii.*
- Pig - *Haemophilus, Pasteurella, Mycoplasma, Bordetella Bronchoseptica, Salmonella.*
- Dog - *Bordetella bronchoseptica, Klebsiella, Pseudomonas, E. coli.*

- Cat - *Streptococcus, Staphylococcus, Haemophilus, Mycoplasma*

II. Viral agents

- Cattle - viral pneumonia of calf, parainfluenza, adenovirus, rhinovirus.
- Horse - Equine influenza, equine infectious pleuropneumonia, adenovirus, equine viral rhinopneumonitis
- Sheep/ goat - Sheep and goat pox, progressive interstitial pneumonia (maedi), influenza virus, reovirus and adenovirus
- Pigs - Swine influenza, viral pneumonia of pigs
- Dog/ cat - Feline viral rhinotracheitis, canine distemper, canine parainfluenza, canine adenovirus type-2, reo and herpes virus, fading puppy complex syndrome in dogs

III. Fungus

- *Aspergillus fumigatus, Histoplasmosis,* Blastomycosis, Coccidioidomycosis, Cryptococcus

IV. Parasites

- *Dictyocaulus viviparous* (cattle)
- *Dictyocaulus filariai* (sheep/goat)
- *Dictyocaulus arnfieldi* (horse)
- *Metastrongylus apri* (pigs)
- *Ascaris* spp.(calf and pigs)
- *Toxoplasma gondii* (sheep, dog and cat)

V. Physical Agents

Faulty drenching of fluids, drugs, chemicals, inhalation of dust, smoke, gas, medicinal vapor, dipping of animal for ectoparasitic treatment during hot summer.

Pathogenesis

The Process of development of pneumonia varies with causative agents, their virulence and portal of entry into lungs parenchyma. The classification based on entry of pathogen is as follows

1. Tracheobronchogenous - This is the most common route for infectious agents like *Aspergillus fumigatus, Streptococcus, Staphylococcus, E. coli, Corynebacterium pyogenes*.
2. Systemic infections spread via blood vascular system and carry *Pasteurella, Salmonella* and parasitic larva to the lungs

3. Penetrating wounds caused by bullets, knives, foreign bodies, accidental injury, may penetrate lungs and carry infectious agents like bacteria producing pneumonia. Similarly, foreign bodies through rumen and reticulum may reach lungs causing pneumonia.
4. Lymphogenous - Certain bacteria like *Mycobacterium tuberculosis* may reach lungs via lymphatics.

Clinical Signs

1. Bacterial pneumonia

- Moist, painful and productive cough
- Serous, mucoid, mucopurulent to purulent nasal discharge
- Rapid shallow respiration leading to abdominal type/respiration
- In later stages, dyspnoea and labored breathing
- Rise in temperature, anorexia, dullness and increased pulse rate
- Gradual loss of body condition, unable to move and tendency to lie down
- Stands with abducted elbow with extension of head and neck
- Pain on palpation and percussion.
- Dull sound is heard in cases with lungs consolidation.
- In early stages, vesicular murmur is very prominent. In chronic stages, dry rales and neutrophilia are the prominent findings.

2. Viral pneumonia

- Dry unproductive cough, which may be hacking in nature.
- Serous to mucopurulent nasal discharge, shallow respiration, high rise in body temperature
- Food refusal, rapid dehydration, and emaciation
- Neutropenia and lymphocytosis are the common feature.

3. Parasitic pneumonia (verminous pneumonia)

- Frequent cough with mucous, sometimes mixed with adult worms.
- Seromucoid nasal disacharge, may cause severe itching of skin around nares and excoriation due to rubbing.
- Gradual loss of body condition, temperature is usually normal, labored respiration, emaciation and anaemia
- Diarrhoea is observed frequently.
- Edema of sub-maxillary region, eyelid or anterior part of the head.

- Auscultation reveals moist rales, animal becomes weak, may fall down leading to death due to asphyxia.

4. Mycotic pneumonia (Fungal)
   - Moist cough, thick mucoid nasal discharge with emaciation, dyspnoea and loss of body condition.
   - Haemorrhagic nasal discharge with expulsion of greenish yellow masses.
   - Dehydration and anaemia
   - Temperature may increase due to secondary bacterial infection with harsh respiratory sound
5. Aspiration pneumonia
   - Mostly fatal.
   - History of faulty drenching within few hours to few days
   - Elevated temperature, rapid pulse, labored respiration
   - Thick nasal discharge, mucopurulent and rusty
   - Anorexia and rapid loss of body condition
   - Reluctant to move and standing with abducted elbow
   - Pain on palpation and percussion
   - Protrusion of tongue and open mouth breathing

Clinical Pathology

- Culture of nasal discharge
- Aspiration of tracheal and bronchial exudates
- Haematological examination for total and differential leukocyte count, total erythrocyte count, erythrocyte sedimemtation rate and haemoparasites
- Neutrophilia in bacterial infection, neutropenia in viral infection and eosinophilia in parasitic infection
- Increased ESR in chronic wasting disease
- Serological test for viral infection
- Examination of faeces for any parasitic ova or eggs
- Radiography

Treatment

Use of specific antibacterial agents- ceftriaxone, cefotaxime, ampicillin and cloxacillin by intravenous route. Sulfa drugs like sulfamethazine 33.33% solution or sulfadimidine 33.33% @15-30 ml/50 kg body weight intravenously give good result in Pastuerella pneumonia and haemorrhagic septicemia. In parasitic pneumonia, drugs like levamizole, fenbendazole may be given. Fungal pneumonia is treated with griseofulvin and nystatin. Amphotericin-B @ 0.05 mg/kg may be given with 5% DNS slowly in dogs and cat. Ketoconazole @10 mg/kg thrice a day is also effective. A course of anthistaminics should be given along with analgesics. In some cases, a course of steroid may be used. Sedative expectorant along with vitamin-B complex, vitamin-C and calcium may be used to rejuvenate pulmonary parenchyma.

Pneumothorax

Accumulation of air in pleural space is called pneumothorax, which causes respiratory distress, where atmospheric air enters during inspiration, but cannot be expelled out.

Causes

Air may come into pleural space

1. through visceral pleura from lungs or bronchus like rupture of lungs due to excessive coughing and rupture of lung abscess.
2. through mediastinum like rupture of oesophagus during manipulation.
3. through chest wall by injury resulting from accident, fracture rib by kicking of other vicious animal, injury by horns etc.
4. through diaphragm like sub-diaphragmic abscess and organism producing gas in pleura.

Clinical Signs

1. Usually appears suddenly leading to asphyxia within 24 hrs.
2. Animal remains in a state of collapse
3. Abdominal respiration, which is very painful.
4. Bulging of affected side of chest.

Diagnosis

Palpation which reveals fractured rib and radiography

Treatment

1. In closed pneumothorax, mustard plaster may be used. Removal of air by needle and canula which helps in decompression and haemorrhage should be checked. To prevent shock and pain, steroid and analgesic may be given.
2. Open type wound should be closed along with oxygen supply.

Haemothorax

Accumulation of blood in the pleural sac is called haemothorax that causes compression of lungs parenchyma and dyspnoea.

Cause

1. Post traumatic and post surgical effect
2. Spontaneous rupture of thoracic vessel
3. Adhesion of pleural and pulmonary vessel
4. *Spirocerca lupi* infection in dog
5. Presence of neoplasm

Pathogenesis

Rupture of intrathoracic artery causes blood accumulation in pleural sac. Ruptured pulmonary artery causes expansion of pleural cavity and the expanding hemothorax compress the lungs leading to collapse.

Clinical Findings

Signs may be dangerous because of loss of blood accompanied by respiratory insufficiency caused by concurrent pleural and pulmonary haemorrhage. Signs of shock due to haemorrhagic anaemia.

Diagnosis

Clinical signs like rapid progressive anaemia, pale mucous membrane, tachycardia, muffled heart and lung sound. Identification of pleural fluid by aspiration

Treatment

Emergency thoracotomy and aspiration of fluid is necessary along with blood transfusion and antibiotic therapy.

Hydrothorax

Accumulation of transudate or fluid in thoracic cavity is called hydrothorax.

Causes

1. General and right side congestive heart failure
2. Renal disorder
3. Hypoproteinemia due to less synthesis of protein or protein loosing disease
4. Injury to vagus nerve

5. Liver disease
6. Pulmonary neoplasia, pleural neoplasia
7. Diaphragmatic hernia

Clinical signs

Fluid usually accumulates on both the sides of lungs. Dyspnoea without fever and edema in other parts of the body may be seen

Diagnosis

Radiographic evidence of fluid, and identification of the nature of the aspirated fluid

Treatment

- Repeated aspiration of fluid
- Surgical intervention
- Correction of etiological factor

11

Diseases of Urinary System

Diseases of bladder and urethra are most commonly reported in farm animals than diseases of kidney. Knowledge of the physiology of the urinary secretion and excretion is required to understand the urinary tract diseases. The functions of kidneys are to excrete the end products of tissue metabolism except CO_2 and to maintain homeostasis with respect to fluid and solutes including acid base balance by selective excretion of these substances. The kidney maintains homeostasis by varying volume of water and the concentration of solutes in the urine. In general, renal tubules maintain homeostasis, while the glomerulus controls excretion of metabolic end products. Diseases of kidney and in some instances of the ureter, bladder and the urethra reduce the efficiency of the kidney function. Disturbances in protein, acid base, solute and water homeostasis and excretion of metabolic end products are observed in renal in insufficiening. When the kidneys can no longer regulate body fluid and solute composition, renal failure occurs.

Renal Insufficiency and Renal Failure

Renal function depends on the integrity of the individual nephron, the structural and functional unit of kidney. Insufficiency can occur from an abnormality in the rate of renal blood flow, glomerular filtration rate and efficiency of the tubular re-absorption. Circulatory emergency may lead to marked reduction in glomerular filtration, but they are extra renal in origin and can't be considered as true cause of renal insufficiency. However, prolonged circulatory disruption can cause renal ischaemia and renal insufficiency. The progress and end result of any type of renal disease tends to be very similar. In glomerulo-nephritis, the primary reduction is seen glomeruli function but secondary involvement of tubules mostly occurs. When assessing kidney function clinically, it is convenient to consider renal blood flow and glomerular and tubular function independently. The clinical and clinico-pathological signs of renal dysfunction often depend on anatomical location of lesion and on imbalance of function between glomeruli and tubules. Renal dysfunction tends to be a dynamic process so the degree of dysfunction varies with time. If renal dysfunction is so severe that the animal existence is not possible, it is said to be in a state of renal failure and clinical syndrome of uremia develops.

Clinical Features of Urinary Tract Disease

The major manifestations of urinary tract diseases are abnormalities of urine composition and volume, pain and dysuria, rupture of renal pelvis, bladder and urethra and defect of nervous control during urination.

Abnormal Constituents of Urine

1. **Proteinuria:** Protein may be present in urine in different conditions like haemoglobinuria, myoglobinuria and haemturia and also in urinary tract infections.
2. **Cast and cells:** Cast occurs when kidneys are involved in disease process.Casts are not seen in all cases of renal diseases.
3. **Haematuria:** Blood in urine can result from prerenal causes when vascular damage occurs such as trauma to kidney and septicemia. Post renal haematuria occurs particulary in urolithiasis and cystitis.
4. **Haemoglobinuria:** Presence of haemoglobin in urine in K/a haemoglobinuria. False haemoglobinuria occur in haematuria, when RBCs are lysed releasing haemoglobin In this case, RBC can be detected only by microscopically by examining the urine sediments for cellular debris. True haemoglobinuria causes a deep red to brown dis colouration of urine and gives a positive reaction to biochemical test.
5. **Myoglobinuria:** Presence of myoglobin in urine is an indication of severe muscle damage (azoturia in horses). Myoglobin molecule is much smaller than haemoglobin and passes more readily through glomeruli, so a detectable dark brown staining of urine occurs without very high plasma level of myoglobin.
6. **Pyuria:** Leucocytes or pus in urine indicates inflammatory exudates at some point in urinary tract, usually renal part or urinary bladder. Pyuria is usually accompanied with presence of bacteria in urine.
7. **Crystalluria:** Crystals in urine of herbivore animals have no special significance unless they occur in very large number and are associated with clinical signs of irritation of urinary tract. Calcium carbonate and triple phosphate crystals are commonly present in normal urine of herbirores. If they occur in large number, it suggests that urine is concentrated and possibility of development of urolithiasis in future.
8. **Glycosuria and ketonuria:** glycosuria in combination with ketonuria occur only in diabetes mellitus, a rare disease of large animals. Glycosuria may occur in association with enterotoxemia due to *Clostridium perfringens* type-D and may occur after parenteral treatment

with dextrose solution and adrenocorticotropic hormone. It also occurs in acute tubular nephrosis. Ketonuria is a more common findings in ruminants which occurs in starvation and acetonemia in cattle, pregnancy toxaemia in ewes and does. A small amount of ketonuria is normally present in dairy cows.

Urine Flow

Care should be taken to differentiate between increased daily flow and increased frequency without increased flow. Normal urine production is highly variable in large animals. In healthy adult horse, normal urine production ranges from 15-48 ml/kg/day. In neonatal foals, it is 150 ml/kg/day. Polyuria occurs when there is an increase in volume of urine production. It can result from extra-renal causes, when horse habitually drinks excess quantity of water. When polyuria is suspected, a urine sample should be collected to determine the osmolality. If urine with a constant specific gravity of 1.008-1.012 is produced, then the presence of renal disease should be considered. If urea and creatinine are within normal limits, a water deprivation test may be performed in horses to access their ability to produce concentrated urine. Animals unable to conserve water due to renal disease can be rapidly dehydrated, and develop pre-renal uremia. If the specific gravity of urine is below 1.008, it indicates production of dilute urine. Low specific gravity may occur in diabetes insipidus following excessive water intake or fluid on fusion or following diuretic administration. Neonatal animals on fluid administration often produce dilute urine.

Oliguria and Anuria

Reduction in daily output (oliguria) and complete absence of urine (anuria) occurs in some conditions and varies only in degree. In dehydrated animals, urine flow naturally decreases to conserve water as plasma osmotic pressure increases. Congestive heart failure and peripheral circulatory failure may cause such a reduction in renal blood flow leading to oliguria. Anuria occurs commonly in uretheral obstruction. Oliguria occurs in terminal stages of all forms of nephritis. Anuria and polyuria lead to retention of solutes and disturbance in acid base balance that aids in pathogenesis of uremia.

Pain and Dysuria

Abnormal pain and dysuria are both expression of discomfort caused by many diseases of urinary tract. Acute abdominal pain from urinary tract disease occurs rarely, usually associated with sudden distension of renal pelvis or ureter or infarction of kidney. None of these conditions is common in animals, but occasionally noticed with pyelonephritis. Painful or difficult urination occurs in cystitis, and uretheritis and is manifested by frequent or scanty urine.

Grunting may occur with painful urination and animal may remain in typical posture after urination is completed.

Clinical Feature of Acute and Chronic Renal Failure

Signs of urinary tract disease vary with rate of development and stage of the disease. In most cases, clinical signs are those of the initiating cause, Acute renal failure causes signs of uremia. In horses, most common signs are depression, colic and diarrhoea with oligouria or polyuria. Cattle show similar signs besides being recumbent frequently. In chronic renal disease of all species, there is severe loss of body weight, anorexia, polyuria, polydypsia and ventral edema.

Uremia

The clinical signs of uremia are anuria or oliguria. Oliguria is more common unless there is complete obstruction of urinary tract. Chronic renal disease is usually manifested by polyuria, but oliguria appears in terminal stages, when clinical uremia develops. Uremic animals are depressed and anorectic with muscular weakness and tremor. In chronic condition, there is poor body condition, loss of protein via urine, dehydration etc. The respiration is usually increased in rate and depth, but is not dyspnoeic. In terminal stages, it may become periodic in character. Heart rate is markedly increased due to dehydration and myocardial ischemia. An ammoniacal or uriniferous smell of the breath is rarely noticed. Animals become recumbent and comatose in terminal stage. The temperature falls below normal leading to death.

Principles of Treatment of Urinary Tract Disease

Treatment of acute renal failure in all species is aimed at removing the primary cause and restoring the normal fluid balance by correcting dehydration, acid base disorder and electrolyte abnormality. Prognosis for acute renal failure depends on initiating cause and severity of lesion. If acute disease process can be stopped, the animal may be able to survive on its remaining functional renal tissue. As fluid deficit is corrected, the patient should be observed for urination. If anuria or oliguria is present, rate of fluid administration should be monitored to prevent over-hydration. If patient has oliguria after correction of fluid volume deficit, then a diuretic should be given to restore the normal urine flow. Frusemide @1-2 mg/kg every 2 hr or mannitol @0.25-2 gm/kg in 20% solution can be used. Diuretic should not be used until dehydration is corrected. After urine flow is restored, the resulting dialysis will increase the maintenance fluid requirements. Animals that remains anuric have a grave prognosis and can only be managed with peritoneal or vascular dialysis. The treatment of chronic renal failure will depend on stage of disease and cost of the animals. Selection of antibiotics for treatment of urinary tract infection should be based on quantitative urine culture. The ideal antibiotic for treatment of urinary tract infection should have antibacterial against causal bacteria, be excreted and concentrated in kidney and urine, be active at pH of the urine, has low toxicity, be easily administered and low cost. It should not have harmful interaction with other concurrently given drugs. Antibiotic therapy for lower urinary tract infection should continue for at least 7 days. For lower urinary tract infection, 3-4 weeks of treatment is often necessary. Success of therapy is evaluated by repeating urine culture 7-10 days after last treatment.

Diseases of Kidney

Nephrosis

It includes degenerative and inflammatory lesion primarily affecting renal tubules. Nephrosis can occur as a sequale to renal ischaemia and following affection of kidney. Nephrosis is the most common cause of acute renal failure. In nephrosis, uremia may develop acutely or may occur in terminal stages of chronic renal disease.

Renal Ischaemia

Reduced blood flow through kidney usually results from general circulatory failure. There is transitory oliguria followed by anuria and uremia, if circulatory failure is not corrected.

Etiology

It may be acute or chronic. Acute renal ischaemia occurs due to shock, dehydration, hemorrhagic anaemia, acute heart failure, embolism of renal artery particularly in horse, extreme ruminal distension in cattle. Chronic renal ischaemia is seen due to chronic heart failure.

Clinical Signs

There is oliguria, azotemia and acute renal failure.

Clinical Pathology

Analysis of urine as well as blood urea nitrogen and creatinine level are most commonly used for diagnosis. Serum biochemistry of collected sample may also be used to monitor the response to therapy. Proteinuria is an early indication of renal parenchyma damage. Passage of large volume of urine of low specific gravity after a period of oliguria is usually a good indication of normal glomerular and tubular function. Diagnosis in made based on symptoms and laboratory findings.

Treatment

Treatment must be done for correcting fluid, electrolyte and acid base disturbance as soon as possible. In case of renal damage, supportive treatment like antibiotic (ceftriaxone, cefotaxim) as well as antihaemorrhagic drug (botropase, vitamin K, chromostat, etamsylate) should be given.

Glomerulonephritis

It can occur as a primary disease or as a component of diseases affecting several body functions as seen in equine infectious anaemia and chronic swine fever. Primary and secondary glomerulo-nephritis is not common cause of clinical disease in farm animals. Proliferative glomerulonephritis is relatively common cause of chronic renal failure in horse. Immune system plays a major role in pathogenesis of glomerular lesion. Glomerular injury can be initiated by an immune response wherein antibody is directed against intrinsic glomerular antigen or foreign antibody present in glomerulus, more commonly circulating antigen antibody complex may deposit in glomerulus. As the complexes accumulate they stimulate an inflammatory response that damage the glomerular filtration system. Inflammatory damage to glomerulus alters the selective permeability of filtration system allowing plasma protein particularly albumin to pass into glomerular filtrate.

Clinical Pathology

Commonly, tachycardia, conjuctival edema, nystagmus, walking in circle, convulsion are noticed. Kidneys are enlarged and tender, severe proteinuria, low plasma albumin is present. Blood urea nitrogen is increased with hypo-phospatemia and hypocalcemia.

Interstitial Nephritis

It is rarely recognized as a cause of clinical disease in farm animals, which may be diffused or have focal distribution. In calves, focal interstitial nephritis (white spotted kidney) occurs as a sequel to bacterimia. In pigs, diffused interstitial occurs as a nephritis is observed following infection by *Leptospira* spp. and is important clinically due to destruction of nephrons. Horses with chronic interstitial nephritis have the clinical syndrome of chronic renal failure with uremia.

Pyelonephritis

It develops by ascending infection from lower urinary tract characterized clinically by pyuria, suppurative nephritis, cystitis and ureteritis.

Cause

1. Bacterial infection of lower urinary tract.
2. Septicaemia in cattle caused by *Pseudomonas* spp.
3. Specific pyelonephritis caused by *Corynebacterium renale* in cattle and *Eubacterium suis* in pigs.

Signs

Initially renal pelvis and medulla are affected and infection may extend to cortex. Pyelonephritis causes systemic signs of toxemia and fever. Extensive uremia may develop with bilateral renal involvement. Pyelonephritis is always accompanied by pyuria and haematuria due to inflammatory lesion of the ureter and bladder. In sows, there may be as initial period during which vaginal discharge is noticed, but most affected animals die without showing prior symptoms.

Clinical pathology

Erythrocytes, leucocytes and cell debris are present in urine on microscopic examination. Urine culture in necessary to identity the causative bacteria.

Diagnosis

Presence of pus and blood in urine may suggest cystitis as well as pyelonephritis. Laboratory examination confirms pyelonephritis.

Treatment

General principle of treatment of urinary tract infection should be followed.

Diseases of Bladder, Urethra and Ureter

Cystitis

Inflammation of bladder is usually caused by bacterial infection showing the symptoms of frequent and painful urination and presence of blood, inflammatory cells with bacteria in urine.

Cause

1. Cystic calculus
2. Difficulty in parturition/dystocia
3. Contaminated parturition
4. Late pregnancy
5. Sequale to paralysis of bladder particularly when horses graze on sudan grasses

Pathogenesis

Bacteria frequently gain entry to bladder, but are usually removed by the flushing action of voided urine before they invade the mucosa. Mucosal injury facilitates invasion, but stagnation of urine is the most important predisposing cause.

Symptoms

Frequent, scanty and painful urination is sometimes associated with grunting Acute case of cystits is associated with abdominal pain, kicking at belly. Acute retention of urine may develop if urethra becomes blocked with pus or blood. In chronic case of cystits, signs are less marked. Frequent urinations and feel thickened bladder wall on rectal examination In acute cases, no palpable abnormality may be detected, but pain may be evidenced and feel of thickned bladder wal on per rectal examination have been recended in cystitis.

Clinical Pathology

Blood and pus in urine is a typical in acute cases and urine may have a strong ammonia smell. In less severe cases, no abnormality is noticed on gross inspection. Microscopic examination of urine sediments will reveal erythrocytes, leucocytes and desquamaled epithelial cells. Quantitative bacterial culture is needed to confirm the diagnosis and for therapeutic measures.

Diagnosis

Cystitis syndromes resemble with pyelonephritis and cystic urolithiasis. Pyelonephritis is commonly accompanied by bladder involvement, which may be determined by per rectal exam in ation. However, prognosis in pyelonephritis is less favourable than cystitis. Thickening of bladder wall may suggest a diagnosis of cystitis. Presence of calculi in bladder can usually be detected by per rectal examination, radiographic examination or by ultra-sonography. In small animals, urethral obstruction may also cause frequent attempts of urination, but urine flow is greatly restricted, urine comes only drop by drop and distended bladder can be felt on per rectal examination.

Treatment

Antibiotic therapy should be given for minimum of 7-14 days. Repeated bacterial culture of urine should be done before giving antibiotic therapy. Recurrence of infection is usually seen due to failure in elimination of infection in the accessory gland and bladder wall. Prognosis in chronic cases is poor because of the difficulty for eradication of infection completely and secondary involvement of kidney. Free access to water should be permitted at all times to ensure a free flow of urine.

Urolithiasis in Ruminants

Urolithiasis is a common sub-clinical problem among ruminants raised in managemental system, where the ration is composed of primarily grains or where the animals graze on a certain pasture type. In this situation, 40-60% of animals may form calculi in their urinary tract. Urolithiasis is an important clinical disease of castrated male ruminants. Calculi cause urinary tract, usually, urethral obstruction, characterized by complete retention of urine, frequent unsuccessful attempt to urinate and distension of bladder resulting in urethral perforation and rupture of bladder. Mortality is high in case of urethral obstruction and treatment is mostly surgical. So, prevention is important to limit loss from urolithiasis.

Cause

Urinary calculi or urolithis are formed when organic or inorganic urinary solutes are precipitated out of the solution. The precipitates occur as crystals or as amorphous deposits. Several factors affect the rate of urolith formation including some condition that affect the concentration of specific solutes in urine.

Clinical Signs

The exit from renal pelvis is blocked and acute distension results in pain accompanied by stiffness of gait and pain on pressure over the loins. Calculi in bladder may cause cystitis. In steers and withers, the clinical signs of abdominal pain are kicking at the belly, repeated twitching of penis, strenuous effort to urinate, grunting resulting in voiding of few drops of blood stained urine are observed. On rectal examination, the urethra and bladder are distended and painful on palpation. A heavy precipitate of crystals is often visible on prepucial hairs or inside of the thigh. The passage of a lead wire into the urethra after relaxing the penis with epidural anaesthesia may make it possible to locate the site of obstruction. Cattle with incomplete obstruction frequently pass small amount of blood stained urine. Occasionally, a small strip of urine will be voided followed by a complete blockage, which confuses the diagnosis. If obstruction is not relieved, perforation of urethra or rupture of bladder occurs in 48 hours. In first instance, urine leaks into the connective tissue of the ventral abdominal wall and causes an obvious fluid swelling, which may spread to thorax. Urine is often infected and severe cellulitis may occur with development of toxemia. When bladder ruptures, there is an immediate relief from discomfort. But anorexia and depression develops and uremia appears.

Animals may continue in this state for as long as 2-3 days before it dies in coma. In occasional cases, death occurs soon after rupture of bladder due to sever internal haemorrhage.

Clinical Pathology

Laboratory examination may be useful for diagnosis in early stages, when a calculus is present in kidney or bladder. The urine usually contains erythrocytes, epithelial cells and a higher number of crystals. Bacteria may also be present in secondary invasion of traumatic cystitis, and pyelonephritis is commonly noticed. Blood urea will be increased before rupture of either urethra or bladder.

Diagnosis

Diagnosis can be made from clinical signs. But radiological examination and ultrasonographic examination give 100% confirmation.

Treatment

Treatment of urolithiasis is primarily surgical. In general, calculi can't be dissolved by medical therapy. It may also be difficult to prevent a further increase in size of existing stone or the development of new one, once urolithiasis becomes clinically apparent in animals. However, preventive measures are useful for others exposed to same risk factors. In early stages or in case of incomplete obstruction, treatment with smooth muscle relaxant may be given to relax the urethral obstruction and permit the passage of the obstructing calculi. Animals treated medically should be observed closely to ensure that urination occurs and complete obstruction doesn't occur. Surgical treatment includes urethrostomy, which is necessary to relieve bladder pressure and for removal of calculi.

12

Diseases of Lymphatic System

The lymphatic system is an extensive drainage system that returns water and proteins from various tissues back to the blood stream. The system consists of a network of very fine vessels or tubes called lymphatics that drain lymph from all over the body, and lymphnodes. Lymphatics are found in every part of the body except the central nervous system. Lymph nodes are round or kidney-shaped, and are usually found in groups in different places throughout the body, including the neck, limbe, thorax, abdomen, pelvis, and groin. About two thirds of all lymph nodes and lymphatic tissue are within or near the gastrointestinal tract. Numerous lymph nodes exist within the thoracic and abdominal cavities that cannot be palpated easily, and their enlargement does not show up on routine examination. The major organs of this system include bone marrow, spleen, thymus gland, lymph nodes, and the tonsils. Other organs including the heart, lungs, intestines, liver, and skin also contain lymphatic tissue.

Lymphocytes in the lymph nodes are white blood cells that helps the body to fight infection by producing antibodies. T-cells and B-cells are two types of lymphocytes. B cells produce immunoglobulin responsible for hunoral immunity and T cells confer cell-mediated immunity. Lymph is a clear watery fluid composed of water, protein molecules, salts, glucose, urea, lymphocytes, and other substances. The lymphatic drains the fluid from various body parts.

Disease Conditions of Lymphatic System

Lymphadenopathy: Enlargement of peripheral lymphnodes (LNs) cause visible and palpable swelling resulting in obstruction to lymphatic drainage and subsequent local oedema. Example - Sporadic lymphangitis, particularly in horse and enlargement of prescapular lymphnode in theileriosis in cattle. Enlargement of internal lymph nodes may cause obstruction of esophagus, pharynx, trachea or bronchi. Enlargement may occur as a result of invasion and localization of infectious agents or due to neoplasia of the affected lymphnode.

Caseous lymphadenitis is a chronic inflammatory condition of lymphatic system seen in ruminants, including sheep, goats and cattle. Generally, it causes both external and internal abscesses, and may result in emaciation and death of the animal. It is caused by *Corynebacterium pseudotuberculosis*. The causative bacteria typically enter the animal through an open skin wound, or through the mucous membrane in the mouth or lungs. The draining abscesses are the major source of infectious agent for disease transmission within a herd. The carriers of the disease may appear healthy. Transmission can also occur from contaminated feed, bedding and equipment.

The disease is manifested by abscesses in the lymph nodes, especially around the head and neck. Abscesses may look like chronic acne, or as large abscesses in the pectoral area. These may clinically manifest as open draining sores, or as closed and swollen abscesses. Internal abscesses specifically found in the liver and lungs may result in weight loss, and ultimately emaciation. In affected heifers and cows, abortion and mastitis may become more prevalent.

The disease is diagnosed by physical examination of external lesions, followed by identification of the pathogen in the abscess aspirate. There is no treatment for individually infected animals. The best herd treatment is culling of infected animals, and completing annual vaccination.

Epizootic lymphangitis is a contagious, chronic disease of horses and mules and donkeys. The disease is manifested by suppurative, ulcerating pyogranulomatous dermatitis and lymphangitis. The lesions are more commonly seen in the neck regions, extremities including legs and chest region. It can also be present as an ulcerating conjunctivitis of the palpebral conjunctiva, or rarely as a multifocal pneumonia. The disease is otherwise called as pseudofarcy, pseudoglanders or equine histoplasmosis.

The disease is caused by *Histoplasma capsulatum var. farciminosum.* This fungal causative agent is thermally dimorphic, and a soil-saprophyte. The contact with infected material with traumatized skin, biting of infected flies and ticks or inhalation transmit the disease. The organism may also invade open lesions including ruptured abscesses in strangles and castration wounds.

The clinical form of the disease largely depends on the route of entry of pathogen. The traumatized skin is either infected directly by infected pus, nasal or ocular discharges or indirectly by soil or contaminated harnesses, grooming equipment, feeding and watering utensils, or flies. Ticks may play a role in the transmission of this agent. The conjunctival form of the disease is believed to be spread by flies of Musca or Stomoxys genera. The pulmonary form of the disease is infrequent and is presumed to occur by inhalation of the organism.

The causative agent can be identified in exudate smears or in histological sections of the lesion material. The yeast form of the organism is present in large numbers in well established lesions, and appears as pleomorphic ovoid to globose structures, approximately 2–5 μm in diameter, located both extracellularly and intracellularly in macrophages and giant cells. Organisms are usually surrounded by a 'halo' when stained with Gram stain, haematoxylin and eosin, Periodic acid–Schiff reaction (PAS) or Gomori methenamine–silver stain. The mycelial form of the organism grows slowly under aerobic conditions at 25–30°C on a variety of media including Mycobiotic agar, enriched Sabouraud's dextrose agar, brain–heart infusion agar. Conversion to the yeast phase at 37°C must be demonstrated.

The incubation period is about 3 weeks to 2 months. In all cases, the lesions are nodular and granulomatous. There is often thickening or cording of lymphatics with the formation of pyogranulomatous nodules. Regional lymph nodes may by enlarged and inflamed. Lesions usually heal spontaneously after 2–3 months, resulting in stellate scar formation. However, extensive lesions with high mortality rates can occur in nutritionally deficient animals.

Serological and other tests: Antibodies to *H. capsulatum var. farciminosum* develop at or before the onset of clinical signs. Several assays techniques have been used for detection of antibody, including fluorescent antibody, enzyme-linked immunosorbent assay, and passive haemagglutination tests. Skin hypersensitivity test has been described for identification of the disease.

The disease is to be differentiated from glanders (farcy) caused by *Burkholderia mallei*, ulcerative lymphangitis due to *Corynebacterium pseudotuberculosis*, sporotrichosis caused by *Sporothrix schenckii*, and the skin lesions caused by *Histoplasma capsulatum var. capsulatum*.

Treatment and control: Injection of Amphotericin B with both antibacterial and antifungal properties with local wound drainage and application of inorganic iodides are used to treat early cases. Killed and live vaccines have been used on a limited scale in endemic areas, but they are not readily available.

Lymphosarcoma is a cancerous condition clinically characterized by progressive weight loss, and is seen in adult cattle from 3-6 years of age. The disease in cattle is caused by oncogenic retrovirus, bovine leukemia virus (BLV). The virus was first identified in 1969 and transmissibility was confirmed in 1972. The virus mostly remains attached to lymphocytes. Therefore, transmission of the disease occurs by transfer of BLV infected lymphocytes. Blood, milk and colostrum are the major source of infection. Bovine leukemia virus has been identified in the milk and colostrum of positive cows. Natural service or artificial insemination hardly transmits the virus. Once infected, the animal carries the virus for life.

The prevalence is higher in North America than Europe, particularly in dairy cattle than beef cattle. The prevalence of the disease is influenced by susceptibility of animals to BLV infection, and managemental practices. The susceptibility of cattle to BLV is influenced by genetic factors. Bovine major histocompatibility complex (BoLA) alleles confer either resistance or susceptibility. Age is another factor in acquiring BLV infection, and the prevalence increases with age, and relatively new infections occur in cattle older than 3 to 5 years. Cattle in herds with a high prevalence of BLV infection appear to become infected with BLV at an earlier age. In general, no breed or sex predilection appears to be reported.

Approximately, 70% of cattle positive for Bovine leukemia virus do not show any clinical signs of disease during their lifetime. Twenty-five to twenty-eight percent of those positive for BLV will not display clinical signs, but will develop a persistent lymphocytosis. Of these, roughly 5% of them will go ahead and develop solid tumors. Only 2 to 5% of animals positive for BLV will develop lymphosarcoma. Only approximately 1 in 10,000 cows have lymhosarcoma without BLV infection.

The clinical signs depend on the organ involved in the disease process and the development of solid tumors. The right atrium, abomasum, peripheral or internal lymph nodes (sublumbar), uterus, kidneys and retrobulbar lymph nodes are the most common organs involved in lymphosarcoma. The common clinical signs irrespective of organ involved include varying degree of anorexia and weight loss. Cattle with right atrial involvement show signs of congestive heart failure. Distended abdomen, melena, diarrhoea and anorexia with weight loss are the common signs with involvement of the abomasum. Sub-lumbar lymph node involvement may lead to hind limb ataxia and recumbency. Retrobulbar lymph node enlargement is characterized by exophthalmia. Uterine involvement can often be appreciated by rectal palpation of a thickened uterus with multiple masses.

Complete blood count is of help in diagnosis provided the lymphosarcoma is associated with persistent lymphocytosis. Presence of abnormal lymphocytes in peripheral blood smears with concurrently elevated counts is suggestive of malignant lymphoma A mild, non-regenerative anemia may be observed in some cases. Cytological examinations of fine needle aspirates on enlarged peripheral lymph nodes for predominance of large lymphoblastic cells with large, prominent nucleoli with a high nuclear-to-cytoplasmic ratio are indicative of lymphoma. One or more of the isoenzymes of LDH are significantly elevated in cases of lymphosarcoma associated with solid tumors. Serologiced testing for the gp-51 and p-24 antigen can provide evidence for the definitive diagnosis of BLV infection.

The basic strategies for the control of BLV infection include test and slaughter, test and segregation, and test and implementation of corrective management. Testing and implementing control strategies to decrease the transmission of the disease are viable in most incidences.

13

Emergency Medicine and Critical Care

Emergency medicine deals with patients those are critically ill and requires immediate healthcare for survival. Every life threatening disease is presented for emergency management and the clinician is required during emergenices to successfully manage these with strong working knowledge, quick assessment and appropriate action. Emergency handling is truly triage as the clinician is expected to manage both the animal and the animal owner during the crucial times. Emergencies and critical care units pay emphasis in pre-hospital management, emergency procedures and expanded emergency management of specific conditions

Emergency conditions

- Cardiac emergencies
- Respiratory emergencies
- Anaphylactic shock
- Electric shock
- Bleeding disorders
- Burns
- Ear emergencies
- Gastrointestinal emergencies
- Hypertension
- Emergencies of female reproductive tract and genitalia
- Anaesthesic complications and emergencies
- Angioneurotic edema and utricaria
- Fractures and musculoskeletal trauma
- Metabolic emergencies
- Neurologic emergencies
- Occular emergencies
- Poisonous and Toxins
- Urinary tract emergencies

The emergency patients before being presented to veterinary hospitals may require first aid for survival. First aid refers to immediate assistance administered in cases of injury or sudden illness by a bystander or other lay person prior to treatment by a trained person. This step involves simple procedure and application of the common senses, and the procedure adopted depends on the kind of injury or illness.

The First aid must be provided to a critically ill patient with the objectives

- to save the animal's life
- to prevent further harm to the patient

  Example - Stopping bleeding by applying pressure on the wound
- to promote recovery

  Example - Applying bandage to a small wound may help in recovery process
- to reduce immediate pain and suffering

The following questions (ABC) are to be addressed for the First aid measures

- A - Is there any open airway?
- B - Is the animal breathing?
- C - Is there a heart beat & a pulse (Circulation)?

Examination of Airway is required to ensure that it is patent, as obstruction can be fatal. Steps should be taken if the airway is not clear. Harness and collar should be removed and the tongue is moved forward and then to one side to ensure passage of the air.

Breathing-If airway is not obstructed, then determine the adequacy of breathing and if necessary, rescue breathing (mouth to nose resuscitation) is provided. Immediate assistance is given after a rapid evaluation with special attention to "ABC". Breeding can be confirmed by watching the chest movement, listening sounds of breathing, and feeling the air of exhalation on first aider's cheek.

If animal is not breathing, chest compressions (regular, intermittent gentle pressure to the chest) and rescue breathing, should be performed. The first aider needs to check the patient's pulse, ABC have been assessed and necessary actions are taken. Severe hemorrhage is controlled by applying pressure using a bandage, a towel or even hand after. The level of consciousness checked and treatment for shock is given by keeping the animal warm. This is best done by covering the animal in a blanket to conserve the body heat. An emergency can be classified into three types.

- **Life-threatening emergencies.** Require immediate action by the owner or first aider at home, and clinicion at veterinary his portal. It unconsciousness, conscious collapse with dyspnoea or cyanosis, severe haemorrhage, severe burns, poisoning come under this category.
- Emergencies requiring **prompt attention** where life is not immediately threatened. Conscious collapse, Dyspnoea, Fractures / dislocations, haemorrhage, gaping wounds, severe dysuria and
- **Minor,** where telephone advice and first aid enables the owner to keep the animal comfortable until an appointment with a veterinary surgeon is achieved. E.g. insect stings, minor wounds (where the haemorrhage is easily controlled by bandaging), minor burns, abscesses, slight lameness and haematuria.

Criteria for Management of Critically Ill Patients

1. Initial survey of the patient

- Is the patient conscious or in unconscious state?
- Is there a patent airway? Is there any abnormal airway noises?
- Signs of breathing should be examined
- Whether there is any abnormality in pulse, capillary refill time?

Primary Diagnostic Aid:

Mucous membrane

Pale - anaemia, shock

Blue - cyanosis

Muddy/Brown - sepsis

Hypermic - hyperdynamic shock cyanide toxicity, heart stroke

Capillary refill time: (CRT)

- Normal CRT – 1-1.5 sec
- Rapid CRT - (< 1sec) suggests shock, hyperdynamic shock, hyperthermia, sepsis, hyperthyroidism
- Slow CRT > 1.5s - indicates dehydration, hypovolemia, cardiac disease, peripheral vasoconstriction, hypothermia.
- CRT (3sec) Very slow - indicates serious vasoconstriction and poor perfusion. Synthetic colloid fluids (hetastarch, dextran 70, or oxyglobin) can be administered as an initial resuscitation from shock at the dose rate of 5-10 ml body weight.

2. Blood pressure

The systolic pressure should remain at or > 90-100 mm Hg, and the diastolic pressure should remain at or> 40mm Hg. In case of cardiogenic shock, vasodialators to decrease vascular resistance (Dopamine @ 5-25 μg/kg/min) should be given. Low dose morphine (0.05mg/kg) should be given to dilate splanchnic vessels and reduce pulmonary edema. Furosemide (1mg/kg/hr) is administered to dilate pulmonary vasculature to potentially reduce edema.

3. Heart rate, rhythm, contractility, pulse quality

- In bradycardia – anticholinergic drug such as atropine @ 0.04mg/kg or glycopyrrolate (0.02mg/kg) is adminstered.
- Ventricular and supraventricular tachycardias Lidocaine @ 1-4mg/kg intra venously and slowly, then 50-100 μg /kg/min, propranolol @ 0.02-0.06 mg/kg intravenously.

4. Albumin- Albumin synthesis can decrease during various forms of shock. Fresh frozen plasma (20ml/kg) is adminstered to maintain serum albumin > 2.0 g/dl

5. Oncotic pressure – Colloids like hetastarch and dextran 70 (20-30 ml/kg/day), plasma (20ml/kg) can be administered intravenously to maintain oncotic pressure.

Management of Specific Emergency Conditions

Shock: Different shock types (hyprovolomic, septic or cardiogenic) evaluated by different parameters as given below:

	Parameters	Traumatic/ Hypovolemic	Septic	Cardiogenic
1	Heart rate	Increased	Increased	Increased
2	Pulse character	Weak	Strong early and weak late	Weak
3	Mucous membrane	Pale	Injected early	Pale
4	CRT	Prolonged	Rapid-early, prolonged late	Prolonged
5	Respiratory rate	Increased	Increased	Increased
6	Core temp.	Low/normal	Elevated early, low late	Low, normal
7	Peripheral temperature	Low	Low/elevated	Low
8	Urine output	Low	Low	Low
9	Blood pressure	Normal to high early	Low	Low

Management of shock patient:-

Fluid therapy:- Rapid administration of large volumes of crystalloid or colloid fluids. One fourth of calculated dose (90ml/kg/hr) of fluid administered.

6. Oxygenation and ventilation

Oxygenation and ventilation can be evaluated by arterial blood gas analysis or by pulse oximetry and capnometry. Supplemental oxygen can be administered as floro-by, nasal or naso pharyngeal catheter, O_2 hood or case. Supplemental oxygen should be humidified and delivered @ 50-100 ml/kg/min.

7. Cocorticosteriod & antiprostaglandins

Management of Critical Burn Cases

- Cool the burn areas with topical cool water.
- Burns affecting >15% of total body surface area requires more fluid therapy.
- In first 24 hours, fluid therapy is given to maintain the metabolic fluid requirements. The urine output should be monitored @ 1-2 ml/kg/hr.
- The calculated out put of fluid should be given i.e 1-4ml/kg x % total body surface area. Half of this calculated dose is adminstered over first 8 hours and the remaining over next 16 hours. Ideally, the patients serum albumin should be kept > 2g/dl and total protein between 4-6.5 g/dl. Colloidal support can be provided in form of hetastarch.
- Serum K+ should be maintained within 3.5-4.5 m Eq/dl using potassium chloride. $MgCl_2$ @ 0.75 mEq/kg/day is adminstered to retain K+
- Dry bandages soaked in silver-sulfadiazine or nitrofurazone ointment should be placed over the wound. Partial or total escharotomy is in performed leaving the wound to heal or reconstruct using skin advancement flaps or grafts.

Snake Bites

Vomiting, mental confusion, hypotension, respiratory distress, weakness, rapid heart rate, shock, high body temperature, bleeding disorders, hematuria, pigmenturia and cardiac arhythmias are the common clinical sings in case of snake bite depending on the type of poison. Treatment includes intravenous administration of 1 vial of antivenom in 200 ml of crystalloid fluid Number of vials of antivenom to be used depends on clinical signs, size of the patient and location of the bite. Generally, 1-3 vials are recommended for dogs. Diphenhydramine 2mg/kg body weight is slowly administered intravenously if there is hyperemia.

Corticosteroids, dexamethasone given intravenously @ 0.1 mg/kg. Broad spectrum antibiotics is adminstered to check secondary bacterial infection. Pain modulators such as Butor-phanol @ 0.2-0.4 mg/kg, Fentanyl @ 3μg /

kg intravenous, morphine @ 0.1-0.2 mg/kg. may be used. Surgical debriment may be necessary to remove necrotic tissue.

Bleeding disorder

Emergency conditions	Blood products to be used
• Coagulopathy with active haemorrhage Disseminated intravascular coagulation (DIC), thrombocytopenia, massive acute haemorrhage)	Fresh whole blood
• Massive acute or ongoing haemorrhage, hypovolemic shock	Stored whole blood
• Non-regenerative anaemia, immune mediated haemocytic anaemia, acute or chronic blood loss	Packed red blood cells
• Factors depletion associated with active haemorrhage (congenital A, Haemophillia-B, rodenticide intoxication, acute or chronic hypoproteinemia,burns, wound, hepatic renal or gastrointestinal loss)	Fresh frozen plasma
• Thrombocytopenia	Platelet rich plasma
• Congenital factors, deficiencies, haemophillia A, B, hypofribinogenpenia	Cryopreserved (Core of factors VIII, as VM-vilebrands factor and fibrinogen)

Toxins and Poisoning

Intoxication and poesoning are medical emergencies necessitating following line of treatment

Emetics: Apomorphipe @ 0.02 – 0.04 mg/kg intravenously, Xylazene @ 0.5 – 1mg/kg intrculenously every 15 min. Orogastric lavage is performed within 1-2 hours of ingestion of poison. Following successful passage and lavage, a slurry of artivated charcoal is administered through orogastric tube. The endotracheal tube is kept cuffed and in place until the animal is semiconscious.

Enemas is useful when poison is solid material (eg. Compost, snail bait, garbage), lukewarm water is best used as enemas Cathartics are use ful for hastening gut elimination of toxins and are useful in solid toxicants (eg. Compost, garbage). It can be used in combination with activated charcoal, and includes sodium sulfate 250-500 mg/kg p.o in 10 times volume of water, Sorbitol (70%) @ 3ml/kg p.o and mineral oil @ 5-15ml/kg in dog. If the toxin or poison can be identified, specific antidote should be used. Urine acidification and alkalization is attempted to facilitate renal clearance of poison or toxin.

14

Diseases of Skin Conjunctiva and External Ear

Pityriasis/ Dandruff

This is a condition characterized by presence of bran like scales on the skin surfaces.

Causes: Dietary causes like hypovitaminosis A, nutritional deficiency of vitamin B complex, linoleic acid. Iodine poisoning. Parasitic causes like flea, lice, mange infestation, ring worm.

Clinical findings: Accumulation of scales without itching or others superficial skin lesions. They accumulate most readily where the coat is long and luster less. Secondary pityriasis is usually accompanied by lesions of primary diseases.

Treatment: Correction of primary cause. Non specific treatment should start with a thorough washing with shampoo followed by alternate application of emollient ointment and alcoholic lotion. Salicylic acid or whitefield ointment is incorporated into lotion or ointment.

Parakeratosis

It is a condition of skin in which keratinization of the epithelial cells are incomplete.

Cause: Non-specific chronic inflammation of cellular epidermis causing faulty keratinization of horny cells. Dietary deficiency of Zn and Se may be cause parakeratosis.

Clinical signs: The lesions may be extensive and diffuse but are often confined to joints. Initially, there is reddening of the skin followed by thickening and development of a grey coloration. The lesions usually crack with formation of fissure.

Treatment: In nutritional parakeratosis, the deficiency must be corrected. The abnormal tissue is removed by use of keratolytic ointment like salicylic acid or by vigorous washing with soap followed by application of astringent preparation frequently for sometimes till the lesions disappears.

Hyperkeratosis

It is a condition in which excessive keratinization of the epithelial cells is seen which accumulate on the surface of the skin.

Cause: It may be local on the pressure points like elbow when animal lie habitually on the hard surface. Generalized hyperkeratosis may be caused by poisoning with highly chlorinated naphthalene compounds used in industry. Chronic asernic poisoning and inherited congenital ichthyosis or fish scale diseases in cattle may result in hyperkeratosis.

Clinical signs: Skin becomes thicker than normal, usually corrugated and hairless. Dryness, scalyness of external surface are characteristic finding. Fissure develop giving a scaly appearance. Secondary infection may occur if area is continuously wet.

Treatment: Use of keratolytic agents like salicylic acid may give some improvement.

Pachyderma

It is the thickening of the skin affecting all the layers, but frequently the subcutaneous layer of the skin may be afected.

Cause: Non-specific chronic or recurrent inflammation in major cases.

Clinical findings: The hair coat is thin or absent. Affected skin is thicker and tougher than normal. Skin appears tight and there is discontinuation of the skin surface.

Diagnosis: In pachyderma, thickening of skin is usually confined to localized area. There is no superficial skin lesion and no cell debris.

Treatment: Administration of cortisone preparation locally or parenterally in early stages. When small area is involved surgical removal may be undertaken.

Impetigo

It is a superficial eruption of thin walled usually small vesicles surrounded by a zone of erythema. The vesicles develop into pustule and rupture to form scab.

Cause: In human beings, impetigo is a superficial *Streptococcal* infection, but lesions are invaded secondarily by *Staphylococcal* organism. In animal, the main organism involved is *staphylococcus*.

Clinical signs: Vesicles appear mainly on the hairless part of the skin. In early stages, zone of erythema is present around vesicles without irritation. Rupture of vesicle occur readily. Vesicles may persist and become pustule forming yellow scab. Involvement of hair follicle is common and leads to development of acne. Individual lesion heals rapidly in about a week, but successive vesicles may occur prolonging the disease.

Treatment: Daily bathing with an efficient germicidal skin lotion.

Urticaria

It is an allergic condition characterized by appearance of wheals on the skin surface which is mostly noticed in horses and occasionally in cattle.

Cause

1. Primary urticaria: insects stings, contact with stinging plants, ingestion of unusual food, administration of penicillin drugs and during blood transfusion.
2. Secondary urticaria: respiratory infection in horses, erysipelas in pigs.

Clinical signs: Urticaria lesion develop very rapidly in large number, which are elevated with flat top and are tense to touch. There is no itching except when the causes including plant and insect sting. No exudation occurs. Other allergic phenomenon including diarrhoea and slight fever may accompany the eruption. Lesions subside within few hour, but disease may persist for 3-4 days.

Treatment: Spontaneous recovery is common. Antihistaminic drugs provide the most rational treatment for relief of pruritus. Parenteral injection of epinephrine may also be useful. The lesion are washed with a cooling astringent lotion like white lotion or dilute solution of $NaHCO_3$. In large animal practice, parenteral inj of calcium are used with apparently good results.

Dermatitis

It includes conditions characterized by inflammation of dermis and epidermis.

Causes

1. Mycotic dermatitis due to Dermatophilus spp., ringworm.
2. Photosensitive dermatitis.
3. Chemical irritation topically.
4. Arsenic poisoning
5. Mite infestation.
6. Dermatitis dut to *Stephanofilarial* spp., *Strongyloid* spp..

Clinical Findings

Affected skin area show erythema. There may be development of vesicular lesion, edema of skin and subcutaneous tissue involvement may occur in severe cases. The next stage may be healing stage and scab formation. Spread of infection to subcutaneous tissue result in diffuses cellulitis. A systemic reaction is likely to occur when affected skin area is extensive. Toxaemia due to absorption of tissue break down products or septicemia due to invasion via unprotected tissue may occur in later stage.

Treatment

Removal of physical or chemical agent from environment or supplementation of diet to repair a nutritional deficiency case is an essential basis for treatment. For bacterial infection suitable antibiotic both parenterally as well as locally is helpful. Antihistaminic drugs may be given in allergic dermatitis. If pain or itching persists anaesthetic agent may be applied locally. Local application of astringent powder or lotion may be given. If shock is evident, intravenous fluid therapy should be given. High protein diet with amino acid combination should be given in valuable animal along with skin tonic like vitamin-A both parenterally as well as orally to facilitate skin repair.

Conjunctivitis and Keratoconjunctivitis

It is the inflammation of covering membrane of the eye that covers the orbit and the inner surface of eyelid. The inflammation commonly extents to layers below the conjunctiva resulting in keratoconjunctivitis extends.

Causes: Parasites like Thelazia, onchocerca, Habronema and other viral and bacterial disease.

Non-specific Conjunctivitis: Inflammation caused by foreign body or chemical or secondarily keratitis and ant bite conjunctivitis etc.

Clinical signs: There is blepharospasm and weeping from the affected eye. The watery tears are followed by appearance of mucopurulent and purulent occular discharge. If the lesion expands below the conjuctiva there is opacity of the conjuctiva with pus. At later stage, there is considerable vascularisation of the cornea. During the recovery stage, there is often long lasting diffused opacity of the eye and may terminally leave a white scar mark.

Treatment

1. The eyes should be washed with the normal saline solution
2. Topical antibiotic drugs may be applied.

3. Steroidal application may be given to facilitate the spread of infection.
4. Vitamin- A therapy either oral or intramuscular should be given.

Dermoid cyst

Occular dermoid cyst are solid skin like masses of tissue adhered usually to the anterior surface of the eye causing irritation and interfering vision. The eye lid, third eye lid and canthus may also be involved and lesion may be unilateral or bilateral. Surgical intervention are recommended.

Otitis Externa

Arthropod parasite, foreign body and other infection may cause irritation of the ear accompanied by robbing of the head against objects and frequent head shaking. When the syndrome occurs in large number of herd, it is necessary to look for a specific causative agent. *Rhabditis bovis* is the common cause in the cattle. Affected animals are depressed, anorectic and appears to express pain while sallowing and shake their head frequently. Both ears are affected in most cases swallowing a patch of alopecia below the ear. The area is painful to touch. The external meatus of the aural canal is inflammed and parotid lymphnode are enlarged. Topical treatment with ivermectin and a broad-spectrum antibiotic is recommended.

15

Diseases of Musculoskeletal System

The major functions of the musculoskeletal system to provide support to organs and help in physical activities including locomotion, prehension, and mastication. The clinical manifestations of the diseases of muscles, bones and joints are much in common, and are generally characterized by lameness, failure of support, in coordination of movement and deformity.

Principal manifestations in musculoskeletal disease are

1. Lameness
2. Abnormal posture and movement.
3. Deformity.
4. Fracture.

Classification

1. **Degenerative diseases**: Muscles (Myopathy), Bones (Osteodystrophy), Joints (Arthropathy)
2. **Inflammatory Diseases**: Muscles (Myositis), Bones (Osteomyelitis), Joints (Arthritis)

Special Examination of Musculoskeletal System

1. Analysis of gait and configuration
2. Physical examination of cause: Fracture, dislocation, pain on movement
3. Radiography
4. Muscle biopsy
5. Arthrocentesis and arthroscopy
6. Serum biochemistry and enzymology: CPK, Aspartate Aminotransferase (AST), Serum levels of calcium, phosphorus, alkaline phosphatase, Muscle enzymes like Creatine phosphokinase (CPK), Serum glutamic oxaloacetic transaminase (SGOT) are elevated
7. Nutritional History
8. Environment and housing

Diseases of Muscle

Myasthenia (Skeletal muscle asthenia)

Paresis, paralysis and incoordination are the distinctive features, and are reversible states common causes of myasthenia are

- Ischemia- Recumbancy in cows as in parturient parasis, myo necrosis
- Metabolic effects on muscle fibers due hypokalamia, hypocalcemia, hypophosphatemia, hypomagnesemia and lactic acidosis.
- Poisons such as plant toxins and neurotoxins.

Myopathy

This is a non-inflammatory degeneration of skeletal muscle, characterized clinically by muscle weakness and pathologically by hyaline degeneration of muscle fibre. Serum levels of muscle enzymes like creatinine phosphokinase (CPK), glutamic oxaloacetic transaminase (SGOT) are elevated. Myoglobinuria is common finding.

Etiology and Epidemiology

- Enzootic nutritional muscular dystrophy due to vitamin E and selenium deficiency, which is common in young calves, lambs, kids etc
- Congenital myopathy
- Degenerative myopathy that occurs in new born calves infected in utero by Akabane virus
- Chemical agents/ myopathy causing drugs
- Ischaemia
- Neurogenic myopathy
- Neoplasma

Clinical Findings

- Nutritional myopathy due to vitamin E and selenium deficiency occurs in young growing animals that may occur in outbreak form in calves and lambs.
- In acute primary myopathy sudden onset of weakness and pseudoparalysis of affected muscles causing paresis, recumbency, respiratory and circulatory insufficiency.
- Affected animals remain bright and alert, but may appear to be in pain
- Temperature is elevated in severe cases of primary myopathy.
- Cardiac irregularity, tachy cardia, myoglobinuria
- Death occurs within 24 hours in acute cases.

Clinical Pathology

- CPK level rises indicating both myocardial and skeletal muscle degeneration.
- SGOT level also rises

Necropsy Finding

Affected areas of skeletal muscles have white, waxy, swollen appearance like fish flesh.

Diagnosis

- Seen in rapidly growing young animals
- Typical clinical findings of sudden onset of acute muscular weakness, pain on exercise.
- History of vitamins and mineral deficiency.
- Rising serum levels of CPK and SGOT

Treatment

- Vitamin E & selenium is adminstered in case of nutritional muscular dystrophy.
- Maintenace of adequate renal perfusion by intravenous administration of large quantities of polyionic balanced electrolyte fluids
- Sodium bicarbonate solution is preferred in case of myopathy with systemic acidosis.
- Supportive therapy includes thick bedding and provision of soft ground.
- Fluid therapy to prevent myoglobinuric nephrosis.
- Provision of paltable nutritious diet.

Myositis

Myositis refers to inflammatory condition of muscle, which is cause due to

- direct and indirect trauma to muscle
- Specific diseases such as black quarters, foot and mouth disease, blue tongue, ephemeral fever, swine influenza, sarcosporidiosis, trichinosis
- Sporadic cases of localised infectious myositis of skeletal muscle is caused by *E. coli* in calves

Clinical Sign

- Severe lameness
- Swelling, heat and pain on palpation

- Accompained by toxemia and fever
- In chronic myositis, wasting of affected muscle is a common symptom

Treatment

- Use of Antimicrobials in systemic infection
- Anti inflammatory drugs are used to reduce pain and swelling

Diseases of Bones

Osteodystrophy

It is a general term used to describe those diseases of bones in which there is failure of normal bone development or abnormal metabolism of already matured bone and is manifested by enlargement, susceptibility to fracture and interference with gait and posture.

Etiology

1. Nutritional cause
   - i. Ca, P, Vit-D deficiency.
   - ii. Cu deficiency.
   - iii. Inadequate dietary protein
   - iv. Hypo and hyper vitaminosis-A
   - v. Prolonged feeding of diet high in Ca. which cause nutritional hypercalcitonism
   - vi. Multiple vitamin and mineral deficiency
2. Chemical agents.
   - i. Chronic lead poisoning-Osteoporosis in lambs, and foals
   - ii. Chronic fluorine poisoning – characteristic lesions of osteoporosis and exostoses of bones

4. Poisonous plants
   - Grazing of certain poisonous plant as in case of horse causing osteodystrophy.

3.Chronic parasitism

4. Inherited and congenital cause

Clinical Findings

There is weakening and bending of bone due to defective mineralization, osteoporosis and lameness with pain. Distal end of long bone is commonly enlarged at the level of epiphyseal plate and circumscribed swelling of soft tissue around epiphyses may be prominent that is painful on palpation. Persistent recumbency due to pain will indirectly affect feed intake. The rib cage tends to become flattened. Any age group may be affected, but is common in young cattle. Thickening of the bones may be detectable clinically. If the deposition of osteoid or fibrous tissue is excessive, compression of spinal cord or nerve leads to paralysis. Calcinosis in cattle is characterized clinically by chronic wasting, lameness, ectopic calcification of cardiovascular system, lung and kidney, ulceration of joint cartilage and extensive bone calcification.

Clinical Pathology

1. Imbalance in serum calcium and phosphorus level
2. Serum alkaline phosphatase level elevated
3. Chemical analysis for bone ash
4. Histopathology and radiographic examination

Diagnosis: The disease is diagnosed based on typical clinical signs of lameness, stiff gait, long period of recumbency, failure to perform physical work normally, progressive loss of body weight, contortions of long bones of rib, head and vertebral column and radiographic examination

Treatment

Oral administration of calcium and phosphorus combined with parenteral inj of vitamin D is recommended. Oral administration of dicalcium phosphate@1 gm/kg body wt. 3-4 times daily for six days followed by a reduction to a daily requirement by 10th day combined with one inj of vitamin D /kg body wt. is recommended.

Affected animals are given a diet which contains the required level and ratio of calcium and phosphorus and vitamin D along with adequate bedding. Copper deficiency will respond gradually to Cu supplementation.

Osteomyelitis

a) Inflammation of bone, called osteomyelitis, may occurs due to infection introduced by traumatic injury or through haematogenous route. Specific diseases such as actinomycosis and brucellosis are associated with osteomyelitis
b) Epiphyseal type – new junction Salmonella infection may affect subchondral bone causing osteomyelitis of epiphysis.

Calves and foals under one month of age and growing cattle from 6 to 12 months age may be affected by osteomyelitis in one or more bone. Inflammation of bone is uncommon in farm animals except when infection is introduced by traumatic injury or by hematogenous route. Bacteria can reach into bone by 3 routes like hematogenous or by extension from an adjacent focus of infection or by direct inoculation via trauma or surgery. Specific diseases which may be accompanied by osteomyelitis include actinomycosis, brucellosis, and rhinitis in pigs. The infection is commonly seen in metaphysis, physis and epiphysis which are sites at long bone growth, and are susceptible to blood borne infection. The common clinical findings are lameness, swelling of soft tissue, erosion of bone and pus discharges into surrounding tissue causing cellulitis. When jaw bones are affected the teeth are often shed interfering with mastication. Involvement of vertebral bones may lead to secondary involvement of meninges and development of paralysis. Lameness and local swelling are the major manifestation of involvement of limb bones.

Clinical Findings

1. Lameness, generalized soft tissue swelling and inflammation
2. Pain on palpation of affected areas
3. Chronic persistent damage
4. Secondary muscle atrophy
5. Erosion of bone, pus discharge into surrounding tissues causing cellulitis and phlegmon.

Treatment

Clinical management of osteomyelitis is difficult. Veterinary management alone is rarely successful because of poor vascularity of affected solid bone and inaccessibility to infection. In case of long term infection or those with extensive bone necrosis, surgery is generally recommended. Good results are obtained when affected bone is removed and affected area is irrigated through a temporary drainage tube. Selective antibiotics should be given parenterally for 4-6 weeks following daily dressing.

Diseases of Joints

Arthropathy

Non inflammatory lesions of articular surface of joints characterized by degeneration and erosion of articular cartilage, hypertrophy of bone surrounding articular cartilage, leads to limping and spur formation (tiny pointed outgrowth of bone) at joints margin. The following causes are attributed for arthopahy.

1. Nutritional causes
   - Secondary to rickets and osteomalacia due to deficiency of calcium & Vitamin D3

- Coxofemoralarthropathy in cattle due to hypophosphataemia inadequate intake of phosphorus in cattle)
- Copper deficiency
- Manganese and magnesium deficiency arthropathy in calves

2. Poisoning:
   - Chronic zinc poisoning
   - Fluorosis in Cattle
3. Prolonged intra articular injection of Corticosteroid
4. Trauma
5. Congenital

Classification of Arthopathy

1. Primary osteoarthropathy
   - Normal ageing process and ordinary joint usages
2. Secondary osteoarthropathy
   - Initiated by injuries or congenital, conformational defects which cause greater shearing stress
3. Osteochondrosis: Disturbances in normal differentiation of cells in growing cartilage

Clinical Signs: Major clinical characteristic is chronic lameness which usually does not respond to treatment and long period of recumbency

Diagnosis

- Chronic lameness does not respond to treatment
- Stiff, disuse muscle atrophy, bony prominence of joint are more prominent
- Examination of synovial fluid
- Radiography

Treatment

- Immobilization
- Physical therapy
- Intraarticular injection of corticosteroid, non-steroidal anti-inflammtory drug, joint lavage etc.

Arthritis

Inflammation of synovial membrane and articular surface occurs most commonly in farm animals due to infection, and is characterized by varying degree of lameness and joint pain. Synovial fluid is usually abnormal containing increased leucocyte count and pathogens causing arthritis.

Cause

Specific bacterial infections of the joint are common in new born farm animals in which localization of infection occurs in joints following bacteremia or septicaemia. In calves *Corynebacterium pyogenes*, *Salmonella*, *Mycoplasma* are the common pathogens. In cattle *Mycoplasma, Brucella*, Ephemeral fever virus, bovine virus diarrhoea (BVD) virus are the common pathogen.

Calves: Non-specific joint ill from omphalophlebitis caused by *Actinomyces pyogens, Fusobacterium necrophorous, Staphylococcus, erysipelothrix inside, Salmonella*

Cattle: *H. somnus, Mycoplasma, Brucella*

Sheep: Mycoplasma, as a part of melioidosis

Clinical Findings

Arthritis is manifested by pain and lameness of the affected limbs, swollen joint fever, anorexia and loss of body weight. In neonates arthritis may be accompanied with omphalophlebitis and lesions of other organs particularly in liver, meninges and endocardium. Joints that are most commonly involved are hock, stifle and knee. There is ankylosis of the joints. Crepitus may be detected in joints where more erosion is present. In new born and young animals involvement of several joints may be noticed. Joints become inflamed simultaneously leading to suppurative arthritis.

Diagnosis

- Swollen joint, painful and warm to touch
- Lameness with varying degree of severity
- Volume of joint fluid is marginally increased and leucocyte count is increased with high percentage of neutrophils.

Treatment

Antibiotic therapy is given parenterally for several weeks along with intra articular administration of antibiotics. Drainage of the affected joints is helpful in removing the suspected pathogen. Antihistaminic drugs along with analgesics should be given parenterally. Local application of hot fomentation may be given to reduce pain and local swellings. Parenteral or intra articular administration of corticosteroid. Parenteral administration of phenyl butanone is used to reduce pain and facilitate healing process.

16

Diseases of Nervous System

The role of nervous system in animal is the maintance of bodies, speical relation with the immediate environment. Such functions are acomplished by several sections of the nervous systsm. The sensory motor system is responsible for maintaing normal posture and gait. The autonomic nervous system controls the functioning of smooth muscles and endocrine glands,and thus, the internal environment of the body. The sensory system section is responsible for special sences whereas the psychic system controls the mental state of animals. the nervous system is considered as a reactive platefrom to the reception of internal and external stimuli and translate into activity and consonants.

The clinical neurology and their aplication to animal practice is not well advanced over the years compared to medical counterpart. This is attributed to failure in establishing releationship between clinical science and neuro-anatomical location of the leglesion, adverse environmental conditon to interprete the findings of neurological disorders. However the clinicians attempts to recognize the common diseases of the nervous system by co-relating the clinical findings with the location and nature of lesion. Few diseases of nervous system has major public health implications. Rabies is a dreaded disease of nervous system that necessitates an early diagnosis to minimize further human contact. Incidence of bovine spongiform encephalopathy has given a momentum to clinical neurology in domectic animals. The clinicians lay more emphasis on the history and epidemiologial findings because of limitations constrains in the neuological examination of large animals. For example, lead poisoning is more common in calves allowed to graze on pasture, and polio encephalomalacia is recorded in grain fed ruminants.

The functional capacity of the nervous system largely depends on other system. As the brain depends on adequate oxygen supply for its optimum functioning cardio-vas cular disease alters the cerebral function due to prevalant hypoxia. Therefore it is necessary to differentiate between primary and secondary diseaes of nervous system. The lesions in primary diseases are seen in the nervous system itself, whereas in secondary diseaes the changes are functional in nature at least in early stages and is more responsive to treatment.

The suspicion for neurologial disturbances arises in abnormalities in the three main functions of the system, posture and gait, Sensory perception and mental state. The functioning of the musculo-skeletal system and efficiency of nervous system enables the animal to maintian normal posture and locomotion, through co-ordinated nervous activity. The sensory perception in animals are only objective in nature and never subjective. That is one of the limitations of clinical neurological examination in animals.

Nervous disfunction can be divided into two forms i) depressed activity ii) exagarated activity which can further subdivided into four common modes of nervous dysfunction, excitation signs, release of inihibition signs, paresis or paralysis is due to tissue damage and nervous shock. The excitability of nerve cells can be increased by stimulant drug, inflamation and mild hypoxia. However, severe hypoxia causes depression of the function or even death of nerve cell. Depression of the nerve cell results from reduced metabolic activity of the cells that occurs due to failure in supply of oxygen and other essential nutrients. An acute lesion of the nervous system may lead to cessation of functioning of a part of the nervous system results in nervous shock, thus flaccid unconsciousness.

The important clinical signs of nervous system dysfunction are altered mentation, involuntary moments, abnormal posture and gait, paresis or paralysis, altered sensation blindness and abnormalities of the autonomic nervous system. Excitation and states are the manifestation of cerebral cortex dysfunction and include mania, frenzy and agressive behaviour. Mania is a exctatory sign, observed in encaphatitis, degenerative diseases of brain, toxin and metabolic diseases affecting nervous system. Depressive mental states include somnolence, lassitude, narcolepsy, syncope and coma. Depression leading to coma results from encephalomyelitis and encephalomalacia, toxic and metabolic diseases affecting brain, hyproxia of the brain due to principheral circulatory failure, heart stroke, methyl alcohol poisoning. Syncope characterized by sudden onset of fainting, may occur as a result of acute cerebral hypoxia as seen in acute circulatory and heart failure, spontaneous cerebral haemorrhage, traumatic concussion, lighting stroke and electro-cution. Involuntary movments are one of the important clinical mainfestations of nervous system disfunction that occurs due to involuntary muscle contractions varying in gradations from fasciculations, shivering, tremor, kekoni, seizures and convulsions.

Encephalitis

It refers to inflamation of the brain; clinically characterised by signs of involuntary movements and loss of nervous funcitons. Involvement of the meningesandspinal-cordalongwithbrainistermedasmeningoencephalomylitis.

Etiology

All species: Viral infection- Rabies, Pseudo, rabies, japanese B-encephalitis.

Bacterial infection in nenatal farm animal

Parasitic Toxoplasmosis and sarcocystosis

Cattles: Bovine spongiformencephalopathy

Viral infections: Bovine malignant catarrh, bovine herpes virus.

Bacterial infection: Listeria monocytogenes, *histophilus somni*, clostridial infections.

Sheep

Prion disease: Scrapie

Viral infections: Louping -ill, visna

Bactrial infection: Histophilus somni,

Parasite infection: Migration of *oestrus ovis*

Goat

Prion disease: Caprine arthritis encephalits virus

Pig

Viral infection: Cholera, african swine fever, swine vesicular disease

Bacterial infection: Salmonella,erysipelas, listeria monocytogenes

Horses

Viral infections: Infectious equine *encephalomylitis*, equine herpes virus, equine infections anemia.

Verminous encephalomyelitis due to *Strongylus vulgaris.*

Encephalitis caused due to an infectious agent is manifested by clinical signs of fever, anorexia, depression and increased heart rate. However, the signs are not seenin chronic diseases such as scropie and bovine spongiform encephalitis are combination of subtle to marked changes in behaviour, depression, scizures, blindness, compulsive walking, leaning on walls and stanihione, circling and ataxia. In young ones, there is lack of suck reflex, weakness, altered gait, and depression, but hyperasthesia to auditory and tactile stimuli. Opisthotonus is seen on later stages. There is initial period of mania, viciousness and on controlled activity. Excessive drooling and laryngeal paralysis are common findings in rabies.The loss of function of nervous system varies from parasis with knuckling at lower limb joints, to spasticity of the limbs with ataxia. Recumbency and inatrilits toxise are seen in some cares of encephalitis from the begining. Clinical Signs referable to certain anatomical site include rotation of head, circling and in coordination.

Clinical pathology: Acute and convalscent sera samples are collected to identify infectious agent responsible for encephalomyelitis. Cerebrospinal fluid can be examined for clear content and specific pathogen.

Necropsy finding: Gross lesions in the brain are not commonly noticed in common encephalits. However extensive areas of haemoragic necrosis maybe seen in histo-pathological examination. Brain tissue is used for culture and transmission experiment to identify the pathogen.

Treatment: Anti-microbial are indicated for bacterial mening on encephalomyelitis. Sedation during the excitement state may prevent injury to animals. Nervous system stimulants are administered during the period of depression.

Encephalomalacia

This is a degenerative disease of the central nervous system characterised by softening of the brain. It includes all degenerative changes such as leuko-encephamalacia and polioencephasomalacia, referring to softening white and grey matter, repectively.

Etiology

All species: Hepatic encephalopathy due to high blood level of ammonia associated with advanced liver disease.

- Multifocal encephalopathy and progressive mild-encepalopathy
- Poisoning by organic mercurials and in some instance lead and selenium poisoning.
- Congenital hypomyelinogenests and dysmyelinogenesis

Ruminants: Bovine spongiform encephalopathy

Plant poison: Astragalus species, oxytropis, vicia species, Kochia scoparia

- Intoxication with clostridium perfringens type-D toxins
- Thiamine (Vitamins B-1) deficiency
- Sulphur toxicosis in cattle

- Abiotrophic lysosomal storage disease
- Cerebral hypoxia

Horse: Feeding of mouldy corn infested with *Fusarium moniliforme*

- Feeding of yellow star thistle (*Centaurea solstitialis*)
- Poisoning by bracken and horsetail causing deficiency of thiamine
- Vitamin-E deficiency

Clinical Findings

Encephalomalicia is characterised by weakness of all four limbs, dullness,blindness, ataxia, head-pressing, circling, involuntary signs like tremour, opisthotonos, nystagmus, convulsion terminal coma.

Clinical Pathology

Some specific disease can be diagnosed with help of clinicopathological test.

Necropsy Findings

Gross lesions include areas of softening, cavitation and necrosis.

Treatment: Thiamine deficiency can be corrected by treating with adequate amount of thymine (Vitamin B-1) However there is no specific treatment of encephalomalicia and the prognosis of the disease is very poor.

Traumatic Injury to the Brain

The sign and the extent of the injury determines the effect of trauma to the brain. However nervous-shock may occur initialy followed by death or recovery.

Etiology

Direct trauma due to accident, collision, falling down, spontaneous haemorrhage into brain, migration of parasitic larvae.

Clinical Findings

Traumatic injury to brain follows a specifc pattern of clinical findings with greatest severity initially followed by quick recovery but incompletely leaving behind residual defects. Cerebral shock or nervous shock may occur following several injury. During the period of unconsciousness, clinical examination reveals pupillary dilation, absence of eye preservation and pupillary light reflexes, slow and irregular respiration. There may be bleeding from nose and ears. Hemiplegea may be associated with lesions in mid brain.

Necrospy Findings

Gross haemorrhagic lesions may be seen in necropsy. In concussion and nematodiasis, the lesions are detected on histological examinations.

Teatment: The prognosis of the disease is poor, if coma presist for more than 3 to 6 hours. The cerebral edema can be treated with intravenous administration of mannitol solution.

Brain Abscess

Brain abscess is commonly seen in young animal below one year of age and rarely in older animals, and produce variety of clinical sings depending upon the location of this space occuring cession in the cranial cavity.

Etiology

The abscess in the brain may originate by spread of the infectious agents into cranial cavity through hematogenous route or via injury. The pathogens responsible for brain abscess *Actinobacillus mallei, Streptococcus zooepidemicus, Mycobacterium bovis, Fusobacterium necrophorum, Staphylococcus aureus* etc.

Clinical Findings

Brain abscess is clinically manifested by mental depression, clumsiness, head-pressing, excitement, uncontrolled activity and convulsion. Location specific signs include cereberal ataxia, deviation of head with circling, hemiplegia. Terminally there is opisthotonus, nystagmus, loss of balance and recumbency.

The functional capacity of the nervous system largely depends on other system. As the brain depends on adequate oxygen supply for its optimum functioning, cardio-vascular diseases alters the cerebral function due to prevalant hypoxia.

Clinical Pathology

Cerebrospinal fluid may be examined for leukocytes protein and bacteria. Blood hematological examination is performed for total leukocytes count and differential leukocyte count. Serum bio-chemical test is carried out to estimate protein and fibrinogen level. Imaging of the brain shows the sight of the abscess and extend of damage.

Necropsy Findings

Gross examination of brain at necropsy may reveal the site of the abscess. Micro-abscesses are only visible on histiological examination.

Treatment

Anti-microbial are used parenterally but the results are generally unsatisfactory because of the inacessibility of the lesion.

Coenurosis

It is caused by invasion of the brain and spinal cord by the intermidiate stage of Taenia-multiceps, and is otherwise called gid and sturdy. The intermediate stage of this tape-worm is called coenurus cerebralis. The adult tape-worm is found in the intestine of dogs and wild cannids. Eggs ingested, contributed by faces of infected dog hatch in the intestine and pass into the blood stream. The embryo that reaches brain or spinal cord continue to grown to coenurus stage

Clinical Finding

The migration of the intermediate stage shows signs of blindness, ataxia, muscle tremor, nystagmus, excitability and collapse.

Treatment: Surgical drainage of the cyst or surgical removal helps in complete recovery. Gid can be controlled by breaking the lifecycle of the tapeworm Periodic treatment of the dogs with taenicide is essential to control gids in ruminants.

Meningitis

Meningitis refers to inflamation of the meninges and is associated with pre-existing bacterial infestion, manifested clinically by fever, cutaneous hypersthesia and rigidity of muscles. Meningo-encephalitis, involving meninges and brain, is common in neo-natal farm animals and rare in adult animal with the exception of listerosis and *Histophilus somni.*

Epilespy is called acquired or secondary when it occurs in a previously healthy dog whose brain has become seizureprone for some specific reason.

Etiology

Cattle: Viral disease -Bovine malignant catarrh sporadic bovine encephalomyelitis.

Bacterial diseases -Listeriosis-*Histophiluas somini,* rarely tuberculosis caused by *Mycobacterium bovis*

Horse; Strangles, *Pasteurella haemolytica Streptococcus* equi, *Actinomyces* spp. *Klebsiella pneumoniae*, *Staphylococci* spp. *Sphingobacterium multivorum Cryptococcus neoformans*

Sheep: Melioidosis, *Staphylococcus aureus, Pasteurella multiocida*

Clinical Findings

Clinical signs produced by menigitis results from irritation of both central and peripheral nervous system including muscle tremor and convulsion. Fever and toxemia may prevail as meningitis is usually bacterial in origin. The pupillargy light reflex is usually much slower than normal and may produce breathing pattern characterised by a period of apnea followed by a gradual increase in rate of resperiation (Cheyne - Stokes breathing) or unpredictable irregularity (Biot's-respiration).

Clinical Pathology

Examination of cerebrospinal fluid reveals higher protein concentration, high cell count and presence of bacterium and turbidity. Blood examination reveals leukocytosis.

Necropsy Finding: Presence of haemorhage, thickening and opacity of meninges are the usual macroscopic findings.

Treatment

Parenteral treatment with anti-microbials is necessary. Culture and anti-biotic sensitivity test on cerebro-spinal fluid identifies anti-microbials of choice. As the blood brain barrier and blood CSF barrier are not intact in meningitis minimum inhibitory concentration (MIC) of some drugs are achived.

Seizures

Seizure is defined as a brief disturbance of brain function, characterized by random muscle movement and loss of consciousness. Synonyms for seizure includes convulsion, ictus, and fits. The word epilepsy refers to a series of frequent seizures or convulsion that does not identify the disease, rather describes a clinical sign. It is one of the top three concerns among more than 80 health issues in dogs, according to survey conducted by American Kennel Club, and affects anywhere before 0.5 to 5.7 percent of canine population. Many a times, the word epilepsy is used interchangeably with seizures, convulsions, attacks or fits. A seizure presents as a terrifying episode especially because the dog seems to have no awareness of the surrounding. Most seizures are not life threatening and end in a matter of seconds, although it may seem like hours. However, the dog with seizures may require immediate and critical veterinary intervention if the seizures continues to persist for more than 30 minutes without relapse. Seizures occur due to the malfunction of brain resulting in firing a barrel of electrical signals through the nervous system that is manifested as convulsion either in a specific body part, or more commonly, many areas at once. The dog may paddle his feet, or become rigid and violently thrash about.

There are many possible reasons why a dog might have a seizure. Anything capable of changing the nerve function within the brain may produce a seizure. Known causes of seizures include infectious diseases (distemper), metabolic diseases (hypoglycemia), toxic substances, neoplasia (tumors), and certain bacterial and fungal organisms. A metabolic disorder, such as hypoglycemia (low blood sugar), is often the cause in toy breeds. Hypocalcemia (low calcium) can cause seizures in bitches nursing puppies. Puppies with distemper are also prone to seizures. Sometimes, a dog can develop seizures after an accident or a blow to the head. A post traumatic scar may develop and result in seizures. Encephalitis, a convulsions. Brain tumors, more often found in older dogs, can cause malfunctioning in the nervous system inducing seizures. Other causes of seizures include heat stroke, congenital malformation of the brain, and ingestion of toxic chemicals. The problem is reported to be more common in adult males than younger dogs and females. Extra-cranial causes noted, in such problem in dogs include strychnine toxicosis, hypocalcemia and hypoglycemia drug intoxication. Intracranial causes include viral encephalitis, canine distemper etc. Diagnosis of idiopathic epilepsy is generally made when all other factors that might cause seizures, have been ruled out. It is the most common cause of recurrent seizures in dogs and the age of onset is usually between 1 and 3 years. Some practitioners use a broader range, from 6 months to 5 years. Epilepsy is called acquired or secondary when it occurs in a previously healthy dog whose brain infection that causes inflammation, can lead to convulsions. Brain tumors, more often found in older dogs, can cause malfunctioning in the nervous system inducing seizures. Other causes of seizures include heat stroke, congenital malformation of the brain, and ingestion of toxic chemicals. The problem is reported to be more common in adult males than younger dogs and females. Extra-cranial causes noted, in such problem in dogs include strychnine toxicosis, hypocalcemia and hypoglycemia drug intoxication. Intracranial causes include viral encephalitis, canine distemper etc. Diagnosis of idiopathic epilepsy is generally made when all other factors that might cause seizures, have been ruled out. It is the most common cause of recurrent seizures in dogs and the age of onset is usually between 1 and 3 years. Some practitioners use a broader range, from 6 months to 5 years. Epilepsy is called acquired or secondary when it occurs in a previously healthy dog whose brain has become seizure-prone for some specific reason. Epilespy is called acquired or secondary when it occurs in a previously healthy dog whose brain has become seizureprone for some specific reason.

Breed Predisposition and Inheritance

The genetic basis of idiopathic epilepsy in dogs has received considerable attention in recent years. Certain breeds seem particularly prone to developing it, suggesting the role of a genetic factor. Among the breeds, most commonly affected are Beagles, Dachshunds, Dalmatians, German shepherd dogs, Keeshonds, Boxers, Cocker and Springer spaniels, Collies, Golden and Labrador retrievers, miniature Schnauzers, Poodles, Saint Bernards, Siberian Huskies, and Wire-haired terriers. The increased manifestation of seizures in some subpopulation and the repeated occurrence in different families of the same sire suggests genetic basis of epilepsy.

Pathophysiology

A seizure is a transitory disturbance of brain function. It has a sudden onset, ceases spontaneously, and tends to recur. A seizure results from a sudden and uncontrolled electric discharge of neurons in the cerebral cortex of the brain due to paroxysmal depolarizing shift of neurons. Neurons can spontaneously discharge for several reasons, including decreased inhibitory neurotransmitter activity, increased excitatory neurotransmitter activity or combination of both. Neurotransmitter activity can be altered by a change in the cell membrane or the internal cell metabolism. At the beginning of a seizure, only a few highly unstable neurons may spontaneously discharge. This initial discharge can cause surrounding neurons or neurons in the opposite brain hemisphere to discharge as well and spread the seizure activity by a process referred to as kindling and mirroring, respectively. Spontaneous discharge can be triggered by almost any alteration in a neuron's environment. Neuronal changes influence the threshold for depolarization that causes seizure activity. High frequency and low amplitude paroxysmal discharge with either a focal or generalized distribution have been observed in majority of cases of idiopathic epilepsy. There are many evidences justifying the role of immediate early gene c-fos in physiological and pharmacological properties in the central nervous system. Astrocytes support the neuronal function and helps in altering the seizure susceptibility through ATP production and aconitase activity.

Clinical Manifestation

Most seizures occur in three stages, each stage is characterized by specific clinical signs. The first part of a seizure is called the aura. This often goes unnoticed but the dog shows changes in the behaviour signaling an impending seizure, and is clinically characterized by apprehension, restlessness, nervousness, and salivation. The period of aura lasts from few seconds to few days. The aura is followed by the actual seizure, called the ictus. Although it seldom lasts for more than one minute, it can be a very disturbing event to the owner. During the seizure, the animal usually collapses onto its side and experiences a series of violent muscle contractions associated with paddling of the feet and rigidity of the body. Loss of consciousness, excessive salivation, and involuntary urination and defecation may also occur in more severe seizures.

The period immediately following the seizure is known as the postictal phase. It usually lasts less than one hour but may last as long as one or two days. The animal may show signs of confusion, disorientation, restlessness, and temporary blindness. In cases of repeated seizures, the inter-ictal period denotes the interval between seizures. Some animals are normal during this period but others are not, depending on the cause of the seizures.

Behavioural changes associated with seizures include loss of memory, lack of consciousness, altered muscle tone or movement, alteration in visual, auditory, or olfactory hallucinations and salivation, urination, defecation, or other autonomic nervous system disruptions.

Thus, depending on the severity of the seizure and the duration of different stages, it is termed as Grand mal, when the seizure is severe. The term petit mal refers to a generalized seizure with a specific EEG pattern. However, the above two terminologies are no more used. A series of seizures within a short period of time, with the dog regaining consciousness between seizures is termed as Cluster seizures. Status epilepticus refers to rapidly repeating seizures with no period of consciousness between them. Seizures are classified as either partial or generalized. In the former case, neurons discharge in a specific area. In case of generalized seizures (also referred to as tonic-clonic seizures) there is involvement of animal's entire body. During the first (i.e. tonic) phase, which usually lasts between 10 and 30 seconds, an animal falls to the ground, looses consciousness, and rigidly extends the legs. It may also stop breathing. In the second (i.e. clonic) phase, the animal's legs make running or paddling, its mouth makes chewing motions, and it may continue to shake. In addition, an animal may urinate, defecate, have dilated pupils, salivate excessively, vocalize, or vomit during enttre phase. A seizure may alternate between tonic and clonic phases once or repeatedly for the duration of the seizure. The entire seizure usually lasts between 1 to 2 minutes.

Management of Seizures

There is no cure or standard protocol for treating idiopathic epilepsy. However, seizures can be controlled with anticonvulsant drugs. The purpose of the treatment is to decrease the frequency, duration and severity of the seizure. Treatment is individualized for each animal based on its history and physical examination. No single drug is always effective; several drugs or a combination of drugs may have to be tried before a successful treatment is found. Also, it may take several weeks to establish a therapeutic dosage that works for an individual dog. This may indicate a need to change medication or alter the dose. It may be necessary to medicate the dog several times daily for the rest of its life and the medication schedule must be closely followed. Variance from the schedule may potentiate a seizure or series of seizures.

The etiological factors in cases of secondary epilepsy should be given due attention and therapy should be instituted to minimize or eliminate the problem that gives rise to seizure. However, in such cases anticonvulsants are to be given to suppress the motor activities. Blood tests have to be performed to identify metabolic disorders, toxic chemicals in the dog's system, infection or inflammation. A fasting blood glucose test can reveal certain metabolic causes for seizures. A neurological examination can point towards an underlying disease of the central nervous system, which may be confirmed by tests done on the dog's cerebrospinal fluid. More advanced tests, such as electroencephalograms (EEG) and brain scans are rarely carried out due to lack of facility and well trained personnel with sound knowledge on interpreting the findings. They are performed only when a dog's epilepsy proves to be difficult to treat, and they are generally available only at well-equipped animal hospitals.

The two most popular medications for long term seizure control are phenobarbital and potassium bromide. Each is an effective anticonvulsant, which can be used either alone or in combination. However, 10 to 50% of the dogs having seizures are found refractory to Phenobarbital sodium. Bromide is a halide anticonvulsant that offers an effective alternative to Phenobarbital and other barbiturates for treatment of epilepsy in dogs. The use of potassium bromide (KBr) as an anticonvulsant in dogs with severe signs (seizures) has been very helpful, particularly in cluster seizures. The drug is not metabolized by the liver and has fewer drug interactions than phenobarbital. Primidone, one more frequently prescribed, is no longer recommended, as it seems to cause greater liver toxicity than phenobarbital. Its administration needs to be carefully monitored by veterinarians to ensure that a therapeutic dose has been achieved. Long term control of psychomotor seizures can be achieved with carbamazepine.

Control and Awareness of Pet Owners

While epilepsy can't be cured, it can be controlled. It is important to brief the dog owner that it is a chronic condition and needs lifelong management and the dog can have a good life even if it has epilepsy. The foremost important tips the dog owner should be advised is to remain calm and to remove objects that the dog might knock into and to place a towel or mat under the dog's head if it is banging against the hard floor.

There is little danger if the dog swallowing it's tongue. Of greater concern is a dog aspirating vomit if it throws up during an attack, so owners should quickly move a dog away from anything it could inhale. The owner should be advised to sit with dog and soothe it during the period of recovery. It may sometimes take a dog several minutes or longer to recover from a seizure, and the comforting presence of the dog owner really matters.

17

Metabolic Diseases

Metabolic diseases assume the greatest significance in dairy cows and buffaloes during transition period, and occur due to imbalance in input and output of production. The main reasons of occurrence of metabolic diseases are an imbalance between the rate of 'input' of dietary nutrients and 'output' of production. Persisting imbalance leads to depletion of reserves of certain metabolites or their throughput giving rise to signs of production diseases. Classical example of the outcome of the process are ketosis caused by hypoglycemia, tetany caused by hypomagnesemia and milk fever caused partly due to hypocalcaemia.

The first few days postpartum are the most critical time in dairy cows. The body's metabolism remains under severe stress due to its transition from pregnancy to lactation. The cow has a high nutrient demand to meet the requirement of production. Therefore, incidence of production diseases is more in the period beginning at calving till the peak of lactation. Under the stress of higher production system, there is relatively high turnover of fluids, salts and soluble materials. Sudden variation in excretion or secretion of sodium, potassium, calcium, phosphorous, magnesium, chloride, etc. in the milk or by other tissues and sudden change in their intake due to altered ingestion, digestion or absorption may cause disruption in the internal environment of the animal. The additional nutritional demand during pregnancy or lactation is exacerbated by a sub-optimal nutrient supply during dry period leading to high incidence of production diseases. Stress, breed, age, season and management practices are important predisposing factors for production diseases. The management of metabolic and deficiency diseases has been possible to some extent by forecasting occurrence of these diseases by using modern tools such as Compton metabolic profile test, micro-mineral profile of soil-plant- animal and by using specific preventive approaches such as calcium gel therapy, hormonal therapy and use of area specific mineral mixture.

Production diseases are those diseases that occur due to imbalance between input and output of production. The transient change that occurs during parturition and at the onset of milk production till peak production creates metabolic stress resulting in metabolic diseases such as milk fever, ketosis, hypomagnesemia tetany, downer cow syndrome, post-parturient haemoglobinuriea, pregnancy toxaemia in ewes, fatty liver syndrome etc. Metabolic diseases differ from deficiency diseases as in later cases, there is absolute deficiency of particular nutrient resulting in manifestation of clinical signs of deficiency. On supplementation of different nutrients if clinical signs disappear (not all), then those diseases are confirmed as deficiency diseases. Anatomical changes, those have take place dut to deficiencies, mayn't get corrected.

In metabolic diseases, there may be deficiency, but the body reserve of that particular nutrient hasn't been completely depleted. Thus, deficiency diseases, there is absolute deficiency whereas in production diseases, there is transient deficiency Metabolic diseases occur due to imbalances in input and output. Body tries to utilize the throughputs (body reserve) to meet the increased demand of outputs. Where the input fails to meet the output needs, metabolic stress prevails. Such metabolic stress is very common in cows from parturition to peak lactation and in ewes during the later part of pregnancy. During this period, there is a rapid turnover of fluid, salts and soluble organic matters and the changes are voluminous resulting in metabolic diseases. Metabolic and production diseases are interchangeably used. International Dairy Federation (IDF) has defined production diseases as those diseases that hampers the quality and quantity of production. So, it includes all metabolic diseases and other diseases that reduce production and quality of the produce viz. metritis, mastitis and other infectious diseases that significantly reduce the level of production.

The factors influencing the occurrence of metabolic diseases is influenced by genetic make up, managemental practices, climatic condition, season of the year and level of production. The dairy animals have been used as a production machine to increase production, pushing the production forward without considering the metabolic turnover in the body system. This has resulted in increased incidences of metabolic diseases in dairy animals. A cow yielding more than 18 liter of milk/day can't meet its glucose requirement by feeding only concentrate ration. The output of glucose is so high, that the animal will have glucose/ carbohydrate deficiency. This results in mobilization of fat depots and sub-clinical ketosis. This is the reason of sub-clinical ketosis in high yielding animals.

The animal at the time of parturition (1st stage of lactation) remains under serious hormonal influences that doesn't support reduction/ caesation of production in spite of the fact that particular nutrient is deficient. Therefore, there are two major factors responsible for occurrence of production disease such as rapid rate of turnover and volume of turn over.

Compton Metabolic Profile Test (CMPT)

It is based on the principle that measurement of certain blood constituents reflects the nutritional status of the animal. It is used for forecasting the metabolic diseases, and the nutritional status of the animal is measured either by growth rate, body condition score, production performance etc or by measurement of blood constituents such as glucose, protein, blood urea nitrogen (BUN), albumin, Na^{+}, K^{+}, Mg^{++}, Ca^{++} and P, Haemoglobin, PCV. So, these constituents of blood have been analyzed in CMPT in a population of dairy animals to forecast the incidence of matbolic diseases. Blood samples are collected from 3 different groups of animals (dry period, during peak lactation and in mid lactation) and in 3 different seasons (Summer, Winter and Autumn). Samples are collected at least from 7 animals of a particular group in a particular season and samples are analyzed for the above parameters to assess the nutritional status and forecasting of diseases. The limitations of this test include cost of processing and analysis and physiological variations of the animals. So, blood should be collected from animals those are physiologically of same nutritional status. There is another Mini Profile Test to minimize the cost wherein blood glucose, blood urea nitrogen (BUN), Ca, Mg, Na and K are being analyzed to forecast the metabolic diseases.

Milk Fever

Milk fever is also known as parturient paresis, parturient apoplexy or calving paralysis. It is characterized by weakness, recumbency, shock and death. Hypocalcaemia (low blood calcium) resulting from inadequate calcium metabolism is common among fresh cows, and can lead to milk fever, most commonly during periparturient period.

Etiology

Milk fever occurs due to low level of ionised calcium in blood (below 5.2 mg/dl) and tissue fluid due to inadequate mobilization of Ca from bone, decreased concentration of 1,25 $(OH)_2$ cholecalciferol and decreased parathyroid (PTH) activity. A cow producing 10 kg of colostrum will loose around 23 g of calcium in a single milking. Increase in age, high level of production, dry period nutrition, housing and environmental condition are the risk factors for the occurrence of milk fever. Host factors responsible for development of this disease are high body condition score, decreased plasma level of 1,25 $(OH)_2$ D_3, decreased receptor for 1,25 $(OH)_2$ D_3 in intestine and decreased osteoclast cells with increasing age. Common dietary factors causing this disease include feeding of more than 100 g calcium daily during the dry period which suppress the active transport of calcium from the diet and bone calcium resorption, high dietary phosphorous which inhibits the secretion of renal enzyme that catalyzes the production of 1,25 $(OH)_2$ D_3. Dietary cation-anion difference (DCAD) is the most important factor involved in this disease. Dietary cations like K+ or Na+ increase the pH and causes metabolic alkalosis which decrease the absorption of calcium and is responsible for development of milk fever. On the contrary, dietary anions like Cl^- and sulphates decrease the pH causing metabolic acidosis which facilitates absorption of calcium from intestine, thus reduce the incidence of milk fever.

Epidemiology

High yielding dairy cows of 3rd to 7th lactation and 5-10 years of age are most susceptible. Among different breeds of cattle, Jersey most susceptible to milk fever. Lactating beef cows are less commonly affected. Mature ewes 6 weeks before and 10 weeks after lambing and goats before kidding to 3 weeks after kidding are more susceptible.

Pathogenesis

Normally, falling calcium levels in blood cause increased parathyroid hormone (PTH) secretion from the parathyroid gland, which increases the bone calcium resorption by stimulating the osteoclastic activity, enhances the calcium reabsorption in kidney and stimulates the production of calcitriol in kidneys which enhances the absorption of calcium by the digestive tract. In contrast, when blood calcium level rises, thyroid gland secrets calcitonin which increases the excretion of calcium by the kidney and also promotes the osteoblastic activity resulting in calcium deposition in bone.

In hyocalcaemia, there will be increased secretion of parathyroid hormone (PTH), stimulating calcium mobilization from bone and absorption of calcium from gastrointestinal (GI) tract in presence of Vitamin D_3. Once the required amount of calcium is achieved in blood, calcitonin hormone is secreted which prevent further absorption of calcium from the intestine.

Clinical Signs

The clinical signs of milk fever are exhibited in 3 stages: Stage excitement Stage I: is Manifested by hypersensitivity, tetany, shaking of head and limb, inappetance protrusion of tongue, grinding of teeth, bellowing, fear to move, ruminal stasis, stiffness of the limb and falling down easily.

Stage II: Stage of sternal recumbency is manifested by sternal recumbency with lateral bending of head towards flank, protrusion of tongue on with extended head, unable to rise, dry muzzle, hypothermia, weak pulse with low pressure forced, expiratory grunt, dilated pupil, absence of pupillary light reflex, relaxation of anus, low intensity but high heart rate and prolapse of uterus.

Stage III: Stage of lateral recumbency is characterized by lateral recumbency, complete struck out of limbs with complete flaccidity, weak pulse and inaudible heart sound. Death occurs due to cessation of respiration.

Clinical Pathology

Total serum calcium level comes to as low as 8 mg/dL (2.0 mmol/L) and clinical signs appear below 5mg (1.2 mmol/L). Serum magnesium level is usually moderately elevated to 4-5 mg/dL (1.65-2.06 mmol/L). Serum inorganic phosphorus level is usually depressed to 1.5-3.0 mg/dL (0.45-0.97 mmol/L). There will be increased level of creatinine phocphouinase (CPK) indicating muscular damage due to recumbency.

Treatment

The treatment of milk fever aims at elevating blood calcium level. Intravenous administration of 8 to 10 g of calcium as calcium borogluconate solution helps in immediate recovery. Calcium borogluconate IV (500 to 1000ml containing, 100-200 g Ca at 20-30% solution is administered intravenously. Calcium gels are fed to the affected cows to sustain blood calcium level. The gels are typically $CaCl_2$ or calcium propionate. However, calcium chloride causes ulceration of the mouth and digestive tract, induces severe metabolic acidosis, and may reduce dry matter intake. Calcium propionate has the advantage of containing propionate, a readily available energy source. Vitamin D_3 and phosphorous should also be given parenterally following calcium therapy.

Control

The vitamin D metabolite 1,25 dihydroxyvitamin D3 is supplemented in large quantities orally before calving to reduce hypocalcemia and milk fever because of its in role in calcium absorption and resorption. Intravenous or intramuscular injection of parathyroid hormone may reduce incidence of milk fever.

Eclampsia in Bitch

It's otherwise known as acute parturient hypocalcaemia in bitch. It usually occurs from 3rd litter onwards especially in small breeds with large litter size. The disease occurs mostly in the 3 week after whelping but sometimes after 30 days or more in a bitch with sucking large litter. It occurs rarely during late pregnancy or at the time of whelping.

Etiology

Calcium deficiency in blood stream due to abnormal function of endocrine glands is precipitated by some systemic upset or stress. However, oral therapy of Ca has been observed to be a common predisposing cause of the outbreak of hypocalcaemia. Apparently, feeding Ca has a negative feedback effect on the parathyroid, depressing its action of mobilizing Ca into blood stream from the skeleton.

Clinical Signs

A good mother first neglects her pups and then becomes restlessness with rapid respiration and hanging out tongue. Bitch becomes staggering, goes down and suffers from violent contraction of muscle groups all over the body. In some cases, bitches are exited and crying. There is increase heart beat and temperature may rise to 108°F or more during this state of excitement. In some bitches, the very first sign are restlessness and barking, later walk with a stiff, uncertain gait, the typical tonic – clonic convulsion with rapid respiration, increased body temperature and pulse rate, dilated eyes and finally collapse. Convulsion may be seen as produced by hypoglycaemia which also occurs before or after whelping.

Differential Diagnosis

Clinically, hypocalcemia may easily be confused with hypoglycemia unless a ketone test is done. Epileptic form convulsion that may arise from canine distemper gastrointestinal irritation, presence of foreign body, lead poisoning, nervous disorder (Tetanus, strychninc poisoning, rabies etc.) may resemble eclampsia.

Treatment

Calcium sandoz -(10ml) should be given intravenously every alternate day along with Arachitol (vit-D3) intramuscularly for 5-7 occasions. Oral calcium syrup along with Vitamin B complex should be continued for maintenance therapy. In case of hypoglycemia, intravenous glucose therapy may be given along with glucose powder orally with water. Sucking puppies should be removed from bitches for around 24 hr to decrease drainage of milk. When bitch is on full dosage of Ca & Vit-D, puppies should be provided the nourishing food carefully. If there is too much excitement, Sodium phenobarbital – 10 ml (30mg) may be slowly given intravenously until dog is sedated. Oral adminstration of cortisone or hydrocortisone has good effects.

Lactation Tetany in Mares

It was a common occurrence when a draught horse breeding was widely practiced but is observed rarely now a days. Mortality rate is high in untreated animals. Most cases occur in lactating mare at about 10th day after foaling or 1-2 days after weaning. Mares which are grazing on lush pasture and have an exceptionally heavy flow of milk appears to be more susceptible Prolonged work or prolonged transport appear to precipitate the attack. Occasional cases occur without any apparent cause. Many mild cases which recover spontaneously occur after transport. Severely affected animals sweat profusely and have difficulty in moving because of tetany in limbs and incoordination. There is stiff gait and tail is slightly raised. There is rapid violent respiration and wide dilatation of nostrils with distinct thumping sound from chest and spasmodic contraction of diaphragm. Affected animals are not hypersensitive to sound but handling may precipitate the tetany. Temperature remains normal or slightly elevated. Pulse is normal in early stage, later becomes rapid and irregular. Mare may attempt to eat and drink but fails to swallow. Within 24 hour animal goes down, tetanic convulsions occur and become more or less continuous in 48 hour after onset of illness. The tetany and excitement in early stages may suggest tetanus but there is no prolapse of 3rd eye lid.

Treatment: Intravenous injection of Ca salt causes rapid and complete recovery. One of the earliest signs of recovery is the voiding of urine in large volume.

Downers Cow Syndrome

Downer cow syndrome is a metabolic disease of high producing dairy animals which usually occurs as a complication following hypocalcaemic parturient paresis and is characterised clinically by prolonged recumbency even after two successive calcium therapy, recumbent at least for 24 hrs without any apparent reason, traumatic injury to limb muscles and nerves, ischemic necrosis of limb muscles, myocarditis, and fatty infiltration and degeneration of liver.

Etiology

- **Primary Recumbency due to Primary Disease**
  a) Metabolic disease: Hypocalcemia, Hypophosphatemia, hypomagnesemia, hypokalemia, fatty liver disease
  b) Starvation
  c) Trauma during calving or when struggling to get up and rupture of gastrocnemius tendon

d) Fractured pelvis, long bones, dislocated hip
e) Nerve damage: Sciatic and/or obturator nerve paralysis
f) Septic/Toxic shock: Mastitis, metritis, right side displacement of abomasum

- **Secondary Recumbency**

a) Prolonged recumbency causes pressure damage
b) Ischemic necrosis of semitendinosus muscles caudal to stifle
c) Edema, swelling, cellulitis, venous thrombosis
d) Primarily gastrocnemius and semitendinosus muscles affection
e) Common peronial branch of sciatic nerve damage leading to loss of function of digital extensor muscle

- **Tertiary Recumbency**

a) Repeated struggling to get up may cause musculoskeletal damage and hemorrhage resulting in long-term recumbency:
b) Fractures
c) Rupture of muscle, ligaments

Pathogenesis

Prolonged recumbency leads to ischemic necrosis of semitendinous muscle and muscle caudal to stifle joint. Prolonged compression of muscles leads to tissue anoxia, cell damage and inflammatory changes. Further swelling limits the tissue perfusion.

Clinical Findings

In the typical case, affected cows either make no effort or are unable to stand following treatment for parturient paresis. The animals which are unable to stand after 24 h and after two successive treatments are termed as under downers. Downer cows are classified as alert or non-alert based on clinical signs.

Alert Downers

- Bright and alert
- Appetite is reduced but downers eat and drink moderately
- Normal body temperature and heart rate or elevated to 80-100 beats per minute
- Normal defecation and urination
- Proteinuria indicating muscle damage

Non-alert Downers

- Lateral recumbency with head drawn back
- Hyperaesthesia or stiff limb on lateral recumbency
- Complete anorexia

Creeper cows: Frequent attempt to stand up with "frog leg" posture but unable to stand

Clinical Pathology

- Enzymes like CPK, AST and LDH, total protein, fibrinogen are important indicators for prognosis of downer cows
- In experimentally induced downer cattle, creatinine phosphokinae (CPK) level remains normal upto 6 hr and 12th increases to 12000-40000 units per L in next 12-24 hour
- Marked proteinuria by 18- 24 h after onset
- Elevation of serum urea, muscle enzymes and laboratory evidence of inflammation are considered indication of poor prognosis.
- Recovery rate is lower in cows with total protein: fibrinogen ratio less than 10:1 and evidence of neutropenia with left shift.

Differential Diagnosis

- Differentiation should be made between primary from secondary causes of recumbency like milk fever, hypophosphatemia, hypomagnesemia, fat cow syndrome
- Musculoskeletal injury (pelvis, hip, long bones, stifle-hock, ruptured tendons)
- Nerve injury (spinal cord lesions, calving paralysis)
- Toxic conditions

Treatment

Treatment is not specific but symptomatic

- Injection of magnesium salts, corticosteroids.
- Stimulant tonics - tripelenamine hydrochloride
- Slow intravenous administration of vitamin E and Se
- Solutions containing K, P, Ca, Mg
- Fluid therapy both oral and parenteral
- Comfortable bedding
- Turning cow from side to side to reduce pressure necrosis

- Physiotherapy to avoid muscle damage
- Antibiotic in septic conditions
- Lifting devices- Danish aqua lift and power cow cradle

Control and Prevention

- Control measures should be followed to prevent milk fever
- Early detection and treatment of milk fever
- Good bedding like straw bedding and for forest 48 hours after calring
- Well bedded box stall for calving and then up to 48 hrs
- Rolling animal from one side to other on hourly basis if possible
- Lateral recumbency should be avoided placing bales of straw to prevent hydrostatic congestion and ruminal tympany
- Exposure to hot sun should be avoided to prevent heat stroke
- Sympathetic approach to the animal; provision of non - slippery surface.

Ketosis

It is a disease of high producing dairy cows during the peripurturient period, characterized by hypoglycemia, ketonemia, ketonuria and ketolactia. Negative energy balance occurring due to nutritional or metabolic insult in high yielding cows in early lactation is the primary and most common cause of ketosis. Failure to provide sufficient glucose when the animals are subjected to heavier demands on their resource of glucose and glycogen leads to incidence of ketosis. In negative energy balance, there will be mobilization of free fatty acids to the liver where they are oxidized to acetyl coA and NADH. This acetyl coA in the presence of oxaloacetate (OAA) is oxidized via TCA cycle. If sufficient OAA is not available then acetyl coA is converted to acetoacetyl coA which is further converted to ketone bodies, aceto-acetate and hydroxy butyric acid (BHBA), which is absorbed to blood leading to elevation of blood ketone levels.

Epidemiology

Ketosis is commonly seen in high yielding dairy cows in early lactation of 3rd or 4th calving. Management practice and nutritional status of herd are the determinants of ketosis in a dairy herd. Reoccurrence may also appear in same lactation.

Classification

(1) Primary Ketosis (Production ketosis)

This type of ketosis occurs in cows in good to excessive body condition and fed good quality ration but are in negative energy balance. Greater proportion of cases remains as subclinical with increased levels of circulating ketone bodies without overt clinical signs. A less proportion of cases appear as clinical ketosis.

(2) Secondary Ketosis

This type of ketosis occurs in cows with concurrent diseases that decreases the feed intake in periparturient periods. The common primary diseases are abomasal displacement, traumatic reticulitis, metritis and mastitis, fever associated with anorexia etc.

(3) Alimentary Ketosis

This type of ketosis occurs when the animal is fed silage with excessive amounts of butyrate. Ketosis occurs due to decreased food intake resulting from poor palatability of high butyrate silage. Silage made from succulent material also contains preformed butyric acid which is highly ketogenic.

(4) Starvation Ketosis

Starvation ketosis occurs in cattle in poor body condition those are fed with poor-quality feed stuffs. There is a deficiency of propionate and protein in the diet and a limited capacity of gluconeogenesis from body reserves. The affected cattle usually recover with correct feeding.

Clinical Signs

Clinical signs of ketosis appear in two forms such as wasting form and nervous form

(A) Wasting Form of Ketosis

- Gradual decrease in appetite and milk yield over a period of 2-4 days.
- Animal refuses to eat grains first, then silage, but may continue to eat hay.
- Depraved appetite with rapid loss of body weight
- Woody appearance due to wasting.
- Loss of skins elasticity due to loss of subcutaneous fat
- Firm & dry faeces

- Moderately depressed, disinclined to move and eat
- Normal temperature, respiration and pulse rate
- Normal frequency but decreased amplitude of ruminal motility
- Characteristic aromatic odour of ketone from breath
- Sharp drop in solid not fat (SNF) content of milk
- Occasional nervous sign with transient bouts of staggering
- Partial blindness

(B) Nervous Form of Ketosis

- Bizarre activity and becoming quite suddenly
- Delirium rather than frenzy
- Walking in circle
- Straddling, crossing of legs
- Head pressing, leaning into stanchion
- Apparent blindness, aimlesss movement
- Wandering, vigorous licking of skin and inanimate object.
- Chewing movement with salivation
- Depraved appetite
- Hyperesthesia
- Bellowing on pinching or when stroked
- Incoordination gait with moderate tremor and tetany
- Short periods of nervous sign lasting 1-2 hrs., reoccur frequently at 8-12 hrs interval.

Subclinical Ketosis

In subclinical ketosis, there is elevation of ketone bodies in the blood but without overt clinical symptoms. Mild decrease in milk yeild with reduction in fertility attributed from ovarian abnormality and endometritis, reduced conception rate and prolonged calving to conception interval are the common manifestation of subclinical ketosis.

Clinical Pathology

- Hypoglycemia, ketonemia and ketonuria.
- Increased plasma free fatty acid.
- Reduced blood glucose level from normal level of -50mg/dl to 20-30 mg/dl
- Blood ketone level increases to 10-100mg/dl from normal 10mg /dl.

- Urinary ketone reaches 80-130mg/dl from normal of 10mg/dl
- Milk ketone level increased to 40mg/dl from 3mg/dl.
- High level of VFA in blood and rumen.

Differential Diagnosis

(A) Wasting form of ketosis should be differentiated from Traumatic reticulitis, abomasal displacement, secondary ketosis from mastitis and metritis, vagus indigestion etc.

(B) Clinical signs of ketosis resembles Nervous form- Listeriosis, rabies, lactation tetany, acute lead poisoning etc.

Treatment

a) Replacement Therapy

- 50 % glucose, 500ml intravenously and 20 % glucose intraperitoneally
- Propylene glycol or glycerine @ 225 g / day for 2 days then 110 g / day for 2 days.
- Sodium propionate 110-225 g/ day, but shows very slow response.
- Calcium or sodium lactate 1 kg initially, later ½ kg / day for 7 days or Sodium acetate 110-500 g/day.
- Anabolic steroids: Effective treatment for pregnancy toxemia of ewes. Trenbolone acetate @ 60 to 100 mg as single injection.
- Insulin with glucose or glucocorticoids 200 – 300 I.U. Repeat every 24 – 48 hrs.

b) Miscellaneous Treatment

- Ketonex boli–2-3 boli twice daily for 5-7 days. (Nicotinic acid & dried yeast.)
- Vit –B_{12} & Cobalt -- for formation of CoA, propionate metabolism.
- Cysteamine @ 750mg –intravenously– 3doses at 1-3 day interval.
- Meboliv as metabolic stimulant, liver tonic (225 ml, 500ml and 1ltr)
- Liver extract injection : 5-10ml daily for 3 -5 occasions.
- Buffered phosphorus injection with inosine and sodium pyruvate.

Control and Prevention

- Estimation of blood glucose level 2 weeks prior to parturition and 2rd-6th week of lactation, below 35mg/dl indicates ketosis to occurs in future.
- Test for urine samples for ketone bodies.
- Rothera test should be conducted for detection of ketone bodies 2 week before parturition and, 2 week after parturition.

- β- hydroxy butyrate level in blood during early lactation, concentration greater than 10mg/dl suggests sub clinical ketosis.
- Feeding ionophore compounds i.e. Monensin @ 25mg daily in grain feed mixture to increase the ratio of propionate.
- Feeding sodium propionate @ 110g daily for 6 weeks commencing from calving.
- Propylene glycol @ 250-350ml daily for 10 days after calving.
- Niacin @ 6-12 g / day from 2 wks. prior to 8 wks. after calving.
- Thus, a balanced feed, adequate exercise and proper scientific rearing and management practice can result in reduced chance of occurrence of ketosis.

Pregnancy Toxemia in Ewes

Ovine ketosis, Twin lamb disease, Ketosis of pregnancy, Kidding sickness

Introduction

Pregnancy toxemia is well known metabolic disease of glucose and fat metabolism in sheep and goat which usually occur spontaneously in the last 4 to 6 week before parturition. Ewes with multiple fetuses are mostly affected. This disease is associated with low plasma concentration of glucose and markedly increases plasma concentration of ketone bodies. It is believed that the disorder is caused by an inability of the pregnant ewe to meet the increased glucose demand of the twin fetuses. Decline plane of nutrition during the last 4th-6th weeks, mostly last 2 weeks of pregnancy results in pregnancy toxaemia. In this period, fetal growth is maximum and demand for energy is more, particularly in ewes carrying twins or triplets.

Classification of Pregnancy Toxemia

According to the cause, it is classified in five types

1. Primary Pregnancy Toxemia

It occur due to fall in the plane of nutrition during the later half of pregnancy and some manage mental procedure in late Pregnancy such as crutching, shearing, change of environment or drenching.

2. Fat ewe Pregnancy Toxemia

It occurs in well fed ewes and over fat conditions in late pregnancy. Fatty ewe will experience a voluntary fall in food intake in late pregnancy due to the reduction of rumen volume by the pressure of intra abdominal and developing fetus. This occurs due to high water contained feed such as silage or root crops and lack of exercise

3. Starvation Pregnancy Toxemia

It is relatively uncommon. Ewes those are excessively thin in prolonged draught period and also in mismanagemental conditions resulting in starvation

4. Secondary Pregnancy Toxemia

It occurs as a sporadic disease as the result of the effect of concurrent diseases such as footrot or abscess which affect food intake, and heavy worm infestation with *Haemonchus contortus*, that affects the glucose metabolism.

5. Stress Induced Pregnancy Toxemia

It is the least common cause of disease. Stress is the principal factor for pragnancy toxaemia. These are several reasons of stress such as housing of late pregnant sheep not used to being housed, transportation of pregnant sheep and outbreak of other diseases, The disease occurs primarily in sheep raised in intensive farming system either grazing or housed during the winter because the sheep used in the intensive farming are more likely to bear twin or triplet. The incidence of the disease varies with the nature and severity of the nutrient deprivation.

Animal Risk Factor

1. Pregnancy

Ewes in the last 2nd-4th week of pregnancy, primarily the ewes having twin or triplet.

2. Parity

Uncommon in maiden ewes because of their low fecundity and increase in prevalence up to 3rd parity.

3. Breed

The disease is more common in British low land breeds and their crosses than the merino because of difference in fecundity and managemental condition.

Pathogenesis

Pregnancy toxemia results from inadequate energy intake in late pregnancy in ewes having more than one fetus. As maximum fetal growth take place in the last 6 week of pregnancy, ewes having ineffective gluconeogenesis response to the continued demand of glucose by the growing fetus results in hypoglycemia, lipid metabolism and accumulation of ketone body and cortisol. Subsequent metabolic changes associated with excessive lipid metabolism with elevated concentration of D-β-hydroxybutyrate suppresses the endogenous glucose production and exaggerate the development of ketosis. Increased plasma concentration of non-esterified fatty acid results in a depression of cellular and humoral immune response in experimentally produced disease. Renal dysfunction is also seen in the terminal stage of ovine ketosis.

Clinical Findings

Earlier stage – Affected ewes remain separated from the group. Ewes are standing near the trough with the group but not eating. Many affected ewes stand in water trough through out the day and lap the water. Faeces are dry and scanty, constipation is usually seen and there is grinding of teeth.

Later stage – tremor of muscle of head cause twitching of lips, champing of jaws and salivation. Dorsiflexion or lateral deviation of head followed by circling. The muscle tremor involves the whole body and the ewe falls with tonic convulsion. In between the convulsions, ewe remains in star gazing posture and there is incordination to walk. Affected ewes recumbent in 3-4 days.

Clinical Pathology

- Hypoglycemia can be used as a diagnostic aid in early stage.
- Elevated blood ketone level.
- Presence of ketone bodies in urine.
- Sheep develops a severe metabolic acidosis, renal failure with terminal uremia and dehydration.
- Liver function test is abnormal. Elevation of plasma cortisol occur in pregnancy toxemia and conc. above 10ng /ml are indicative of pregnancy toxemia

Necropsy Finding

Severe fatty degeneration of liver. Intestine may contain fetid light coloured diarrheic faeces. Twins or greater numbers of fetus are present.

Differential Diagnosis

Pregnancy toxemia is usually suspected in late pregnant ewes which show nervous sign and die within 2-7 days and there may be a history of exertion or sudden deprivation of food.

a) Hypocalcemia – onset is within 12hr of stress and a considerable proportion of flock will be affected at the same time .It has a much shorter course of 12-24hr. and affected animals respond well to treatment.

b) Rabies is associated with mania, ascending paralysis and is always fatal.

c) Cerebral abcess affects only 1to 2 sheep and has a long course and localizing signs.

d) Listeriosis is associated wtih tongue paralysis, facial paralysis, depression and coma

Treatment

Parenteral use

1. 5-7 gm of glucose given I/V, 6-8 time a day.
2. 20-40 unit of zinc protamine insulin given I/M in every other day in 3 day.
3. I/V injection of isotonic sodium bicarbonate/lactated ringer solution [5-10ml / kg body wt.]
4. Treatment with recombinant bovine somatotrophin [0.15mg/kg bw] in conjunction with dextrose and electrolyte.

Oral Therapy

a) Propylene glycol or glycerine (110g/day)

b) Oral drenching of 160 ml of solution containing 45g of glucose, 8.5g of sodium chloride, 6.17 g of glycerine and electrolyte in every 4-8 hr interval.

c) Caesarean section for removal of fetus, it is helpful in early stage of disease.

d) Induction of parturition – dexamethasone 21 isonicotinate or sodium phosphate can be used 16-25mg /ewe.

Control

The flock should be examined daily for any evidence of ketosis and affected animals should be treated immediately with glycerol and carbohydrate intake should be ensured. Minimum change of feed should be made during advanced pregnancy. Care should be taken to avoid over stress and fasting during late pregnancy

Prevention

- Sudden change in type of feed should be avoided.
- Extra feed should be provided during bad weather.
- Ewes should be observed 30min /day for exercise.
- Animal should be provided with vitamin A rich feed during pregnant period.

- Care should be taken to rule out parasitic burden before induction of pregnancy
- Care should be taken to avoid over stress and fasting during late pregnancy
- Provision of concentrate containing 10% protein @ 0.25 kg per day during the last two weeks.

Hypomagnesaemia

The disease is otherwise called as grass tetany, grass staggers, and wheat pasture poisoning. It is manifested by clinical signs of tremor, clonic to tonic convulsion, hyperesthesia (Exaggerated response to external stimuli that means the animal can be easily provoked as is seen in tetanus, rabies, lead poisoning) and death due to respiratory failure. Hypomagnesaemia tetany is termed as a production disease as input and output balance is disturbed due to drainage of Mg in the milk. There is no significant feedback mechanism (unlike calcium homeostasis), that regulates blood magnesium (Mg) level. Therefore, input through ingestion of feed and fodder is the principal source of Mg to maintain its level. Regular supplementation of Mg through feed and fodder is essential. Starvation of 24-48 hours in a high yielding lactating cow may lead to hypomagnesaemic tetany. This disease requires emergency treatment and in many occasions the animals are found dead (the diseases in which animals don't show any notifiable clinical signs before death. Example- per-acute form of hemorrhagic septicemia anthrax, lightening stroke, snake bite, bloat etc)

The disease is highly fatal in all classes of ruminants and is mostly in lactating cows. Partial dietary deficiency of magnesium and other nutritional and metabolic factors reduces the availability of Mg from feed and fodder. Consumption of lush green grass and young green cereal crops leads to deficiency of magnesium. High serum level of potassium (hyperkalaemia) or higher content of K in feed and fodder as seen upon feeding of lush green grass or long cereal crops reduces the bioavailability of Mg. Milk, urine, digestive secretions contain high amount of Mg. In absence of effective feedback mechanism to maintain Mg homeostasis, the animal suffers from this disease with complete starvation for 24-48 hours. A milch cow generally ingests around 20g of Mg daily, absorbs about 4g daily. The pasture should contain a minimum of 0.2% of magnesium on dry matter basis to prevent hypomagnesaemia tetany.

The morbidity in a herd ranges from 2-12% and depends on climatic conditions and managemental practices. Mortality is high. The disease has a short course and found dead is seen 20% of the cases. The manifestation of clinical sign is seen when the serum Mg level drops below 1mg/dl as against normal level of 1.7-3 mg/dl. Deficiency of Mg facilitate quick transmission of impulses to neuro-muscular system that results in tonic to clonic convulsions and tremor. Reduced level of Mg in central nervous system is responsible for central effect of Mg.

Factors Influencing Bioavailability of Magnesium

1. Ammonia production in the rumen- Ingestion of protein rich diet leads to production of large quantity of ammonia in the rumen that interferes with Mg bioavailability. Heavy top dressing of fodder with nitrogen fertilizers also leads to production of ammonia in the rumen resulting in same effect.
2. Chelating agents such as α-ketoglutarate in the plants or ruminal contents also reduces Mg bioavailability.
3. Reduced alimentary sojourn (as in case of diarrhoea) also leads to reduced absorption of Mg because the ruminal contents take a certain time to pass the small intestine and large intestine.
4. High Potassium content of diet and intake of more aluminum also cause poor absorption of Mg.
5. Cold, wet and windy weathers with no shelter and supplementary feed also reduce the Mg availability.

Clinical Signs

The disease is manifested in 3 clinical forms.

A. Acute form

In this form there is sudden cessation of grazing, unusual alertness, discomfort, twitching, of muscles and ear, hyperesthesia, continuous bellowing, frenzied behavior, opisthotonous, nystagmus, champing of jaw, frothing of mouth, retraction of eyelid. The most characteristic feature is that, animal lies quietly between two episodes of clinical signs. Temperature may go up to 105°F due to muscle exhaustion. There will be increased pulse and respiration rate, and death within 1 hour.

B. Sub-acute form

It is manifested by gradual onset of clinical signs. Slight inappetance, exaggerated limb movements, spasmodic urination, frequent defaecation, reduced milk yield, reduced ruminal motility.

C. Chronic form

It is manifested with dullness, unthriftiness and indifferent appetite.

- Clinical Pathology Biochemical examination reveals Mg level below 1mg/dl and is generally associated with hypocalcaemia in lactating cows and may be hypokalemia.
- The CSF Mg level is a good indicator of body Mg status. CSF magnesium level of 2mg/dl is considered as the animal is normal. When it falls to 1.2 mg/dl or below, the animal shows the clinical signs of hypomagnesaemic tetany.

Postmortem Findings

- At necropsy, there will be extravasation of blood into the subcutaneous space, peritoneum, pericardium and into interstitial muscular space.
- Bovine vitreous humor of eye is a true reflection of Mg level even 48 hours after death.

Differential Diagnosis

- The disease should be differentiated from rabies lead poisoning etc
- Rabies occurs mostly due to dog bite that does not respond to treatment. Rabies may occur due to consumption of infected raw meat. There is ropy salivation and saliva hangs till ground. There is ascending paralysis, starts from toe and ends in head and neck.
- Lead poisoning is manifested by diarrhoea, gastro-intestinal disorders. Treatment with antidote for Pb poisoning; Calcium disodium EDTA, alleviates the clinical signs, Bones are considered as lead sink. There will be circling, pressing of head against hard surface, a lot of aimless running by the animal lead poisoning in common in mining areas.
- In tetanus, these is rigidity of limbs (muscles) and death occurs due to respiratory failure

Treatment

- Generally, 500 ml of Ca and Mg salts in combination (25% Calcium borogluconate + 5% magnesium hypophosphate) are injected intravenously, followed by subcutaneous injection of 200-300 ml of 20% solution of $MgSO_4$ gives good result. Intravenous administration of Mg salts alone may cause cardiac embarrassment, medullary depression leading to respiratory failure. So, generally a combination of Ca and Mg are prescribed.

Control

1. Feeding of Mg supplements.
2. Top dressing of pasture with Magnesium limestone @ 5600kg/ha.

3. Spraying of the fodder with 2% solution of $MgSO_4$ at fortnight interval and provision of shelter during difficult weather.

Azoturia/ Paralytic Myoglobinuria

It is a disease of horses particularly race horses, occuring during exercise following a period of inactivity with full ration and is characterised by myoglobinuria and muscular degeneration. This disease is also known as paralytic myoglobinuria, Tying up, Monday morning sickness.

- Large storage of muscle glycogen during a period of about 1-10 days of inactivity with full working ration leads to rapid and overproduction of lactic acid following strenous excercise, that is precipitated by deficiency of vitamin E and selenium.

Pathogenesis

During the period of idleness with full working grain feed, a large quantity of glycogen gets stored in heavy muscles like gluteus, rectus femoris and vastus muscle etc. After the rest period, when the animal is allowed for sudden exercise, there is rapid metabolism of large quantity of muscle glycogen resulting in production of lactic acid within a short period due to anoxia. When the rate of production of lactic acid exceeds the rate at which it can be removed to blood stream and urine, lactic acid accumulates in muscle as sarcolactate and cause degeneration and coagulation necrosis of muscle fibre leading to release of myoglobin in to blood stream. Excess myoglobin in blood is excreted in urine resulting in dark brown colour urine (myoglobinuria). There will be damage to renal tubules, the condition referred to as myoglobinuric nephrosis. This leads to uremia followed by death. Death in this disease may occur due to decubital septicemia, myoglobinuric nephrosis, uremia and degeneration of myocardium.

Clinical Findings

Signs develop within 15 minutes to 1 hour on work. Signs may disappear in few hours if the horse is given complete rest immediately, but the condition usually progress to recumbency. The animal first assume a dog sitting posture followed by lateral recumbency. There is severe pain, restlessness, struggling and repeated attempt to rise. Temperature increases in severe cases. One or all four limbs may be affected; commonly both hind limbs are involved. There is dark brown colour urination.

Clinical Pathology

- High specific gravity of urine due to presence of myoglobin.
- Low renal threshold for myoglobin, Serum does not get discoloured

- Protein and cast may be found in urine.
- Marked polycythemia.
- Increased serum creatinine phosphokinase (CPK) indicates degeneration of skeletal and cardiac muscle
- Increased SGOT reflects damage to muscle and liver.

Treatment

- Further exercise should be avoided.
- Animal should be treated immediately on spot.
- Narcosis with chloral hydrate or ataractic drugs.
- Tranquilization may be given in severe pain .
- Slinging is highly essential .
- Dexamethasone @ 1-3mg/kg body weight - intravenously
- Thimaine hcl @ 0.5- 1g – intramuscular followed by 100-200g orally thrice daily for 3-5 days.
- Antihistaminics may be administered
- Parenteral poly-ionic infusions to prevent myohaemoglobinuric nephrosis.
- Alakalinisers e.g. $NaHCO_3$ – intravenously and orally to combat acidosis and to preventing precipitation of myoglobin in renal tubules.

Osteodystrophy Fibrosa

This is a disease of bone resulting from failure of normal development or abnormal metabolism of mature bone, and is characterised by distortion and enlargement of bone, abnormalities in gait and posture, and sometimes fracture of bone. This disease is common in horse but also occurs in pig, sheep and goat.

Etiology

- Secondary calcium deficiency due to excessive serum phosphorous level.
- Inadequate nutrition
- Both hypo and hyper vitaminosis A
- Chronic interstitial nephritis leading to excess retention of phophorous and sulphate.
- Chronic lead poisoning, fluorine poisoning etc.

Pathogenesis

Imbalance in dietary calcium and phosphorous ratio leads to defective metabolism of bones. There will be laying down of soft cellular fibrous tissue instead of osteoid tissue as a result bone becomes weak and soft. There will be detachment of muscles and tendons from the bones, articular erosions and displacement of bone marrow.

Clinical Findings

- Shifting lameness is characteristic clinical sign
- Arching of back
- Creak badly in joints while walking in different limbs at different times
- Fracture with visible sprains of tendons in severe cases
- Fracture of lumbar vertebrae while racing
- Swelling of lower and alveolar margins of mandible
- Soft symmetric enlargement of facial bones (Big Head)
- Anorexia, difficulty in mastication, drooling of saliva
- Flattening of ribs
- Swelling of joints and curvature of long bones
- Emaciation, anemia and death

Clinical Pathology

- Increased level of serum alkaline phosphatase and phosphorous
- Decreased serum calcium level
- Radiographically increased translucency of bones

Treatment

- Supplementation of Ca, P and vitamin D
- Vitamin D @ 10,000 I.U. /kg
- Di calcium phosphate
- Adequate bedding

Nutritional Hemoglobinuria

It is a disease of high producing animal soon after calving characterized by intravascular haemolysis, haemoglobinaemia, haemoglobinura, and anaemia with passage of red urine. Although the exact etiology of post parturient haemoglobinuria is not known, ingestion of identified haemolytic agents like turpin and other cruciferous plants with high lysine level, ingestion of large quantities of onion making the erythrocytes more sensitive to haemolysis. This occurs due to lipid peroxidation of erythrocyte membrane and making the cell membrane more turgid, rigid and fragile.

Hypophosphataemia is considered as the predisposing factor, however disease may occur with normal phosphorous level. Slight deficiency in Se and Cu may also cause post parturient haemoglobinuria. This disease has relatively low incidence, but case fatality rate may go upto 50%. Adult cows 2-4 weeks after calving, between 3rd-6th lactation generally suffer from this disease. However the disease may be seen before parturition, therefore the disease is termed as periparturient haemoglobinuria. The drain of lactation further depletes the P level creating an imbalance in input and output, therefore the disease comes under production diseases.

Clinically there will be haemoglobinuria, inappetence, weakness, decreased milk production and pica. In some cases, the appetite is normal. The disease runs for a course of 3-5 days. Gangrene and sloughing of tip of tail may occur during the course of disease. Sub-clinical or clinical ketosis may occur concurrently showing the signs of both ketosis and periparturient haemoglobinuria.

The normal phosphorus level is 2-3 mg/dl, but the disease is seen when the level drops to 0.4-1.5 mg/dl.

Differential Diagnosis

1. Leptospirosis- It affects all age groups. There will be rise in body temperature, complete anorexia and abortion. *Leptospira* can isolated from urine and blood sample.
2. Bacillary Haemoglobinuria- It is caused by *Clostridium haemolyticum*. That affects matured cattle. Disease is enzootic in nature.
3. Babesiosis- Intravascular haemolysis and red urine, rise in temperature. It is restricted to particular areas with high tick population. Clinically erythrocytes contain club-shaped piroplasms.
4. Anaplasmosis- There is rise in temperature. Anaemia is a common feature but not red urine. Severe jaundice is recorded as the erythrocytes are trapped in Reticulo-Endothelial System (RES) and destroyed intracellularly.
5. Copper poisoning- It is restricted to areas where the copper content of soil is too high. Continuous ingestion of Cu leads to its accumulation in liver. Spontaneous surge of Cu from the liver and damage to the liver parenchyma leads to intravascular haemolysis and severe jaundice. There mayn't be any fever in case of Cu poisoning. It is more common in sheep than other ruminants.

6. Poisoning due to haemolytic agents- Cruciferous plants, onion, Kale may lead to intravascular haemolysis and haemoglobinuria.
7. Cold water haemolytic anaemia- This occurs following ingestion of cold water after exercise, particularly in young animals. Absorption of water provides hypotonic medium in intravascular space leading to rupture of RBC and release of haemoglobin.
8. Drug induced haemolysis
9. Haemolysis may occur due to blood transfusion reaction

Postmortem Findings

At necropsy, blood will be thin, carcass is jaundiced, swollen liver. Fatty infiltration and degeneration of liver and discoloration of urine in bladder.

Treatment

1. Tranfusion of large amount of whole blood (may be 5 litre to a cow weighing 450 kg).
2. Fluid therapy to flush the urine to prevent haemoglobinuric nephrosis.
3. 60g of sodium acid phosphate in 300 ml of distilled water may be administered intravenously.
4. This may be followed by provision of bone meal or dicalcium phosphate @ 120g twice a day.

Hypothyroidism

It is the deficiency of thyroid hormone i.e thyroxine & tri-iodo thyronine. It is a primary disorder in over 95% of dog population. Adult dogs may be affected from 2 year old onwards but majority are suffering from 4-8 year old and occasionally in older ones. They usually belong to larger or medium sized breeds. Hypothyroidism appears to be minimum in miniature or toy breed dogs. Affected dogs show stunted physical deviation with a broad skull and short legs with dwarf appearance and subnormal mental activities. Most pups with congenital hypothyroidism probably die before weaning. About half of canine species suffering from hypothyrodiosim the disease is attributed to autoimmune thyroiditis (lymphocytic thyroiditis) which eventually results in wide spread follicular destruction & deposition of fibrous tissue. An equal number of cases are due to idiopathic atrophy of follicles and their replacement by adipose tissue

Clinical Signs

Rough hair coat with alopecia in 90% cases. Alopecia mainly affects flank, neck, posterior thigh & tail region. Some times there is floppy coat or even thickening of coat, hyperkeratosis (formation of dandruff). Thickening of skin produces exaggerated skin folds on forehead and neck region showing a worried expression. Slow hair growth and wound healing, increases in sleeping time, inability to take exercise due to muscle atrophy, obesity and intolerance to cold, lack of libido and irregular estrous cycle are common manifestatrans, in severe cases, there is keratoconjunctivities and corneal ulcer, difficulty in walking, stiffness, ataxia and tilting of head.

Clinical Pathology

Mild anemia, elevated plasma cholesterol level, increased CPK level, increased triglyceride level due to liver dysfunction, exceptionally leucocytosis due to pyoderma.

Treatment

Most appropriate drug for oral replacement therapy in all cases is synthetic thyroxine which should be given @ 20 µgm/kg body weight twice daily initially for a minimum of 03 months to provide a fair result. If there's history of cardiac disease, the dose should start @ 5 µgm/kg body weight twice daily and be gradually increases to 20 µgm/kg body weight over 6-8 week.

Diabetes in Dogs

(A) Diabetes Mellitus

It is a disorder of carbohydrate, fat & protein metabolism which results from an inability to produce or utilize adequate amount of insulin. Its diagnosis is based on fasting plasma-glucose level that regularly exceeds 8mmole/lit or on any occasion exceeds 11mg/lit. There must be unusually glycosuria. The incidence of diabetes mellitus is 0.4 – 0.5 % of dog population. Incidence rises with age and it's seen under 01 year old. diabetes mellitus was found to be an inherited disorder in keeshond breed of dogs with onset between 2-6 month of age.

Clinical Signs

Primary polyuria and polydipsia, secondarily polyphagia, weight loss, muscle wasting but initially there must be obesity, cataract, hepatomegaly, rarely alopecia, predisposed to pyoderma and cystitis, inappetance, increase rate & depth of respiration , vomition, dehydration due to oligouria, smell of acetone on breath. Abdominal pain due to acute pancreatitis, ultimately coma and death.

Clinical Pathology

Hyperglycemia, glycosuria, increased plasma cholesterol level, dehydration, causing increased PCV, total protein & albumin level, increased leukocyte count & increased triglyceride and cholesterol level and ketoneuria.

(B) Diabetes Insipidus (DI)

It is a disorder in dog characterized by polyuria or polydipsia arising from defective antidiuretic hormone (ADH) release or defective response to ADH.

Symptoms

1. Polyuria: 3 to 4 litres/day.
    - Urine: Watery with odour: Low specific gravity- 1.001 to 1.002.
    - In early stage: Easy voiding.
    - In Late: Some what painful.
2. Polydipsia: Horse 100 litres; Dog 10-15 lit/day.
3. Appetite slowly decrease.
4. Cataract, abscess in the perenial glands and prostate gland.

Treatment

- Hypoglycemic drugs
- Insulin should be given intra-peritoneal in insulin syringe

18

Diseases Caused by Nutritional Deficiency

Following criteria are suggested for assessment of the importance of nutrition in the etiology of a diseased state in a single or group of animals.

i. If there's any deficiency of a specific nutrient occurring after examination of diet?
ii. Is there any deficiency of suspected essential nutrients causing disease after examination of animals?
iii. If the supplementation of essential nutrients in the diet prevented or cured the disease condition?

Evidence of Existence of Deficiency

General evidence of deficiency include either nutrient deficiency in diet or abnormal absorption, utilization or requirement of nutrient under consideration. Special evidence may be obtained by chemical or biochemical examination of diet.

Diet

Diet for considerable period prior to occurrence of disease must be examined because body stores of most dietary factors may delay the appearance of clinical signs. Specific deficiency is likely to be associated in particular soil types and in many instances, soil and geographical maps may predict the probable occurrence of a nutritional disease. Diseases of plants may also indicate specific soil deficiency. For eg. Reclamation diseases of oats indicate copper deficiency in soil. Farming practices may have a marked bearing on the presence or absence of specific nutrients in a livestock feed. Heavy application of nitrogen fertilisers can reduce Cu, Co, Mb and Mn content of pasture.

On the other hand, many applications of lime reduce plant Cu, Co, Zn and Mn level but increases the Mo content. Modern hay making methods of artificial drying of immature forage tend to conserve vit-A but result in vit-D deficiency. So, local knowledge of farming and feeding practices in a particular area is most important in diagnosis of nutritional deficiency states.

Abnormal Absorption

Some other factors that reduce the absorption of nutrients decrease the dietary supply, even though the diet may contain adequate amount of particular nutrient.

- Eg. Excess phosphate in the diet decreases calcium absorption.
- Excess calcium interferes with the absorption of iodine, lead, zinc and codmium and absence of bile salt prevents proper absorption of fat-soluble vitamins.
- Chronic enteritis decreases the absorption of most dietary nutrients

Abnormal Utilization of Ingested Nutrients

This may also have an effect on the development of conditional deficiency disease Molybdeneum and sulphate reduce copper storage, vitamin-E has a sparing effect on vit-A and thiamine decreases the dietary requirements of essential fatty acid.

Abnormal Feed Requirement

Stimulation of growth rate of animal by improved nutrition may increase requirement of specific nutrients.

Energy Deficiency

i. Causes: Insufficient quantity or quality of feed is a common nutritional deficiency and practical problem of feeding livestock. Protein and energy deficiency occur concurrently in underfed livestock. Supply of feed may be inadequate because of over grazing, draught, snow covering or too expensive.
ii. Available feed may be of such low quality and low digestibility, animal can not consume enough to meet energy requirement. In some cases, forage may contain a high concentration of H_2O which limits total energy content.

Clinical Findings

It depends on age of animal stage of production (Pregnant/Lactating), presence of concurrent deficiency of specific nutrient and environmental influences.

In general, an insufficient supply of energy in young animals results in retarded growth and delay in the onset of puberty. In milch animals there is a marked decline in milk production. A prolonged energy deficiency in pregnant beef heifer will result in failure to produce adequate quantity of colostrum during parturition. The period of anestrous may last up to several months which has marked effect on reproductive performance in a herd and prolonged deficiency of energy during late gestation may result in undersized neonates with high mortality rate. Deficiency of energy during prolonged period of cold weather especially in beet cattle and ewes on poor quality roughage, beef may result in abnormal impacting.

If sufficient feed is not available in cold weather, animal will mobilize energy stored as fat to maintain body temperature and thus loose body weight. In case of ruminants and horses, if feed is of poor quality, such as poor quality roughage, increase in feed intake may result in impaction of abomasum and rumen in cattle and of large intestine in horses.

Cold and wet weather increases the needs for energy resulting in weakness, recumbency and death. A sudden dietary deficiency of energy in fat, pregnant beef cattle and ewes can result in starvation with ketosis and pregnancy toxaemia.

Protein malnutrition occurs in neonates fed inferior quality milk replacer that may contain insufficient energy and protein.

Protein Deficiency

A deficiency of protein is commonly accompanied with deficiency of energy. Insufficient protein intake in young animals results in decreased appetite, lowered feed intake, slow growth rate, and a prolonged time to reach maturity. In mature animal, there is loss of body weight and milk production. In both young and adult animals, there is drop in haemoglobin concentration, packed cell volume, TSP (Total Serum Protein) and serum albumin. In later stage, there is oedema associated with hypoproteinemia. Amino acid composition of dietary protein for ruminants is not critical because the rumen flora synthesizes necessary amino acids from lower quality protein and non-protein sources of nitrogen.

Clinical Symptoms

Protein malnutrition in beef cattle occurs most commonly in late gestation showing the symptoms of weakness, recumbency, marked loss of body weight and desire to live in normal mental attitude. Protein malnutrition is less common in dairy cattle as they are usually fed to meet the requirement of maintenance and milk production. In calf, diarrhoea may occur concurrently that is confused with diarrhoea due to enteropathogenic virus. Affected calves recover quickly when fed with whole milk of cow. Protein malnutrition also occurs in sheep, but is less commonly in goats.

Treatment and Prevention

Marginal deficiency of protein may be detected by the metabolic profile test. Specific treatment of protein malnutrition in livestock is usually not undertaken because of cost and prolonged recovery period.

Parenteral and oral fluid (electrolyte) therapy can be given. Provision of high-quality feed appropriate to the species is recommended. Prevention requires provision of nutrients requirement of the animal according to age, stage of pregnancy and production, and cost of feed.

Body condition and scoring of cattle and sheep can be used as a guide to monitor body condition and nutritional status. Regular analysis of feed supplies will assist in the overall nutritional management programme.

Diseases Caused by the Deficiency of Mineral Nutrient

Magnesium Deficiency

Magnesium deficiency causes lactation tetany in cows and hypomagnesemic tetany in calves. There are complicating factors that may affect absorption and metabolism of the element in both diseases. Mg is an essential constituent in ration for recently weaned pig. Experimentally induced deficiency causes weakness of pastern joint especially in forelegs causing backward boozing of the legs, sickled hock, approximation of knees and hocks, arching of back, hyperirritability, tremor, reluctant to stand, continued shifting of weight from limb to limb and eventually tetany leading to death. The disease cause reduction in growth rate, feed consumption and conversion, and decreased serum level of Mg.

Cobalt Deficiency

In ruminants, cobalt is required for synthesis of Vitamin B12. Cobalt deficiency is characterized clinically by in appetence and loss of body weight. In sheep, there is affection of reproductive performance. The deficiency of cobalt in diet results in deficiency of vitamin B12. Cattle and sheep are similarly affected and the signs are similar in both the species. Cattle are less susceptible than sheep and lamb and calves are more susceptible than adults. Horses appear to be unaffected.

Clinical Sign

Gradual decrease in appetite is followed by loss of body weight, emaciation and weakness. Pica is likely to occur especially in cattle. There is marked pallor of mucosa. Growth, lactation, and wool production are severely retarded, and wool may be tender or broken. Severe lacrimation and profuse out pouring of fluid sufficient to wet the wool of face is one of the most important signs in advance case. Death occurs in 8-12 months after the first appearance of the illness although severe wasting may be precipitated by stress of parturition or abortion. Cobalt deficiency in pregnant ewes can result in reduced lambing percent, increased still birth and increased neonatal mortality

Lambs from cobalt deficient ewes are slower to start suckling, have decreased serum, vitamin B12 and reduced concentration of serum colostral immunoglobulin. The disease has been associated with greyish colour of liver in sheep and clinically, it is manifested by photosensitization in acute cases and anaemia and emaciation in chronic cases.

Management and Control

Affected animals respond satisfactorily to oral dosing with cobalt or intramuscular injection of vitamin B12. Oral dosing of vitamin B12 is also effective but much larger dose is required. Treatment of ovine white liver disease is accomplished by administration of hydroxy-cobalamin that gives immediate beneficial response, and treatment is repeated again after 10 days.

Calves reared in the cobalt deficient pasture require cobalt or vitamin B12 supplementation prior to weaning. Cobalt deficiency in grazing animals is prevented most easily by top dressing of affected pasture with cobalt salt.

Affected animal should be treated orally or parenterally with vitamin B12 to obtain a quick response.

Copper Deficiency

Copper deficiency may be primary due to inadequate intake in diet or secondary because of impaired utilization of copper by the tissues even when dietary intake is sufficient.

In secondary copper deficiency, the amount of Cu in diet is adequate but dietary factors interfere in utilization of Cu. The conditioning factor is known only in some instances but the dietary excess of molybdenum (Mo) is one of the most common causes. A high Mo intake can induce Cu deficiency even when Cu content of pasture is quite high and a higher Cu intake can overcome the effect of molybdenum.

Sheep are more susceptible to Cu poisoning and cattle are prone to excess of Mo. Zn, Pb, Fe & $CaCo_3$ also act as conditioning factors. The administration of Se to sheep on Cu deficient pasture increases Cu absorption and improves the growth rate in lambs.

The use of $ZnSO_4$ for the control of facial eczema may cause a depression of plasma Cu level which could be alleviated by injection of Cu-glycinate. Dietary inorganic sulphate in combination with Mo has a profound effect in uptake of Cu by ruminant. The disease caused by a primary deficiency of Cu in ruminants is known as enzootic ataxia of sheep and licking sickness in cattle.

In pigs, Cu deficiency may cause anemia in suckling piglets and reduced growth rate and a cardiac disease in grazing pigs.

Adult horses are unaffected but foals reared in Cu deficient areas may suffer from abnormality of limbs and joints.

Osteochondrosis is caused by Cu deficiency in young farm rreared deer. Both the primary and secondary Cu deficiency occurs most commonly during spring and summer season coinciding with the lowest level of Cu in the pasture.

Pathogenesis

a) Effect on tissue

Copper is necessary in tissue oxidation process as it is a component of cytochrome oxidase systems. Ceruloplasmin is a copper containing enzyme through which Cu exerts its physiological function resulting in changes of wool quality in sheep.

b) Effect on body weight

In advanced stages of copper deficiency, the impairment of tissue oxidation causes interference with intermediary metabolism and loss of condition or failure to grow.

c) Diarrhoea

Pathogenesis of copper deficiency induced diarrhoea is uncertain. There is little evidence that a naturally occurring primary copper deficiency will cause diarrhoea. Diarrhoea is usually a major clinical finding in secondary Cu deficiency associated with molybdenosis.

d) Anemia

The known importance of Cu in the formation of haemoglobin accounts for anemia in Cu deficiency. The presence of hemosiderin deposit in tissue of Cu deficient animal suggest that Cu is necessary for re-utilization of Fe liberated from normal breakdown of haemoglobin. Anaemia may occur in later stage of primary Cu deficiency but is not remarkable in secondary form unless there is a marginal Cu deficiency.

e) Bone

Osteoporosis that occurs in some natural cases of Cu deficiency is caused by depression of osteoblastic activity.

f) Connective tissue

Cu is a component of enzyme lysine oxidase secreted by cells involved in synthesis of elastic component of connective tissue, and has important. function in maintaining integrity of tissue.

g) Heart

Myocardial degeneration of falling disease may be a terminal manifestation of anaemic anoxia or due to interference with tissue oxidation. Experimentally produced Cu deficiency also causes sudden death. Lesions of pancreas may be present in normal cattle with low blood copper status.

h) Nervous tissue

Copper deficiency interferes with the formation of myelin and causes demyelination in lambs.

I) Reproductive performance

There is no evidence of Cu deficiency causing reproductive failure in diary cows. The presence of Mo rather than low Cu level may affect reproductive performances in cattle

j) Immune system

Copper deficiency results in decreased humoral or cell-mediated immunity. as well as, decrease in non specific immunity regulated by phagocytic cells, macrophage and neutrophil.

Clinical Signs

In cattle, primary Cu deficiency causes unthriftiness, loss of milk production and anaemia in adult cattle. Coat colour is also affected, where red and black hair coat cattles changes to peached rusty red with rough and staring hair coat.

In severe deficient condition, calves grow slowly, and fractures of bone particularly of scapula and limb bones, readily occurs. Ataxia may occur after exercise with a sudden loss of control of the hind limb and the animal falls down or assumes a sitting posture, however, normal control resumes after rest.

Itching and hair licking are also recorded in cattle. There may be increased occurrence of post parturient haemoglobinuria due to Cu deficiency. Secondary

Cu deficiency syndrome include signs of primary Cu deficiency except that, anaemia occurs less commonly and diarrhoea is more common.

Falling Disease

It is an enzootic disease of cattle characterized by behaviour of bellowing and falling down. Death is instantaneous in most cases but some fall and struggle on their sickles for a few minutes with intermittent bellowing, running movement and falling down with attempt to rise. Rare cases show signs up to 24 hours or more followed by death.

Peat scour (Tearts)

The passage of watery yellow, cream to black colour faeces with an offensive odour occur soon after cattle grow on affected pasture or after 8-10 days. Faeces are released without effort or without lifting the tail. Severe debility is common although appetite is normal. Hair coat is rough and de pigmentation is manifested by reddening around eyes, particularly in black cattle. Affected animal usually recover in a few days following treatment with copper.

Unthriftiness (Pine) in Calves

Earliest signs are stiffness of gait and unthriftines, Epiphysis or distal end of metacarpus and metatarsus may be enlarged resembling Ca, P and Vit-D deficiency syndrome. Epiphysis is painful on palptation and some calves are severely lame, unthriftiness and emaciation are progressive and death may occur in 4 to 5 months. Greyness of hair especially around the eyes in black cattle is apparent; diarrhea may also occur in few cases.

Sheep

In primary copper deficiency, first observed sign is the abnormality of wool. Fine wool become limp, glossy and loose alongwith its crimp developing a straight appearance. Black wool shows de pigmentation to grey or white, that is why Merino sheeps appear to have more Cu requirement than mutton sheep. In extreme deficiency condition, there is anemia, scouring, unthriftiness and infertility. Enzootic ataxia is the major manifestation in sheep, Retardation of growth and diarrhoea, delay from marketing time and increased mortality is common.

Clinical Findings in Lamb

Osteoporosis with increased tendency of long bones to fracture is seen in lambs.

Sway Back & Enzootic Ataxia in Lambs & Kids

Sway back is the only authentic manifestation of primary nutritional deficiency of Cu in sheep. This disease occurs in several forms. Congenital form that is cerebrospinal sway back occurs only when Cu deficiency is extreme. Affected lambs are born dead or weak and unable to stand and are suck. In coordination and erratic movement are more evident than in enzootic ataxia and there is spastic paralysis, blindness that occurs occasionally.

There is softening and cavitation of cerebrum, white matter which probably commences about 120 days of gestation. Progressive (delayed) spinal sway back begins to develop some weeks after live birth with lesions and clinical signs appearing at 3-6 weeks of age. Postnatal acute fatal sway back may be a 3rd form of disease which develops suddenly. There is sudden onset of recumbency with death occurring 1-2 days later due to acute swelling of cerebellum.

Enzootic Ataxia

It affects only unweaned lamb in severe outbreak Lambs may be affected at birth but most cases occurs at 1-2 months age group. The severity of paresis (for some time never affected) decreases with increase in age of onset. Lambs after birth usually die within 3-4 days. The disease in older lamb may last for 3-4 weeks and survival is more likely although surviving lambs always show some ataxia and atrophy of hind quarter. There is incoordination of hind limb, respiratory and cardiac rate are gradually accelerated by exhaustion. There is excessive flexion of joint, knuckling of fetlock, wobbling of hind quarter and finally falling. Hind legs are affected first and lamb may be able to drag itself on sitting posture. Recumbency persists with involvement of four legs and lamb dies due to inanition. The lambs able to kick vigorously even in recumbent stage and appetite remains unaffected. Enzootic ataxia due to Cu deficiency has been reported in young goat kids. The disease is similar to that of lamb. Cerebellar hypoplasia is a common finding of goat.

Naturally occurring enzootic ataxia has occurred in growing pig at 4-6 month of age with symptoms of posterior paresis. Adult horses are unaffected by Cu deficiency but foals are affected with limb abnormality.

Treatment

Oral dosing with 4g of Cu SO4 for calf from 2-6 months of age and 8-10 gm for mature cattle at weekly internal for 3-5 weeks is recommended. Parenteral injection of Cu glycinate may also be given @ 120 mg for adults and 60 mg for calves. In sheep, oral dosing of Cu SO4 @ 1gm weekly is adequate. Lambs can be protected after birth by dosing with 35 mg of $CuSO_4$ every 2 week.

Iodine Deficiency

Iodine deficiency may be due to deficient iodine intake or secondarily by a high intake of calcium, diets consisting largely with brassica species, gross bacterial population of feed stuff or drinking water or continuous intake of low level of cyanogenetic glycoside. This deficiency in commonly associated with a high incidence of goitrous offsprings.

Linamarin, a glycoside in linseed meal produces goitre in newborn lamb borne from ewes fed with the lin seed meal during pregnancy.

Rapeseed and rape meal is also goitrogenic. The most common cause of iodine deficiency in farm animal is failure to provide iodine in diet. Congenital goitre has also been observed in foals.

Pathogenesis

Iodine deficiency results in decrease production of thyroxin and stimulation of secretion of thyrotropic hormone by pituitary gland which commonly results in hyperplasia of thyroid tissue and considerable enlargement of gland. Most case of goitre of newborn occurs due to iodine deficiency in diet. Primary deficiency of thyroxin is responsible for severe weakness & hair abnormality of new born. Colloid goitre is less common in animals. Some pasture and fodder plant including white clover, rapeseed, kale etc. are known to have cyanogenetic glycoside. These goitrogenic substances may appear in milk producing a toxic hazard to both animals & humans. Inherited form of goiter in cattle occurs due to increase activity of an enzyme (codtyrosine deiodinase) which inhibit formation of thyroxine. There is evidence of foetal hypothyroidism, characterized by absence of wool growth, delayed skeletal maturation, and delayed parturition in sheep.

Clinical Signs

Loss of condition, decreased milk production and weakness, loss of libido in case of wound, oestrous failure in cows and a high incidence of aborted still birth are seen in animals. Weak calf is a manifestation of hypothyroidism in cattle where as prolonged gestation is reported in mares, cows, & ewes. High incidence of still birth in new born animals is more common clinical findings due to iodine deficiency. Partial or complete alopecia and enlargement of thyroid gland are other signs with varying frequency in different species. Affected foals have abnormal hair coat & a little thyroid enlargement. In most cases, they are unable to stand without support and unable to suck. Defective ossification, deformity of hock and thyroid enlargement has also been observed. In cattle, enlargement of thyroid is much lesser occurring than horses along with alopecia.

In pigs, characteristic findings are birth of hairless, still born, or weak piglets with edema of skin in neck region, less marked thyroid enlargement, poor growth and weakness of limbs.

Adult sheep in iodine deficiency areas may show a high incidence of thyroid enlargement, poor growth and weakness of limbs.

New borne lambs show weakness, alopecia, & thyroid enlargement. Goat kids are more prone to goiter and are alopecic.

Treatment and Control

Treatment of neonates with obvious clinical signs of iodine deficiency is usually not undertaken because of high CFR. When outbreaks of Iodine deficiency occur in neonates, emphasis is usually on providing additional Iodine therapy to pregnant animal. Recommendation for control can be adopted for the treatment of affected animal. Recommended dietary intake of cattle -0.8-10 mg/kg of feed for lactating and pregnant cows and 0.1-0.3 mg/kg for non pregnant cows.

Iron Deficiency

Iron deficiency is usually primary and most likely to occur in new born animals whose source of Fe is milk of dam. Milk is a poor source of iron (Fe). Deposits of Fe in liver of newborn are insufficient particularly low in piglets to maintain normal haemopoesis for > 2-3 weeks.

Fe deficiency states are not common in farm animals except in the very young that are confined to a milk diet. Fe deficiency anemia occurs in nourishing piglets due to following reasons.

i. They don't have access to soil which is the main source of Fe for young farm animals
ii. They grow rapidly and requirement of Fe is high.
iii. Milk is a poor source of Fe.

Administration of *Fe-Dextran* to piglets at a few days of age is preventive and a routine health management practice in swine industry.

Clinical disease occurs usually in 3-6-week-old piglets not supplemented with iron showing piglet anaemia. Under modern swine production system, piglets don't have access to sufficient dietary Fe until they are weaned to a dry diet containing supplemental Fe. Thus, parenteral Fe Dextran should be provided at a few days of age. Fe deficiency anaemia occurs in nourishing lambs that are housed and don't have access to soil, don't consume much feed other than their dam's milk for 7-10 days of life. The parenteral administration of Fe Dextran at 24 hours of age prevents anemia. Continued blood loss by hemorrhage in any animal may result in sub clinical anemia and Fe deficiency.

Cattle heavily infested with sucking lice and other external parasites may develop serious and even fatal anemia. Chronic form is characterized by a non-regenerative anemia with sub normal serum Fe level. Treatment with Fe is necessary for an optimal response.

Horses carrying heavy burden of blood sucking Strongyloid worm often have sub normal haemoglobin levels. Subclinical Fe deficiency anemia also occurs in new born calves and kids. Calcium carbonate ($CaCo_3$) added to the diet of weaned and finishing pigs may cause Fe deficiency leading to moderate anemia but this is not apparent in mature pig. Manganese may exert a similar antagonist effect causing iron deficiency.

Clinical Findings

The highest incidence of Fe deficiency anemia in piglets occurs at about 3 weeks of age but it can occur up to 10th week of age. Affected piglets may be well grown and in good condition but growth rate of anaemic piglets are significantly lower. A mild diarrhoea may occur but faeces are usually normal in form. Dyspnoea, lethargy and marked increase in amplitude of heart beat can be felt after exercise. The skin and mucosa are pale and may appear yellow especially in white pigs. Oedema of head and fore quarters gives the animal a fatty appearance. A lean and a white hairy look is more common. Death usually occurs suddenly. Affected animal may survive in a thin, unthrifty condition. A high incidence of infectious disease especially enteric infection with *E. coli* is associated with anemia. Streptococcal pericarditis is a well recognized complication. A high incidence of still birth is recorded in litter of sows suffering from Fe deficiency anemia.

Treatment and Control

In severe Fe deficiency, treatment is usually parenteral and consists of Fe organic preparations, Fe Dextran, Fe Serbitol, citric acid complex, Fe-saccharate or gluconate, Vit-B12 therapy, both parenteral and oral folic acid or choline orally. Preventive measures should be directed to neonatal piglets because treatment of sows before or after farrowing is generally ineffective. However, feeding of Fe preparation at least 2 week before farrowing helps to prevent piglet anaemia, Fe should be provided @ 15mg/day until wearing in case of indoor housing rearing system. These methods are satisfactory but results are not usually as good as when the piglets are raised outdoor.

Sodium Chloride Deficiency

A dietary deficiency of NaCl is likely to occur:

i. In rapidly growing young animals fed on low Na and cereal based diet.

ii. Under very hot environmental condition where more loss of water and Na occurs through sweating and animals are fed on grass forage and seeds may be low in sodium.

iii. In animals engaged in heavy or intense physical work and allowed to graze pastures on sandy soils heavily fertilized with potash which depresses forage sodium level.

Normally occurring salt deficiency causing illness in grazing animal is uncommon except under certain circumstances. After a period of 10 to 12 month, there is considerable deterioration of animals health, anorexia, haggard appearance, lustreless eyes, rough hair coat and a rapid loss of body weight. High yielding animals are more severely affected and some may collapse and die. Oral administration of NaCl is both preventive and gives rapid cure. In dairy cattle with sodium deficient diet, there is poly uria, salt hunger, pica, including licking dart and other animal's body coat, drinking urine, loss of apetite, body weight and drastic fall in milk production. Urination is frequent with low specific gravity, Urine concentration of NaCl decreases and K increases. Experimental restriction of Cl^- in diet of dairy cows in early lactation results in a depraved appetite, lethargy, reduced feed intake and milk production, scanty faeces, gradual emaciation and severe hypochloremic and secondary hypokalemic metabolic alkalosis.

Diagnosis of salt deficiency is dependent on clinical findings, analysis of feed and water supply, serum level of sodium in saliva, urine and faeces of deficient animals. Experimentally induced Na deficiency in young pigs causes anorexia, decrease water intake and decrease weight gain. Provision of salt in diet at level of 0.5% is considered to be fully adequate for all farm animal species.

Zinc Deficiency

A primary zinc deficiency due to low dietary Zn is rare in ruminants. The risk of Zn deficiency increases when soil pH rises above 6.5 and fertilization with nitrogen and phosphorous increases. Several factors may also affect availability of Zn in ruminants causing a secondary Zn deficiency which include the consumption of immature grass affecting digestibility, feeding of late-cut hay with poor digestibility and presence of excessive dietary sodium.

The contamination of silage with soil during harvesting can also affect the digestibility of Zn. Zn deficiency in young swine can cause parakeratosis which may not be due to a simple zinc deficiency. The availability of Zn in diet is adversely affected by presence of phytic acid, a constituent of plant protein such as soya bean meal.

Use of meat meal in diet will prevent disease, due to high availability of Zn. An excess of dietary calcium can favour the development of parakeratosis in swine but addition of higher level of Zn to such diet can prevent the occurrence of disease.

The level of copper in diet may also bear some significance. Increase of Cu decreases the requirement of zinc. A concurrent enteric infection in diarrhea exacerbates the damage done by Zn deficiency especially in pigs.

Parakeratosis in swine occurs most commonly during the period of rapid growth, after weaning between 7-10 weeks of age. Zn deficiency also occurs naturally in cattle, sheep, goat which respond quickly by supplementation of Zn in diet.

Clinical Symptoms

In pigs, rate and efficiency of body weight gain decreases, circumscribed areas of erythema of skin on ventral abdomen and inside thigh region are seen. Papules develop in the area, which are covered with scales followed by thick crusts, fissures and cracks, rusts that are easily detached from skin. There is little scratching and rubbing. Diarrhoea of moderate degree is common.

Secondary subcutaneous abscess occurs frequently but in uncomplicated cases, the skin lesions disappear spontaneously in 10-45 days. In naturally occurring severe diseases in cattle, case parakeratosis and alopecia may affect 40% of skin area which are more marked on muzzle, vulva, anus, tail head, ears, back of hind legs, flank and neck region. Most animals are below average body condition and are stunted in growth. After treatment with Zn improvement is apparent in 1st week, and complete recovery is seen in 3week.

Natural disease in sheep is characterized by loss of wool and development of thick and wrinkle skin. Wool-eating is also seen in sheep and may be one of the earliest signs noticed in lambs after fed on Zn deficient diet for 4 weeks.

Zn deficient lambs exhibit decreased growth rate, salivation, swollen hocks, wrinkled skin and open skin lesions around the hoof and eyes. Clinical symptoms observed in goat are similar to that of lambs. Zn responsive dermatitis must be differentiated from sarcoptic mange and exudative epidermatitis. Sarcoptic mange is accompined by more itching and rubbing and parasites are found in skin scarping. Exudative dermatitis is similar in appreance but occurs mainly in unweaned pigs. Lesions have a greasy character, grears which is quite different from dry, crumbly lesions of parakeratosis and the mortality rate is higher in excudative dermatitis than Zn deficiency.

Treatment

In outbreak of parakeratosis in swine, Zn should be added to diet @ 50mg/kg body weight. The Ca level of animal should be maintained between 0.65% -0.75%. The parenteral injection of Zn @ 2-4 mg /kg body weight daily for 10 days is also effective. Oral administration of $ZnSO_4$ @ 250 mg daily for 04 week results in a clinical cure of Zn deficiency in goats in 12-14 weeks.

Manganese Deficiency

A dietary deficiency of manganese causes infertility and skeletal deformity both congenitally and after birth. Primary deficiency of manganese occurs endemically in some areas due to geological deficiency in the local rock formation. An excess of Ca and P in the diet is known to increase the requirement of Mn of calves, and is considered to decrease the availability of dietary Mn in cattle generally.

Congenital chondrodystrophy in calves is associated with Mn deficiency & an outbreak of congenital skeletal defects in Holstein calves due to Mn deficiency has been reported.

Clinical Signs

In cattle, manganese deficiency is associated with infertility, poor growth, dry hair coat and loss of coat color. A severe congenital dystrophy has been reported in calves where limbs are shortened and joints enlarged. Pregnant cows fed on apple pulp and corn silage show Mn deficiency. A Mn responsive infertility has been reported in ewes and cows. Bones of affected lamb is shorter and weaker and there are signs of joint pain.

Diet low in Mn causes reduction in skeletal growth, muscle weakness, obesity, irregular, diminished or absence of estrous, agalactia and still born piglets. Leg weakness, bowing of front leg and shortening of bone also occurs in piglets.

Treatment and Control

Fertility improve in young cattle supplemented with 2g $MnSO_4$ daily. Although feeding of 015g of $MnSO_4$ daily is reported to cause no signs of toxicity. Mn is known to interfere with utilization of Co & Zn in ruminants. Very large level of intake in calves can decrease growth rate and haemoglobin level. Recommended procedure is to feed Mn for 9 weeks commencing from 3 week before service. Recommended dietary intake in pigs is 24-57 mg/4-5 kg.

Selenium Deficiency

Selenium acts as antioxidant which helps in defense mechanism of body and protects from eroxidation of tissue, Vitamin-E, Se, and sulphur containing amino acids combinely protect the tissue from oxidative damage. The following clinical disorders may develop due to selenium deficiency.

1. Nutritional muscular dystrophy

This condition is also called as white muscle disease, stiff lamb disease or nutritional myopathy. There are non-inflammatory, degenerative or necrotic changes in cardiac and skeletal muscle. White areas of muscle show Zenker's degeneration. Affected animals decline to move or move with stiffy gait and arched back condition leading to recumbency and starvation.

2. Hepatosis

Commonly noticed in pigs due to deficiency of selenium and Vitamin E. There is muscular dystrophy, heart disorder & hepatosis. There is extensive necrotic changes of liver and a yellowish brown color of body which is called as mulberry heart disease yellow fat disease.

3. Reproductive defects

Selenium deficiency causes reproductive failure leading to infertility. Se deficient dairy cow shows retention of placenta of following parturition.

Treatment

Selenium along with α-tocopherol should be given parenterally.

Calcium Deficiency

Calcium defeciency may be primary or secondary. But, in both conditions, the end result is an osteodystrophy depending largely on species and age of animal affected. Primary deficiency due to lack of calcium in diet is uncommon. A secondary deficiency with marginal Ca intake is aggravated by a high "P" intake. Calcium deficiency is a sporadic disease occurring in a particular group of animal rather than in a geographically limited area. Although death doesn't occur usually, these is considerable loss of function and disability lesions of bone and joints.

Clinical Symptoms

Clinical findings are less marked in adults than in young ones. There is decrease rate or cessation of growth and dental mal development. The later is characterized by deformity of gums, poor development of incisors, failure of permanent teeth to erupt for periods up to 27 months and abnormal wearing of permanent teeth due to defective development of dentine and enamel. Inappetance, stiffness, tendency of bones to fracture, disinclination to stand, difficulty in parturition, loss of body condition and decreased fertility are all non-specific clinical signs recorded in adult animal in primary calcium deficiency. Rickets, osteomalacia, osteodystrophy, fibrosa espeially in horse and pig and degenerative arthropathy in cattle are common syndrome in secondary Ca deficiency. In sheep, rickets are seldom recognized but there's marked dental abnormalities.

Diagnosis

Diagnosis depends upon the proof that diet is absolutely or relatively insufficient in Ca that the lesions and signs observed are characteristic and the provision of calcium in the diet alleviates the condition. The close similarity between dental defects in severe calcium deficiency espacially in sheep, and those occurring in chronic fluorosis may necessitate quantitative estimate of fluoride in on teeth or bone to determine the cause.

Treatment

Response to treatment is rapid. Parenteral injection of calcium salt (Calborol) – LA, Ca Sandoz – SA- 10ml is advisable, if tetany is present. When animals are exposed to dietary depletion of Co, P over a period of time, it's necessary to supplement the diet with Ca & P during dietary mineral repletion.

Phosphorous Deficiency

Phosphorous Deficiency is usually primary and is characterized by pica (intake of unusual things), poor growth, infertility and in later stage, osteodystrophy, Hypophosphatemia in dairy cattle, is associated with increased fragility of RBC and post-parturient hemoglobinuria. "P" deficiency is usually primary in field condition exaggerated by a deficiency of Vitamin D and possibly, by excess of calcium. Primary deficiency of "P" in diet of cattle within the first several weeks of lactation can result in post-parturient hemoglobinuria. Deficiency is most common in animal at pasture during draught season but can also be a serious problem in housed cattle fed on only hays. Sheep & horses at pasture are much less susceptible to osteodystrophy due to phosphorous deficiency than cattle and their failure to thrive on "P" deficiency pasture is probably due to low protein content of pasture. Primary deficiency can occur in swine kept in confinement and not provided with sufficient dietary phosphorous. Lactating sows are more commonly affected than growing pigs.

Clinical Symptoms

Primary P deficiency is common only in cattle. Young animals grow slowly and adults develop rickets. Initial sub-clinical stage is followed by osteomalacia in cattle of all age. A reduction in voluntary intake of feed is the first the effect of P deficiency. Retarted growth, decreased milk and decreased fertility are earliest signs of P deficiency. Infertility is accompanied by anestrous, subestrous, and irregular estrous, and delayed sexual maturity. Development of wearing on teeth are not greatly affected except malocclusion may result from poor mineralization resulting in weakness of mandible.

Clinical Signs

Clinical signs including general unthriftiness, marked body weight loss, decreased feed consumption, reluctance to move, fracture of bone and impaired reproduction. Detectable signs of P deficiency develops in following sequence such as loss of body weight and condition, decreased whole blood "P" level associated with increased calcium level, allotriophagia, abnormal structure, locomotion and recumbency.

Treatment

In cases of urgent need of phosphours as in post-partuent hemoglobin uria and parturient paresis complications intravenous administration of Na-acid phosphate (60 gm in 300ml distilled water) is recommended. In mild deficiency cases, parenteral preparation (Tonophosphan) is given intramuscularly along with oral mineral mixture with feed.

Potassium Deficiency

Potassium deficiency is thought to be rare in animals. However, calves fed on roughage grown on soil deficient in K^+ may show a clinical syndrome of poor growth, anemia and diarrhoea. Supplementation of diet with calcium salt appears to be curative in pigs, some symptoms like poor apetite, emaciation, rough hair coat, and marked cardiac impairment due to degeneration of purkinje fibres of myocardium are noticed. Similar changes of cardiac function are observed in diet deficient with Mg or Vit-E. Hypokalemia in cattle may occur secondary to anorexia, diarrhoea, upper gastrointestinal obstruction. and right side displacement, torsion and impaction of abomasum. In most cases, hypokalemia is not severe enough to cause weakness and recumbency. Hypokalemia resulting in severe weakness and recumbency has occurred in diary cattle treated with isoflupredone acetate for ketosis.

Treatment included intravenous and oral administration of KCl and fluid therapy but response is poor and most affected cattle succumb to death. In

K^+ deficiency, potchlor syrup should be given to small animals and mineral mixture containing K^+ salt is added in feeds of large animals.

Vitamin A Deficiency

It's an essential nutrient required for number of vital functions in humans as well as animals. Signs of this vitamin deficiency are well marked in new born calves, lamb and piglets characterized by under developed skin coat and abnormalities of eye. Signs in patients include anorexia, wt. loss, increased keratinization, decreased salivations from mucous, secretory glands, nervous disorder, reproductive inefficiency, impairment of vision, reduced resistance to infection and finally death.

Clinical Signs

a) Vitamin A is essential for growth of tissues which is related to weight gain in animals. Vit-A deficienct diet causes poor apetite, and emaciation in growing animals.

b) There is impairment in vision that causes corneal xerosis, Biot's spot, conjuctival xerosis, corneal ulceration, keratomalacia, night blindness, xeropthalmia etc.

c) Compression of brain due to deficiency of vitamin A leads to, encephalopathy especially in calf due to increased intracranial pressure & such calf shows convulsive seizures.

d) Neurological disorder: Hypovitaminosis –A may cause neurological disturbances in growing animals characterized by the weakness of limbs in coordination, paralysis of skeletal muscle, facial paralysis and rotation of head.

e) Congenital: Hypovitaminosis – A may bring about certain changes in the fetus.

f) Bone development: Vit-A is essential for normal development of bones. Deficiency may decrease the osteoblastic action during growth stage bone formation.

g) Mucous epithelial cells: Configuration and integrity of epithelial tissue are maintained by vitamin A. Its deficiency leads to poor functioning of epithelial cells.

h) Development of skin: There's thickening and keratinization of skin. Skin becomes dry with bran like deposit due to vitamin A deficiency.

i) Alimentary tract: There are degenerative changes of intestinal epithelium and secretory glands, making animal very much prone to enteritis.

j) Respiratory tract: There is degenerative changes and stratification of epithelium and animal is susceptible to respiratory tract infection.

k) Urinary system: There is degeneration and cornification of epithelial cells that favors the formation of urinary stones. Low vit-A and high Ca diet exacerbates the formation of carbonate on phosphate calculi in urinary blader and kidney.

l) Reproduction: There is degenerative changes of testes and ovary leading to impairment of spermatogenesis and oogenesis, respectively Retention of foetal membrane & abortion are also noticed in vitamin A deficiency.

Treatment: Vit-A @ 400IU/kg is administered orally or parenterally.

Vitamin – D Deficiency

It is usually caused by insufficient UV-solar radiation with showing clinical symptoms of poor appetite and growth in early stages and osteodystrophy in later stages. Vit-D deficiency is uncommon because the diets are supplemented with Vit-D by the manufacturer. More animals suffer in countries with relatively lack of U.V radiation especially during winter months and in animals raised indoors for a long period. Grazing animals especially during winter on lush pasture, including cereal crops leads to a high incidence of rickets especially in young and growing animals. There are variety of Vit-D of which D2 is called as Ergosterol and D3 as cholecalciferol.

Vit-D2 is converted to Vit-D3 under the influence of UV sunlight. Epidermal cells of skin in animal contain large quantity of pro vitamin D which is formed in the gut from cholesterol and is converted to D3 through exposure of skin to sunlight. Vit-D2 and D3 are equally effective in most animal but in poultry, D3 is more effective. Vit-D helps in the absorption of calcium from gut and helps in proper growth of bones.

Clinical Symptoms

Most important effect of vitamin-D deficiency in farm animal is decreased productivity, appetite and efficiency of food utilization, poor weight gain in growing stocks and poor productivity in adults. In late stage, there is lameness, noticed in forelegs, bending of long bones in young animals and joint enlargement. Clinical rickets may occur simultaneously in later stage with cases of osteomalacia in adults. An adequate intake of Vit-D appears to be necessary for maintenance of fertility in cattle especially with low phosphorus intake.

Treatment

Vitamin-D should be provided in diet along with parenteral injection of Vitamin-D. Affected animal should also receive adequate Ca and P in diet due to limited storage of Vit-D in the body of animal compared to storage of Vit-A. It's recommended that daily dietary supplement should be provided for optimum effect.

Vitamin –K Deficiency

Vit-K is adequately available in plants. Therefore, deficiency of this vitamin is rarely noticed in animals. This vitamin exists in three forms, K1, K2, K3 which is fat solubule and heat stable, and thus withstand cooking. Herbivore animals can synthesise this vitamin in their intestine through bacteria but prolonged use of antibiotics can retard the synthesis of vit-K due to decrease or destruction of beneficial bacteria.

Vitamin K helps in formation of prothrombin and bile salts, and play role in normal coagulation process. Due to deficiency, clotting of blood is seriously affected resulting in haemorrhages. Vit-K is normally used in cases of bleeding disorders. Bleeding from nose or other orifices can be controlled by use of vit-K. Haemorrhagic gastroenteritis especially in parvo virus infection can be controlled by the use of this vit K intravenous intravenously. Bleeding due to dicoumarol, warfarin and salicylate can be controlled by use of vit-K.

Vitamin – E Deficiency

There are 3 varieties of tocopherol i.e. α, ß, δ, out of which α-tocopherol is the most effective. Deficient signs include, sterility, fetal death, and muscular degeneration in young calf, and is characterized by weakness and stiffness followed by paralysis. Muscles of affected animal show white streak longitudinally. Death occurs due to cardiac arrest. Other deficiency clinical signs include retention of placenta, arthritis like symptoms in dog, mulberry like heart in pig and nutritional dystrophy in sheep.

Treatment

Vit-E and Se containing drugs should be administered parenterally or orally and tocopherol must be given with feeds.

19

Diseases of Neonates

The diseases that occur during the first one month of life are termed as diseases of neonates. During this period, the animal requires special attention to reduce mortality rate. The clinical examinations that are applied to adult animals are being used for the examination of newborns. Besides special attention should be given for congenital defects and thorough examination should be made to identify problems in liver, joints, cardiac valves and umbilicus. Neonates require special attention as the disease resistance power of newborns are comparatively poor and the animals are not sufficiently immunocompetent. Therefore, a hygienic environment and reduction of microbial load in the feed, milk and in the immediate environment reduces the mortality. It is generally recommended that, the newborn should be provided with milk from its mother or from the dam @ 10% of the body weight and colostrum should be fed within within 4 hours of birth to enhance specific immunity, thereby protecting the newborn from the diseases. During this period the villous pores are open and immunoglobulins can be directly taken into the body system and that poorly occurs 72 hours after parturition. So, feeding of colostrums enhance specific immunity and increases disease resistance. The specific immunity against the disease can be enhanced by vaccinating the dam and feeding colostrum from the vaccinated animals.

Perinatal diseases are classified into 5 groups

1. **Foetal diseases** occur during the intrauterine period, and includes prolonged gestation, congenital defects, abortion, resorption of foetus, mummification and goitre.
2. **Parturient diseases** occur during the process of parturition, and includes dystocia resulting in cerebral anoxia, injury to skeleton and soft tissues.
3. **Post-natal diseases** occur during 24 hours after birth, and include poor mothering, hypothermia, low vigour, navel infection, colibacillosis etc.
4. **Delayed post-natal diseases-** occur within 2-7 days after birth and the conditions include rejection by the mother, mammary incompetence, starvation, hypogammaglobulinemia, may be due to non-feeding of colostrums during first 72 hours of life, colibacillosis, lamb dysentery, foal septicemia.

5. **Late post-natal diseases** include white muscle disease, enterotoxaemia etc.

Diseases of newborn and the neonatal mortality are the major cause of economic loss in livestock sector. Neonatal mortality in cows ranges from 3-30% and averages 10% of the calves born. In well managed dairy herds, the mortality can be reduced up to 5%. Lamb mortality occurs in the first 3 days of life.

The mortality pattern in a particular herd depends on:-

i. Type of housing
ii. Density of rearing calves- generally overcrowding is a predisposing factor for higher calf mortality.
iii. Calving facility
iv. Attendance during calving
v. Weather condition- Cold and winter weathers increase the newborn mortality more particularly in piglets. The mortality is high due to development of hypothermia and poor mothering.

In piglets, the causes of neonatal mortality are more commonly non-infectious in origin and mostly depends on environmental and nutritional factors. Still birth accounts for 4-8% of the piglet death, of which 70-90% occurs due to intraparturient defects. Pre-weaning mortality ranges from 5-48% (average of 12-19%). Congenital defects in piglets are seen in around 5% of the piglets born. Provision of warm and comfortable environment and proper bedding during parturition can reduce neonatal death.

Special Investigation of Neonatal Diseases

In addition to routine practices adopted for diagnosis of disease in large animals, some special attentions should be provided in the following lines while investigating neonatal diseases.

- Attention / investigation should be made to determine the duration of pregnancy.
- Pre-colostral serum samples from the calves should be collected to establish intra-uterine foetal infection.
- Epidemiological investigation to ascertain the abnormalities in the population or in the age group affected.
- The environment in which the animals are kept and some tentative reasons from the owner of neonatal death.
- Postmortem examination of the available dead animals.
- Dispatch of foetal tissues and placenta for laboratory examination for

pathogens like *Brucella abortus, Leptospira pomona, Leptospira hardjo, E. coli, Salmonella* and Rota virus.

- Investigation should be done to examine the managemental practices such as feed supply, maternality of the dam, surveillance by the owner and outer environmental condition.

The congenital defects noticed in the newborn may or may not be inherited and all inherited defects may not be present at birth. Virus responsible for congenital defects include hog cholera virus, blue tongue virus, bovine virus diarrhoea virus and Akabane virus. Congenital defects due to nutritional deficiency include goitre (due to deficiency of iodine), enzootic ataxia (Copper deficiency), limb deformities in calves (due to Mn deficiency), neonatal rickets (due to deficiency of Vit-D), eye defects and hare lips (due to vitamin A deficiency). Some poisonous plants may induce congenital defects. Such plants include *Astragallus, Oxytropis, Veratrum californivum,* tobacco plants etc., Drugs showing congenital defects included parabendazole and cambendazole in sheep, administration of cortisone in early pregnancy, administration of estrogen and estradiol, bismuth, selenium, nitrogen mustard and sulfonamides. Severe exposure to β and γ radiation also results in congenital defects. The common pathogens responsible for neonatal infection include *E. coli, Salmonella, Clostridium perfringens type A, B, C, Cryptosporidium, Leptospira monocytogenes, Pasteurella* and *Streptococcus.* Non-specific infections may occur due to pathogens like *Corynebacterium pyogenes, Spherophorus necrophorus, Streptococcus faecalis, Streptococcus zooepidemicus, Micrococcus* etc.

The principle of control and prevention of neonatal diseases caused due to infectious agents are as follows

a. Removal of the cause of disease from the environment.
b. Removal of the newborn from the infectious environment.
c. Increasing and maintaining non-specific resistance (Innate immunity).
d. Increasing specific resistance or passive immunity through use of vaccines.

20

Common Poisonings

Animals contract poisoning due to a variety of toxic chemicals (inorganic and farm chemicals), phytotoxins, mycotoxins, and zootoxins, which is often fatal. Toxic chemicals and poisonous plants represent a tremendous economic impact. However, more often the poisoning episodes go undiagnosed. In general, poisoning is suspected when number of previously healthy animals show same symptoms and severity of illness at the same time and the same lesions at necropsy. Although infectious, metabolic and deficiency diseases also possess alike epidemiological profile, cases of poisoning are confirmed by information on immidate environment:

Clinical findings and laboratory specimens for diagnosis of environmental pollutants and chemical poisons

Pollutant	Clinical manifestations in animals	Specimen for laboratory testing
Fluoride (Fluorosis)	Stunted growth, exostosis of bones, lameness, dental mottling characterized by chalk like spots, patches or striations, bulging of gingiva, delayed eruption of permanent incisors.	Bone, teeth and urine
Lead (Plumbism)	Apathy and CNS disorders, staggering, respiratory distress, poor growth loss of appetite	Kidney, bone and blood
Arsenic	Involvement of cutaneous, pulmonary and nervous system. Long term exposure leads to carcinogenic growth in these system. Gastro enteritis, muscle tremors, incoordination etc.	Kidney, skin and hair
Mercury	Involvement of CNS, characterized with mental retardation, primitive reflexes, synergy, incoordination, ataxia, distured growth and deformity of skeletal system.	Kidney
Molybdenum	Weight loss, hair coat depigmentation, and anemia due to secondary hypocuprosis and persisteing debiliating, diarrhoea	Blood, urine
Cadmium	Involvement of renal and pulmonary systems. Weight loss, cough, dyspnea, emphysema and cadmium rhinitis, proteinuria, glucosuria and ostemalacia.	Kidney

Pollutant	Clinical manifestations in animals	Specimen for laboratory testing
Selenium	CNS involvement, emaciation, lameness, loss of hair.	Liver, kidneys, wool, hair
Copper	Emaciation, staggering, inappetance, apathy, icterus and haemoglobinura	Liver, kidney
Organophosphate	Salivation, diarrhoea tremor, pupillary contraception (Cattle), abdominal pain, diaarhoea, dyspnea and laryngeal paralysis (horses).	Blood, urine
Strychnine	Restlessness, tremors, stiff neck, intermittent tetanic convulsions	Blood, kidney, urine

Laboratory Examinations

Laboratory tests are often necessary to monitor the extent of hazardous effects and also to understand the pathogenesis of causative agent and underlying organ dysfunction associated with exposure. Exposure to toxic pollutants, particularly at low concentration does not necessarily lead to clinical illness and diagnosis of such cases depends heavily on interpretation of the biochemical findings which are regarded many a times as an early indicator of exposure. For an example, decreased activity of delta aminolevulinic acid in urine is an early indication of lead exposure. Similarly urinary activity of alkaline phosphatase and gammaglutamyl transferase are considered among the earliest and the most accurate indicators of nephrotoxicity caused by mercury. Diethyl phosphorothionate (DETP) estimation in urine is helpful in detecting organophosphate exposure. Besides hematobiochemical tests, other laboratory aids such as radiography and histopathological observations have also been used effectively in diagnosis of pollution exposures as in case of fluoride, cadmium, lead and mercury pollution.

Chemical Analysis

The final diagnosis and confirmation of causative pollutant are usually established by chemical analysis of correctly selected, preserved and transported specimens collected from animals and from the environment. Since laboratory procedure for chemical analysis are quite laborious and expensive, a careful selection of material and its proper preservation and transportation has great significance. Specimen for chemical analysis should invariably include materials suspected as the source of pollutants to the animals such as contaminated feed, water, pasture grass and vegetation, and also clinico pathological samples from the exposed animals. Blood, urine, hair and milk are easily available specimens for chemical analysis from live animals. Samples of gastro-intestinal tract particularly from rumen, and its contents should always be submitted for chemical analysis when animals are suspected to have died due to exposure to pollutants via oral route. Similarly, skin and lung specimens are required when exposure has occurred via skin and respiratory tract, respectively.

Assessment of Pollution Exposure

Diagnosis of health hazards of pollution should be concluded if exposure relationship is established. The history, clinical findings, and clinico-pathological observations determine the adverse effects on the health of exposed population. The presence of pollutants beyond critical levels in animal tissues and organs confirms the diagnosis. However, assessment of exposure is necessary to link the effect with environmental pollution. This process involves consideration of the probable source of pollutant and environmental measurements to determine the average and peak concentration of the pollutants in the environmental samples e.g. air, water, soil and vegetation/food. Exposure can often be assessed by measurement of pollutants in these samples, but it does not necessarily reflect to the intensity of effects, which may be influenced by the number of factors other than concentration of the pollutants in food, water, air or vegetation. Since a host of interacting pollutants are present in the environment in many instances, concomitant or co-exposure to such pollutants can modify the risks to health. The kind and type of compound of pollutant, amount of contaminated food ingested or air inhaled by the animals, amount of pollutant absorbed via respective routes, and concentration of the pollutant at the target organ and presence of interacting agents in host system can alter the magnitude of hazards.

Environmental Monitoring

Environmental monitoring is the most general method of qualitative assessment of exposure. It has been defined as the systemic collection of environmental samples for analysis of pollutant concentration. In general prior to undertaking an environmental monitoring program, it is important to have a complete information on what agents need to be investigated, what should be the frequency of sample collection, source (s) of sample to be drawn, quality of data required and which analytical techniques have to be applied. Both sampling methods and analytical procedures determine the quality of data, therefore it is essential to standardize the methods in a particular laboratory with available technology. A number of sampling instruments and analytical techniques have been developed in the recent years and one can adopt and standardize them as per own requirements.

Plant Poisoning

Plant toxicity is a major cause of poisoning, particularly in farm animals who thrive on pastures. There are more than 1500 species of poisonous plants world wide. The incidence of poisoning in animals due to all these species has not been established. In India list of common poisonous plant was compiled by Chopra *et al* (1969). A plant can be toxic to animals due to natural ingredient present in it or if the plants are contaminated by environmental toxicants. There are certain plant species that are not toxic under normal condition, but they become toxic if soil or water contains higher concentration of a toxicant. Further, certain plants may be toxic at a certain stage of their growth and some plants become toxic to animals due to production of toxic substance in rumen from innocuous substances in the plants. For example, lactic acid is produced by fermentation of starch present in grains and ammonia is produced during protein digestion. The main reason of plant poisoning is, however, due to presence of toxic principle (phytoxins) in plants. The occurrence of nitrate and nitrite and cyanide poisoning, which is commonly seen in India, is linked to the presence of toxic principles in plants.

Nitrate and Nitrite Poisoning

Nitrates and nitrites are generally dealt together as a cause of poisoning in animals. These are the major common causes of plant poisoning in Indian livestock. In fact, nitrate and nitrite poisonings are diagnosed with increasing frequency due to extensive use of nitrogenous fertilizers in cropping system. The nitrate is a precursor of nitrite, which is the main cause of toxic syndrome Nitrate, itself is capable of producing gastro-enteritis but its main effect is due to formation of nitrite from nitrite before or after ingestion. Ruminants are especially vulnerable to nitrate poisoning due to reducing capacity of ruminal microbes converting nitrate to nitrite.

Source of poisoning Nitrates in soil, surface and ground water are produced from natural microbial decomposition of nitrogenous material. The ammonium originating from decomposition are converted into nitrate and nitrite by environmental micro organisms. In the atmosphere, nitrates are found in higher concentration in the urban environment during photochemical oxidation. Plant accumulate nitrates mainly from soil and water. Spraying of forage with 2-4 D herbicide also contribute to toxic quantities of nitrates in sugar beet top. A nitrate concentration of $> 1.5\%$ in plant on dry matter basis is considered toxic to cattle. The most common plants accumulating nitrates arc cereals and root crops, particularly when grown in a heavily fertilized soil and when their growth is rapid during hot humid weather. This type of situation occurs more commonly after first spell of rain and particularly in shorghum (Bazra) and maize grown during summer months as fodder crop. The other plant species that accumulate nitrate are: *Brassica* spp. (Rapeseed, Turnips, mustard. etc.) oat. wheat, sudan grass and white clover.

Diagnosis

General principles for diagnosis of poisoning also applies to the diagnosis of phytotoxicities. Criteria used to establish diagnosis of poisoning are clinical evidence, pathological evidence, circumstantial evidence and chemical analysis.

Clinical Evidence

Nitrate and nitrite poisonings are difficult to diagnose clinically as other conditions such as hydrocyanic acid poisoning, acute bovine pulmonary edema and emphysema (ABPEE), anaphylaxis and cyanobacterial poisoning also produce similar signs. Salivation, Abdominal pain, diarrhoea, respiratory distress, blanching of visible mucosae, rapid weak pulse, and sub-normal temperature are the prominent signs in nitrate/ nitrite poisoning. Blood is dark red to brown in colour in acute nitrate/ nitrite poisoning. Blood is bright red in hydrocyanic acid poisoning. Lack of abnormal lungs sound and chocolate brown colouration of mucous membrane is the differentiating signs between nitrate/nitrite poisoning and ABPEE.

Necropsy Lesions

Dark red to brown coloured blood with poor clotting time and congested gastrointestinal mucosae are common findings in post mortem examination.

Circumstantial Evidence

Circumstantial evidence that should be considered for diagnosis of nitrate and nitrite poisoning is: existence of common sources, predisposing factors contributing to nitrate/nitrite poisoning in the surrounding environment. For example: Immature green oat, barley, wheat, sudan, grass, sorghum, application of excessive nitrogen-containing fertilizers, prolonged drought, industrial pollution, etc. Occurrence of disease in several animals immediately after grazing on new pasture, disease following ingestion of fodder grown after prolonged drought in the vicinity of nitrate releasing units are common circumstantial evidence.

Laboratory Tests for Confirming Diagnosis

Following materials should be sent for confirming diagnosis of nitrate/nitrite poisoning.

Aqueous humor (Frozen) – 1 ml – for nitrate/nitrite assay

Urine (frozen) – 1 ml for nitrate/nitrite assay

Blood in 4 ml phosphate buffer – 2ml – for methemoglobin estimation.

Blood smear – Thick air dried for diphenyl blue test

Ingesta in chloroform/formalin – (100g) or suspected fodder 100 g for nitrate/nitrate content.

Modified Diphenylamin blue test can be applied under field condition for crude estimation of nitrate/nitrite content in fodder/ingesta as detailed below:

Dissolve 0.5 g diphenylamine in 20 ml distilled water and make volume to 100 ml by adding H_2SO_4 (conc.). Place the reagent on the tissues of the inside of stem. Intense blue colour within 10 seconds indicates > 1% nitrate (Toxic dose 0.6-1% nitrate on DM basis).

Cyanide or Hydrocyanic Acid Poisoning

Ingestion of plants containing glycosides leads to outbreaks of hydrocyanic acid (HCN) poisoning in animals. Enzyme β-glycosidase is responsible for liberating HCN from glycosides. The enzyme is present in plant tissues and is also produced by ruminal microorganisms. In monogastric animals, acid medium of stomach inactivates this enzyme. Thus horses and pigs are least susceptible to HCN poisoning and cases occur more commonly in ruminants.

Nearly 120 plant species have been identified to contain enough cyanogenic glycosides Important of these present in India are – Acacia, sorghum, sudan grass, sugarcane linseed, etc. The consumption of large quantities of linseed cake or meal is also associated with HCN poisoning. The minimum lethal dose of HCN to induce poisoning is 2 mg/kg b.w.t. for cattle and sheep and plant material carrying 200 ppm HCN can cause toxicity. The predisposing factors include drought stunted pasture after rain, wilted frost bitten and herbicide sprayed fodder plants, young, lush immature sorghum, plant grown on low phosphorus and high nitrogen-soil, and excessive ingestion of cyanogenic plants by hungry, un-accustomed animals.

Diagnosis

Clinical Signs:

Sudden onset of acute poisoning characterized by dyspnea, tremors, recumbency, convulsion and death in ruminants immediately after grazing on cyanogenic plants suggest acute HCN poisoning Neonatal goitre, or arthrogry posis causing dystokia and cystitis, ataxia (Myelomalacia) are the important signs in chronic HCN poisoning.

Necropsy findings

Bright Red coloured blood in acute poisoning. Blood clots slowly, dark musculature, with bitter almond smell in rumen.

Circumstantial evidence:

Presence of source, predisposing factors as described above.

Laboratory tests for Confirmation:

Investigation in Case of Poisoning

Information on 4 aspects, viz. clinical, pathological, circumstantial and chemical analysis.

Although types of practical approaches to collect information may differ considerably in their time frame, investigations taken to establish a valid and final diagnosis of specific cause (s), source and effects of poisoning include circumstantial evidence, clinical and pathological findings, environmental quality assessment and laboratory analysis of suspected bio-samples. Sometimes as fifth aspect i.e. biological testing is also included to evaluate biological response to toxicants. These investigations are complementary to each other to establish the cause of poisoning.

Diagnosis of Pollution Episode and Chemical Toxicosis

Epidemiological Approaches

These are either *effect oriented* or *agent oriented.* Generally, an unusual distribution of disease or mortality pattern prompts to take up an effect oriented epidemiological investigation. Sometimes, agent oriented studies are taken up when it is thought that some qualitative changes in the environment have induced adverse effects.

The epidemiological studies aimed at investigation of role of environmental pollutants in a particular disease or condition are generally started with 'Exploratory' or 'Descriptive investigation', which are useful in formulating hypothesis that can be followed up by the studies to test them and whenever, appropriate to try to assess relationship between exposure and effect in a quantitative manner. Perusal of hospital records for existing morbidity and mortality statistics in various sub-populations provides necessary information for descriptive study and to develop a hypothesis about the causal factor.

Cross sectional, case control and cohort studies are used to identify a cause by applying Evans postulates on the evidence collected. A relationship between hypothesized cause and disease is established in following motication. The prevalence of a disease is higher in individuals exposed to the supposed cause than those, which are not exposed (Evidence from cross sectional study).

- Exposure to the supposed cause is presented more commonly in diseased animals than those without disease (Evidence from case control study).
- The number of new cases of disease is significantly higher in those exposed to the supposed cause than those not so exposed (Evidence from cohort study).

While considering the observations made through epidemiological studies, consideration should be given to the fact that there may be other variable than pollutant alone to influence the profile of traits used in the study. For example, age, sex, breed, health and nutritional and physiological status of exposed population, topography and prevailing wind direction, etc. can influence the outcome of pollution hazards and hence, need due consideration.

Clinical and Pathological Observations

A case of toxicity or pollution related condition is diagnosed tentatively when large number or a group of animals, maintained in similar management and environment condition, fall sick. In most instances of acute toxicity, the affected animals show identical clinical and pathological signs at a given time. Most animals dying during acute pollution hazards show lesion in the liver and kidneys and in respiratory tract during air pollution. Chlorinated naphthalene, coal tar pitch, paraffin etc. are hepatotoxic causing lesion in liver. Kidney lesions are more common in animals dying due to mercury, lead, cadmium, oxalic acid and ethylene glycol poisoning. Air pollutants such as hydrogen sulfide, ammonia oxides, carbon monoxide, etc. produce changes in respiratory tract.

Rumen content, liver and muscle (each 50 g) in air tight container is collected for cyanide assay. Samples must be collected immediately (rumen content) or within 4 hrs. (liver up to 20 hr of death). Suspected plant material (100 g) for qualitative determination of HCN, qualitative determination of suspected plant material and rumen ingesta is very simple and can be carried out under field conditions. The material is placed in a test tube containing little water and few drops of chloroform is added to it. A sodium picrate paper is hanged with the help of a cork from the top of the tube and the mixture is heated very gently. Change in colour of reagent paper from yellow to red within 5-10 min, indicates the presence of free HCN. Placing a drop of rumen fluid on picrate paper may also give positive result in HCN poisoning.

Management of Some Common Toxicity in Animals

The chemicals used in agricultural practices, emitted from polluting sources in industrial areas and of plant origin are the common cause of toxicity in animals. These chemicals produce more of less similar kind symptoms in a herd and remains by and large undiagnosed in animals. In both the cases, large number of animals shows similar symptoms of illness in a previously healthy stock, and the symptoms and illness are noticed at the same time. Diagnosis of chemical toxicity in isolated case is more difficult, and creates a bigger challenge for veterinarian. It is only the acquaintance with the syndrome produced by the common toxicants and environmental evidence such as distribution of poisonous plant in a particular locality, recent use of pesticides in the agricultural field, particular industrial enterprise in the locality that give clue for diagnosis of the toxicity in animals. So, while investigating the cause of toxicity in a group of animals it is highly essential to thoroughly examine the animal's immediate environment in addition to clinical and physical examination of the animals. Examination of immidiate environment provides the investigator a clue for tentative diagnosis and for further processing of the samples for toxicological analysis for confirmation of the toxicant. Only giving the clinical signs of the problem while submitting the specimen for identification of toxicant rarely solve the problem, as there are thousands of chemicals having potential to produce animal health hazards and the tests for analysis of toxicants is very expensive. So, the toxicity in animals poses a serious problem for its confirmatory diagnosis and, thus, majority cases of the toxicity are being managed not with specific antidote rather with drugs to improve the condition of the animal.

Toxicant / Poison

Any substance that has potential to produce health hazard by its inherent chemical properties is called toxicant. So, the dose or quantity of the substance to which the animal is exposed determines whether a particular chemical is toxic or not. However, only exposure to chemical should not be considered as animal having chemical toxicity as there are biological interactions and body may not accumulate that chemical to a toxic level. There are many ways to classify the toxicants. They are based on origin of the toxic chemicals such as plant or animal origin, use of the chemicals such as herbicides, insecticides and so on and chemical nature of the toxicant like inorganic or organic etc. The more common inorganic toxicants include lead, cadmium, arsenic, selenium, phosphorus, mercury, fluorine, molybdenum, copper, sodium chloride, zinc, sulohur etc. Organic poisons include hydrocyanic acid poisoning, nitrate and nitrite poisoning, oxalate poisoning, strychnine poisoning etc. The farm chemicals that commonly reported to induce poisoning are anthelmintics, insecticides (organophosphorus and carbamates), rodenticides, herbicides, molluscicides etc. Feed additives such as iodinated casein, estrogenic substances, urea, chemically treated natural feed, dried poultry wastes, ionophore antibiotics like monensin and lasalocid can also induce toxicity in animals, if used beyond their safe limit. The other group of chemical toxicants is from poisonous plants such as fern (bracken fern), grasses (*Philaris* spp., rye grass) etc.

Clinical Findings in Some Common Cases of Poisoning

Fluorosis: Stunted growth, exostosis of bones, lameness, dental mottling characterized by chalk like spots, patches or striations, bulging of gums and delayed eruption of permanent incisors.

Lead poisoning: Apathy and CNS disorders, staggering, respiratory distress, poor growth, loss of appetite, tremor, nystagmus, twitching of facial and cervical muscles, blindness, diarrhoea, cramping, abdominal distension and pain.

Arsenic toxicity: Dermatitis, gastroenteritis, muscle tremor, signs referable to pulmonary and nervous systems, carcinogenicity.

Cadmium poisoning: Involvement of renal and pulmonary systems, weight loss, cough, dyspnea, rhinitis, proteinuria, glucosuria and osteomalacia.

Molybdenum toxicity: Weight loss, hair coat depigmentation, and anemia due to secondary hypocuprosis, persisting diarrhoea, debilitating body conditions.

Copper poisoning: Emaciation, staggering, inappetance, apathy, icterus and haemoglobinura

Selenium toxicity: CNS involvement, emaciation, lameness, loss of hair

Organophosphate and Carbamate poisoning: Salivation, diarrhoea tremor, pupillary constriction (Cattle), abdominal pain, diarrhoea, dyspnea and laryngeal paralysis (horses).

Strychnine poisoning: Restlessness, tremors, stiff neck, intermittent tetanic convulsions

Collection and Dispatch of Specimen for Confirmatory Diagnosis of the Poisoning

Materials should be collected in suspected cases of plant or chemical poisoning from animals as early as possible after death or sacrifice for confirmatory diagnosis. Samples should be sent quickly to laboratory through a messenger in ice without using any preservative. Feed, fodder, water or any other material ingested by animal prior to illness and suspected to contain toxic substances should also be collected and sent for laboratory investigation. Complete history and information regarding species, breed, age and sex of the animal, number of animals affected and total population exposed to risk factors, clinical symptoms, treatment given, source of feed, water, post mortem lesions etc should also be noted and sent along with samples.

Biomarkers of toxicity: Instead of relying completely on identification of toxicants responsible for ill health of animals, the recent practice is to monitor some of biological response to an environmental chemical. Biomarker are defined as any measurable biochemical, physiological, or other alteration within an organism that, depending on the magnitude, can be recognized as an established or potential health impairment or disease. In other words, the biomarkers are the changes in cellular and biochemical activities in animals that results from exposure to toxicants. The biomarkers are of particular interest to obtain clear evidence of toxic effects of environmental toxicants in both laboratory and in field studies, and many time these have edge over conventional methods in detecting exposure effects. For examples, traditional residue analysis are of limited value for organophosphate (OP) and carbamate exposure, as their residues are rapidly metabolized by birds and mammals. But inhibition of acetylcholinesterase (ACh) persists for many days and can be used to measure the intensity of exposure as well as degree of hazards posed to exposed population. Birds, for example, show no overt symptoms of toxicity up to 40% inhibition in brain ACh. Characteristic physiologic and behavioral effects occur in the range of 40-75% inhibition and extreme symptoms of neutrotoxicity occur above this range. In cattle, blood ACh levels are depressed for much longer than the clinical signs in organophosphate and carbamate toxicity.

Management of Common Toxicity in Animal

As the diagnosis of toxicity in a particular animal or a group of animals is a challenging job for veterinarian, and is rarely attained with the limited laboratory facility, and specific identification of toxicant is only practicable with advanced laboratory aid that to with complete information on environmental history and proper storage, packing and dispatch of the material to the laboratory. Management practices focus on mainly symptomatic treatment for promoting removal and/ or neutralization of the toxicant and to maintain the vital functions of the body.

Removal of the Poison

Gastric Emptying of the Poison

Removal of the poisonous substance from the gastric tract is very important when the toxic substances have been consumed within preceding 2 to 3 hr and the substance has been consumed in large amount, that has potential to get absorbed quickly from the gastrointestinal tract. This can be achieved by gastric lavage. But, vomition should not be induced if caustics or hydrocarbons have been ingested. Emetics are of no value in farm animals but adsorbents and purgatives have been proved very beneficial. The recommended emetics for use in dogs include apomorphine @ 0.05 – 0.1mg/kg body weight sc or im without any depressant effect. However, this is contraindicated in cats. Even, sodium chloride 1 to 3 teaspoonful in warm water or hydrogen peroxide @ 1ml/kg can be given to induce vomition.

Decontamination of Skin

Some toxicants like hydrocarbons, acids alkalis, agrochemicals contaminate the skin and in such cases, skin should be scrupulously washed with water and dried. The contaminated skin area should not be rubbed nor organic solvent be used for cleaning of the toxicants as they enhance the cutaneous absorption.

Neutralization of the Poison Within the Gastrointestinal Tract

Activated charcoal as adsorbent can be given @ 1-3 gm/kg body weight and should be repeated, if required. It can adsorb chlorinated hydrocarbons, organophosphorous compounds, mycotoxins, plant alkaloids, common feed additives, antibacterial agents and bacterial toxins. But activated charcoal fails to adsorb heavy metals, halogens, nitrite, alcohol, caustics and sodium chloride. Purgative administration is necessary to remove combined adsorbent and poison. The irritant purgative is contraindicated in cases the toxicant itself is irritant in nature and in such cases oily purgatives should be used to remove the poison from the gastrointestinal tract. Oxidizing agents and tannic acid are used to precipitate alkaloids. The toxicant that coagulates protein can be effectively adsorbed by egg albumin.

General chemical antidotes that form complex or insoluble precipitate with poisons and neutralize them in the gastrointestinal tract are used with limited and debatable effects. Milk is generally believed to act as the best general antidote. In fact, it promotes absorption of liposoluble poisons and thus milk should never be used in cases of poisoning without knowing the chemical nature of the poisonous substance. Water containing albumen form complexes with heavy metals and neutralize acid and bases. Tannins and ferric hydrate precipitates heavy metals and alkaloids and thus neutralize their toxic potential.

Renal Elimination

Forced diuresis through increasing glomerular filtration can be attained through slow intravenous infusion of 5% glucose solution @ 2 – 5ml/ kg body weight in large animals and 5 to 20ml/kg body weight in small animals or with diuretics like furosemide @ 0.5 – 1 mg/kg body in large animals and 2.5 to 5 mg/ kg body weight in small animals. Weak base toxicants can be eliminated by forced acid diuresis with ammonium chloride or arginine chloride and weak acids can be eliminated by forced alkaline diuresis with sodium bicarbonates or Ringer's lactate. In dogs and cats, peritoneal dialysis with an appropriate dialysate @ 20 – 50 ml/kg could help remove the toxicants from the blood.

Additional Treatment Measures

Symptomatic treatment of the animals is highly essential to keep the vital functions working properly. Animal should be shifted to a comfortable place with minimal disturbances. Caffeine and theophylline are used as cardiovascular stimulant which also have diuretic action. Nikethamide is used as respiratory stimulant. Large doses of water solubles vitamins and hepato-protective drug should be administered. The later reduce hepatic damage and enhances liver function to detoxify the poisonous substances. Some physiological antidotes based of the clinical symptoms shown by the animal, may be given. For example, in case of sever muscular contraction, muscle relaxant may be administered to prevent respiratory arrest. Besides, pharmacological antidotes should be given as detailed below can use of known toxicant.

Specific Antidotes Against Some Common Chemical and Plant Toxicity

Poisoning due to anions

Fluorosis in animals can be diagnosed easily, particularly in areas with the history of emission of fluoride from industrial activities or high fluoride content in ground water. In cases of fluoride poisoning, aluminum sulfate should be given @ 50 gm/ adult animal at 24 hours interval for 3 to 4 days.

Heavy Metal Poisoning

Calcium versenate ($CaNa_2EDTA$) has been used successfully for the past many decades for chelation of lead from the body. This is given @ 110-220 mg/kg. b.wt. as 1-2% w/v solution twice a day for two days. The treatment is repeated for two more days. Thiamine hydrochloride should also be given @ 25-50 mg/kg intravenously 12 hourly. BAL(2-3-Dimercpato propanol) 5% solution in 10% solution of Benzyl benzoate in peanut oil should be given@ 3-5 mg/kg 1/m at every 4hr interval for 2days, then at 6hr interval for 3 days and at 12hr interval for 10 days Sodium thiosulfate should be given @ 15-30 gm/ animal in 100 to 200 ml of water at 24 hr interval IV followed by 30 to 60 gm /animal in 300 ml water at 6hr interval orally for 3 to 4 days. Mercurous and mercuric chlorides, gold mining, fungicides, paints and mercury broilers are common sources. BAL can be used as antidote in mercury poisoning and should be given @ 6.5 mg/kg body wt at 24 hrs interval IV single doses and 6.5 mg/kg body weight at 6 hrs interval orally for 3-4 days. In molybdenum toxicity, copper should be given @ 5 mg/kg at 24 hr interval orally till complete recovery. In copper poisoning ammonium tetrathiomolybdate should be given @ 2.7 mg/kg at 24 hrs interval IV for 2-3 days interval.

Insecticide Toxicity

Chlorinated hydrocarbons (Aldrin, Hexachloride, Lindane, Heptachlor etc.): These are commonly used in agricultural and animal husbandry practices as contact poisons for insects and ectoparasites. No specific antidote is available. Sedation with triflupromazine or pentobarbital sodium and intravenous glucose and calcium administration are recommended. Sedation is required to prevent self-inflicting injury to the animal. Non-oily purgatives may be given to eliminate poisons from the gastrointestinal tract. A small dose of atropine sulphate should be administered to control parasympathomimetic signs. Organophosphorus compounds and carbamates compounds are considered as contact toxicants that are commonly used to control insect population in plant and animals. The acute cases of these poisoning is controlled by giving atropine sulphate at the dose rate of 2.5 mg per body weight at 2-8 hrs interval IV or IM and it is repeated if the signs reappear.

Rodenticides

Wafarin is a commonly used rodenticide and its accidental ingestion is not uncommon in animals. Vitamin K is the drug of choice to check extravasations of blood in this poisoning.

Plant Toxins

Plant toxicity is commonly encountered in animals during scarcity of feed and fodder where the animals are forced to eat anything available. Cyanide, nitrate and nitrite, oxalate and dicoumarin are the main poisoning compounds under this category. Cyanogenic glycosides present in sudan grass, sorghum, wild cherry, johnson grass etc. are the main source of cyanide to animals and the cases of poisoning are treated with sodium nitrite and sodium thiosulfate at the dose rate of 5 gm sodium nitrite and 15 gm sodium thiosulphate in 200 ml water/ cattle at 24 hrs interval intravensouly on single dose. Methylene blue 1% solution is the drug of choice for nitrate and nitrite poisoning and is given at the rate of 1-2 mg/kg body weight at 6-8 hrs intervals intravenously.

Calcium borogluconate (25%) should be given at the rate of 300-500 ml per adult cattle 24 hrs interval IV as single dose and is repeated, if necessary in case of poisoning oxlate. Vitamin K is the specific antidote aganst poisoning with dicoumarin derivatives from sweet clover and other plants which is given at the rate of 50-70 mg/kg body weight at 24 hrs interval i.m. or i.v. as single dose.

In the field of clinical toxicology, it is highly essential to have knowledge on the animals' immediate environment and possible cause of the poisoning, that helps in further analysis of the samples for confirmatory diagnosis and management of toxicity.

21

Alternative Medicine in Animal Disease Management

The whole plants or their parts have been used as source of medicine and health tonics both in medical and veterinary practice since time immemorial. Many of the active ingredients in chemically manufactured drugs have been originally derived from plant components (e.g. pyrethroids). Despite availability of the modern allopathic medicines, herbal medicines are still used on a very large scale. In the back drop of current global trade of herbal medicine and intellectual property right (IPR) scenario, and to overcome side effects of 'single golden molecular bullet' drug technologies of twentieth century, there is an upsurge of interest in traditional practices. The ethno-veterinary medicine is becoming a growing area of research, and more and more scientists, veterinary professionals and livestock owners are interested in indigenous medicinal therapy. The traditional medicine system appears to be a viable solution for providing cost- effective primary healthcare to animals in rural India, where modern drugs are not readily available. However, the traditional knowledge is required to be more effective-farmers friendly and economically viable in the changing agro-climatic conditions of the country. There is a need to popularize natural drugs and for organic cultivation of medicinal plants to ensure phytochemical consistency and quality. Enforcement of drug quality control and good management practice (GMP), scientific validation of veterinary Indigenous Technical Knowledge (ITKs) and improved availability of quality herbal drugs at competitive price will not only boost the confidence of livestock owners but would help in enhancing export potential of medicinal herbs and herbal products.

India possesses huge animal population including domestic animals. Livestock and pet animals play a vital role in socio-economic structure of the country. Livestock, in particular, are the backbone of agrarian economy contributing approximately over 32% to the total share from agriculture to national gross domestic products (GDP). The animal draught power contributes significantly to agricultural practice of rural India. The value of output from livestock sector is expected to rise further and this can be achieved even with the existing animal resources by addressing certain important issues confronting the animal sector. Poor health of animals is one of the most significant factor that has inimical effects on the production and productivity of livestock. The veterinary healthcare infrastructure has been identified as the most critical constraint to improve the productivity of livestock. Much of losses due to livestock diseases can be reduced by proper veterinary healthcare, particularly by using herbal remedies, which are claimed to be effective and are often regarded safe, easily available and eco-friendly as compared to modern system of therapy. The herbal medicinal knowledge may also be an important way to provide prompt primary health care to the animals in rural areas.

Traditional Herbal Veterinary Medicine

Veterinary medicine is an age-old profession, which perhaps dates back to the period of Neolithic Agricultural Revolution. Archeological evidences indicate that the ancient Egyptian had well developed veterinary profession nearly over 4 millennia ago and used various methods including application of herbs for treatment of animal diseases. It is believed that during the period of *Hamburabi* (2000 BC), the physicians had knowledge of more than 250 medicinal plants and 120 mineral salt.

The veterinary and animal husbandry practices of the ancient India find mentions in *Rigveda* and *Atharvaveda.* Books written by *Salihotra* (1800 BC) and *Charak* (2300 BC), and *Palikapaya* (1000 BC) describe treatment of animal diseases using medicinal plants. The two great *Pandavas – Nakula* and *Sahadeva*, had expertise in treatment and management of horses and cattle, respectively. The ancient Indians also had distinction to establish the first state funded well-equipped veterinary hospital during the period of the Great *Ashoka* (238BC), and *Shalihotra* is considered to be the first known veterinary doctor in the world lived around 1800 BC in Northern India. The significance of herbs in ancient Indian veterinary care is underlined by the edict of King Ashoka, which states that Everywhere the King Priyadarshi, beloved of God erected two kinds of hospitals; hospitals for men and hospitals for animals. Wherever there were no healing herbs, either for men, or farm animals, he commanded that the medicinal plants be brought and planted.

From the *Vedic* period till the end of 19th century, much of the veterinary practice in India was based on the experiences gathered through generations and improved through informal experimentation. This traditional system of medicine, also referred to as ethnoveterinary medicine and defined in simple terms as 'local or indigenous knowledge and methods for caring, healing and managing domestic animals' by locally available traditional healers. However, a paradigm shift occurred in veterinary profession with the introduction of modern system of veterinary education through establishment of veterinary colleges in Lahore, Bombay, Madras and Calcutta, and the Imperial Bacteriological Laboratory (presently IVRI) in Pune, Mukteswar, during British period. Invention of antiseptics, sulfonamide and antibiotics brought revolutionary changes in both human and veterinary medical practices and majority of diseases were being treated with the newly invented synthetic drug molecule. Thus, the existing Traditional Knowledge was pushed to back seat till the advent of the concept of sustainable agriculture and livestock industry in the Indian agricultural scenario in late 1980s. Th herbal remedies are now considered as a potential candidate for developing eco-friendly, safe and cost-effective drugs for human and animal uses.

Healing Herbs for Animals

In many developing countries including India, which possesses a rich treasure of medicinal plants, majority of traditional medicines are plant based containing one or more herbal components. Nearly 750 medicinal plants are used by traditional healers for treatment of animal and human diseases. Most of these plants are used either as green or dried powder form or as water extract or decoction. They can also be refined into tablets, capsules, powder, tinctures and other supplement formulations.

The World Bank funded Mission Mode NATP on 'Collection, documentation and validation of indigenous technical knowledge (ITK), launched by Indian Council of Agricultural Research in 2000. A total of 595 veterinary ITKs have been collected from different sources and recorded. Many of these ITKs which were recommended for scientific validation are found to possess therapeutic and ameliorative potential for treatment of animal diseases, were plants based. In another NATP on 'identification and evaluation of medicinal plants for control of parasitic diseases in livestock, 158 plants have been catalogued and 50 have been evaluated for antiparasitic activity. Number of herbs are also reported to act as free radical scavengers and inhibit lipid peroxidation. They also increase hepatocyte protein synthesis, decrease the activity of tumor promoters, stabilize mast cells, chelate iron and lead and slow down calcium metabolism. The herbs with antioxidant potential are mainly used to ameliorate stress. Common conditions for which the herbal medicines have been used include gastrointestinal disorders such as indigestion, bloat, diarrhoea and constipation, mastitis, internal and external parasites, skin ailments, reproductive disorders, joint swelling, yoke gall, wound, respiratory problems and debility etc. The recent researches have also established antioxidant, immunopotentiating and anti-toxic properties of plants and recommended their use in conditions such as post-parturient disorders, mastitis, and poisoning.

Herb	Parts used	Key constituents	Medicinal use
Acacia catechu (catechu, *katha, khadira*)	Bark, stem-bark, leaves pods	Catechin, quercetin, tannin, catechutannic acid	Bark astringent, ripe pods used in constipation, unripe in diarrhea, wounds, ulcers
Aegle marmelos (bael or Bengal quince, bilva, bael)	Fruits, leaves, root, twigs and stem bark	Coumarins, flavonoids, alkaloids, tannins and fixed oil, vitamin-C	Half-ripe fruit- astringent reduces intestinal irritation used in diarrhea, ripe-friut-demulcent and laxative. Pulp used to treat peptic-ulcer, antipyretic and stimulant. Aegelin is used in bronchial spasm
A*llium sativum* (Garlic, *lasun*)	Bulb, tuber, oil	Volatile oil (alliin, alliinase, allicin), scordinins, Selenium	Carminative, diuretic. Used in bronchial and digestive infections, cough, fever, diabetes, and in heavy metal toxicity.
Aloe vera (Indian aloes, *Ghikanvar, Ghritkumari*)	Plant, dried juice of leaf, pulp, root	Antroquinones (aloin, aloe-emodin), resins, tannins, aloectin-B.	Purgative, skin conditions, colic, ulcers, laxative, burns, scalds, anthelmintic, to improve fertility, etc
Annona squamosa (custard apple, *sitafal*)	Leaf, seed, fruit, root	Amorphous alkaloid in leaf and seeds; andnain alkaloid in bark and sugar in fruit	Leaf- antibacterial, miticidal, astringent, anthelmintic, reduces uric acid; fruit & seeds- insectide, miticidal; bark- astringent. Crushed leaves used for maggot wound, tympany, bloat, FMD lesions, anthelmintic; bark and seed powder as insecticide
Argemone mexicana (Mexican poppy, *shringalakantaka, satyanashi, kali dhaturi,*)	Root, seed, leaf	Isoquinoline alkaloid, mucilage and sachharine matter	Seed- enetic, emetci, expectorant, demulcent, oil- purgative, root-alternative. Yellow used for jaundice, skin infections, Infusion of seeds in small quantities used as sedative in children, Flower used in cough

Table 1: Some herbs valued for medicinal use

Herb	Parts used	Key constituents	Medicinal use
Acacia catechu (catechu, *katha, khadira*)	Bark, stem-bark, leaves pods	Catechin, quercetin, tannin, catechutannic acid	Bark astringent, ripe pods used in constipation, unripe in diarrhoea, wounds, ulcers
Aegle marmelos (bael or Bengal quince, bilva, bael)	Fruits, leaves, root, twigs and stem bark	Coumarins, flavonoids, alkaloids, tannins and fixed oil, vitamin-C	Half-ripe fruit- astringent reduces intestinal irritation used in diarrhea, ripe-friut-demulcent and laxative. Pulp used to treat peptic-ulcer, antipyretic and stimulant. Aegelin is used in bronchial spasm
Allium sativum (Garlic, *lasun*)	Bulb, tuber, oil	Volatile oil (alliin, alliinase, allicin), scordinins, Selenium	Carminative, diuretic. Used in bronchial and digestive infections, cough, fever, diabetes, and in heavy metal toxicity.
Allium cepa (onion, *piyaj*)	Bulb, seeds	Volatile oil, mucilage	Used in prolapse of uterus, to induce heat
Aloe vera (Indian aloes, *Ghikanvar, Ghritkumari*)	Plant, dried juice of leaf, pulp, root	Antroquinones (aloin, aloe-emodin), resins, tannins, aloectin-B.	Purgative, skin conditions, colic, ulcers, laxative, burns, scalds, anthelmintic, to improve fertility, etc
Annona squamosa (custard apple, *sitafal*)	Leaf, seed, fruit, root	Amorphous alkloid in leaf and seeds; andnain alkaloid in bark and sugar in fruit	Leaf- antibacterial, miticidal, astringent, anthelmintic, reduces uric acid; fruit & seeds- insectide, miticidal; bark- astringent. Crushed leaves used for maggot wound, tympany, bloat, FMD lesions, anthelmintic; bark and seed powder as insecticide
Argemone mexicana (Mexican poppy, *shringalakantaka, satyanashi, kali dhaturi,*)	Root, seed, leaf	Isoquinoline alkaloid, mucilage and sachharine matter	Seed- laxative, emetic, expectorant, demulcent, oil- purgative, root- alternative. Yellow used for jaundice, skin infections, Infusion of seeds in small quantities used as sedative in children, Flower used in cough
Asparagus racemosus (*Shatavari*)	Leaf, root	Bitter (asparagine) & steroidal glycosides (asparagoides) falvonoid,	Refrigerant, demulcent, aphrodisiac, tonic, galactagogue, antidiarrheal. Used in skin diseases& maggot wound as tonic and galactagogue

Herb	Parts used	Key constituents	Medicinal use
Azadirachta indica (Margosa tree, *Nimba, neem, nimb*)	Leaf, seed, root, bark, gum, fruit	Meliacins, triterpenoid bitters, tannins and flavonoids	Leaves, seeds and fruits-Antibacterial, antiviral, insecticide, bitter tonic, antiseptic, astringent; Fruits- astringent, purgative, Dry flower- tonic and stomachic.; oil- anti diabetic. Used in skin diseases, FMD (Leaf), leprosy, bronchitis, intestinal worm (seeds), mastitis, rheumatism & diabetes (oil),
Benincasa hispida or *B. cerifara* (Wax guard, *petha*)	Fruit, seeds and fruit rind	Saponins and guaridine	Seeds are used in cough, fever, and excessive thrust. Fruits are diuretic laxative and aphrodisiac and are used for peptic ulcer and debility. Fruit juice mixed with lemon used to prevent bleeding
Bignonia catalpa (Indian bean tree)	Bark and fruit	Bark- catalpine	Sedative and narcotic (Bark). Used in asthma, and spasmodic cough, and as eye wash in conjunctivitis
Boerhavia diffusa (Spreading hogweed, *punernava, gudparna*)	Plant, root	Alkaloid, potassium nitrate	Bitter stomachic, root- diuretic, purgative, laxative, anthelminitic, and expectorant, febrifuge. Used in asthma, kidney diseases, jaundice & liver enlargement.
Butea monosperma or *B frondosa* (Bastard teak, *palas*)	Seed, flower, stem bark, leaf, gum	Tannins, gallic acid, glucosides	Anthelmintic, (seed), astringent, tonic aphrodisiac, diuretic (leaf and plants). Used in acid indigestion, sore throat, vaginitis, diarrhea, fever, ringworm, septic wounds, and intestinal worm.
Caesalpinia bonducella (Nikkar nut, *karanj, katkaranj*)	Seeds, bark, leaves	Fixed oil, non-alkaloid bitter- bonducin and tannins	Antispasmodic, bitter tonic, anthelmintic, febrifuge, antidiabeteic. Used in intermittent fever, colic, diabetes and asthma
Calotropis gigantica (swallow wart, *manelara, akonda*)	Root, plant, root bark, flower, juice	Mudarin, glycoside, usenarin calotoxin, calotropin	Caustic and astringent, cardiac tonic, astringent, antispasmodic, expectorant. Leaves used in tympany, FMD, chronic rheumatism, skin diseases, leprosy
Calendula officinalis (Marigold, *Genda*)	Flowers	Triterpenes, resins, bitter glycosides, volatile oil, sterols, falvonoids, mucilage, carotenes	Anti-inflammatory, astringent, antiseptic, checks bleeding, detoxifying, mild estrogenic. Used in wound healing, skin inflamamtion, and as infusion for digestive disorders and liver tonic

Herb	Parts used	Key constituents	Medicinal use
Cassia tora (Foetid cassia, *chakramarda, panever, takala)*	Seed, leaves, root	Glycoside, emodin,	Antifungal, laxative, anthelmintic, antipyretic. Useful in cough, constipation, diarrhea, pains in joints and skin diseases
Centella asiatica (Indian Pennywort *Gotu kala, Mandukparni, brahmi)*	Plant, leaves	Triterpenoid saponins, alkaloid, bitter principle	Alternative, tonic. Used in dysentery, as tonic, improving memory skin problems and wounds. Reduces fertility and blood sugar.
Cinnamomum cassia, C. verum, C aromaticum, C. sinense (Cinnamon, *Gudatvak Dalchini*)	Stem bark, twigs, oil	Volatile oil, tannins, coumarins, mucilage	Carminative, antiseptic, antiviral, antispasmodic. Used for cold conditions, digestive problems, aching muscles treatment of debility, and toothache
Curcuma longa, C. domestica (Turmeric, *Haridra, Haldi)*	Tuber, rhizome	Volatile oil, Curcumin, bitter principles, resin,	Carminative, cooling, antiseptic, antioxidant, antibacterial, anti-inflammatory (stronger than hydrocortisone), stomchic. Used in bronchitis, skin infections, arthritis, allergies, mastitis, wound
Dalbergia sissoo (Black wood, *Shingshupa, shisam)*	Stem bark, root, leaves, mucilage	Mucilage, tannins, alkylphenol, dalberginone, dalbergin	Stem bark- alternative, root- astringent, leaves- bitter, astringent and stimulant. Used in haemorrhages, boils, eruptions, skin affections. Leaves in diarrhea
Elettaria cardamomum, E. major(Cardamom, *Chandrika,* elachi)	Root, seeds,	Volatile oil (borneol, camphor, pinene, humulene, carbophyllene, etc)	Strong antispasmodic, carminative, stomachic, stimulant, diuretic. Used as laxative, tonic, asthma, kidney stone, and in digestive problem and as aphrodisiac.
Eucalyptus globulus (eucalyptus, blue gum, *Nilgiri*)	Leaf gum, oil from stem	Volatile oil, Flavonoids, tannins, resins	Antiseptic, expectorant, febrifuge, carminative. Useful as sialogogue, appetite and digestion and in respiratory problems, fever, cystitis.
*Eugenia caryophyllata or Syzgium aromaticum, (*Clove, *lavang)*	Flower buds (fresh & dried)	Volatile oil, gum, tannin	Antiseptic, carminative, analgesic, anti-emetic, antispasmodic, anthelmintic. Used in toothache, to treat infections, in colic, fever, neuralgia, fungal skin infections
Ficus bengalensis (Banyan tree, *Vata, bargad, vad)*	Fruit, bark, leaves latex, aerial roots	Ficusin and bergaptin	Astringent, tonic, cooling. Used in diarrhoea, dysentery, in joint pain, leaf poultices applied in abscesses

Herb	Parts used	Key constituents	Medicinal use
Hibiscus rosasinensis (Chinese rose, *Jalpuspa, Jasund)*	Root flower, seed	Quercetin, cyanidin, kaempferol	Leaf and flower- emollient, demulcent, anti-inflammatory, refrigerant, aphrodisiac, anodyne and laxative. Used in fever, cough, and diarrhoea.
Leptadenia reticulata *(*Corkwort, *jivanti, doodhi)*	Plant, leaf	Tocopherol, Phytosterols,	Stimulant, tonic, galactagogue, estrogenic. Used in agalactia and decreased milk, prolapse of uterus and vagina, repeat breeding and to induce heat and milk let down
Moringa oleifera (drum stick*, sobhanjana, sahajan*)	Root, bark, flower, seed, oil, gum	Alkaloids, Volatile oil	Stimulant, carminative, stomachic, abortificient. Used in paralytic afflictions, intermittent fever, epilepsy, chronic rheumatism, liver diseases.
Ocimum basilicum (sweet basil, bisva tulsi, manjarika, bantulsi)	Leaf, root, flower, seed	Volatile oil, Flavonoid, triterpene	Flower- carminative, diuretic, stimulant, demulcent; seed- diuretic, demulcent; plant juice anthelmintic, root- febrifuge. Seed used in chronic diarrhoea, dysentery, nephritis, cystitis; leaf in cough and FMD

Herb	Parts used	Key constituents	Medicinal use
Ocimum sanctum (Holy basil, *vishnu-priya, tulsi*)	Plant, leaf	Volatile oil, Flavonoid, triterpene	Antidiabeteic, antibacterial, expectorant, antipyretic, adaptogenic, anti-inflammatory. Useful in relieving pain, fever, cardiac problems and stress, diabetes, respiratory problems joint pains, wound healing , mastitis
Phyllanthus emblica or Emblica officinalis (Indian goose berry, *Amalalai, Amla)*	Plant, stem bark, leaf, root, flower, fruit, seed	Fixed oil, volatile oil, tannins, vitamin-C	Refrigerant, astringent, laxative, carminative, stomachic, aperient, anthemintic, antioxidant. Used as tonic, strengthen pancreas and in diabetes, anemia, jaundice, infusion of young shoots in dysentery, ulcers
Terminalia arjuna (White murdah, *Arjuna)*	Leaves, root, bark, fruit	Tannins, triterpenoid saponins, flavonoids, sterols	Cardiac tonic, febrifuge, astringent, expectorant. Useful in heart diseases, earache, cough, sore throat, and asthma
Tinospora cordifolia (Amrita, guduchi, geloi)	Stem root, plant fruit	Berberine- bitter substance, giloin, gilonin	Tonic, antipyretic, alternative, aphrodisiac, diuretic, antirheumatic. Useful in chronic diarrhea, dysentery, liver diseases, fever, and in mastitis
Vitex negundo (Five leaves chest tree, *Nirgundi, Nirgandi*)	Root, fruit, flower, leaf, bark	Volatile oil, Resin, Alkaloids	Aromatic, vermifuge, anodyne, ectoparasiticide, febrifuge, nervine tonic, astringent. Useful in inflammatory swelling, rheumatism.
Withania somnifera (Withania, *Ashwagandha)*	Leaves, root, berries	Alkaloids, steroidal lactones, iron	Adaptogenic, tonic, antioxidant, sedative. Used as tonic restorative, anti-stress, nervine tonic and in anemia, rheumatic swelling
Zingiber officinale (Ginger, *Adarak, Wishvabhesaj)*	Rhizome (fresh and dried)	Volatile oil, oleoresin	Anti-emetic, carminative, circulatory stimulant, stomachic, lactagogue anti-inflammatory, antiseptic. Used in digestive problems including GIT infections and some types of food poisoning, cold, flu fever, nausea and high blood pressure

Table 2: Some veterinary prescriptions containing herbal component

Condition	Traditional practices/ITK used
Anorexia	• Mixture of powdered fennel seed (*Foeniculum vulgare*) + jaggery 60 g each + black salt 20g applied as electuary • Mixture of powdered seed of Bishop weed or Ajowain (*Carum copticum)* + salt 20 g each in 20 g molasses given twice daily orally
Rumen indigestion	• Magnesium sulfate 500 g + Common salt 200 g + ginger powder 10 g in 500 ml lukewarm water orally for adult cattle
Constipation/ purgation	• Vegetable oil 500 ml orally for adult cattle • Mixture of Bishop seed powder + black salt in equal part orally • Decoction of 100 g turmeric powder / liter water daily for 2-3 day • Ground leaves of *Arictolochia indica* 250 g + molasses 50 g given three times at ½ hrly interval
Bloat	• Vegetable oil 500 ml orally for adult cattle • Asafetida 10g+ black salt 20 g+ Tulsi seed 5g + ginger powder 5 g in little water given orally • Asafetida 5g+ black salt 100 g+ *soova dana* (*Anethum sowa*) seed 50g + ginger powder 25 g + ajma (*(Trachyspermum ammi*) + jaggery 500 g boiled in 1000 ml water to reduce volume by half. Decoction is given orally
Diarrhoea	• Powder of shisam (*Dalbergia sisso*) leaves @ 70-100 g per 100 kg body weight orally in calves • Powder of half ripe Bael fruit (*Aegle marmelos*) @ 15-25 g per kg b .wt orally in calves • Kaolin 5g + Prepared chalk 5 g + catechu 0.8 g + *Aegle marmelos* 1 g + Alum 0.8 g + *Cyprus rotundus* 2g + *Holarrhena antidysentrica* 3g. Give 10-20 as a drench twice daily for 5 days
Intestinal parasites	• Powder of *Holarrhena antidysenterica* + *Veronia anthelmintica* + *Embelia ribes* + *Azaadirachta indica* + *Cyprus rotundus* + *Caeselpinia bonducela* in equal part and one forth part of *Gardenia gummifer* given as electuary or drech preferably in empty stomach @ 10-100 g
Pneumonia	• Inhalation of steam of mixture of Tea leaves + Margosa leaves with eucalyptus or turpentine oil • Massage of liniment of Camphorated oil (250 ml vegetable oil + 50 g camphor) or turpentine on either side of chest
Wound	• Paste of fresh peach (*Prunus persica*) leaves applied on wound and bandaged • Crushed leaves of *Ocimum sanctum* or Margosa applied on wound and bandaged • After cleaning the wound, powder of *Margosa* and *Annona* leaves (2:1) + jack leaf powder in oil applied on wound • Paste made from *Moringa oleifera* (Shahajan) leaves applied as poultice • Paste of fresh ridge gourd (*Luffa acutangula)* leaves applied on wound after cleaning
Joint swelling and yoke gall	• Mixture of powder of snail shell 10 g + Alua (*Aloe vera*) 10 gm, *Moringa oleifera* (Shahajan)gu 10g + geru 30 g in 150 ml caster oil. Mixture is heated and after cooling at warm stage applied on the affected part twice or thrice a day.
FMD lesions	• Decoction of babool+ jamun bark or paste of peach leaves or bantulsi applied on foot lesions

Source: Anjaria et al, (2000) and Anon (2002)

Active phyto-constituents: The medicinal properties of plants is attributable to the active ingredients comprising of flavonoids, phenols, tannins, steroids, polysaccharides, mucilage, anthocyanins, coumarin, anthroquinones, saponins, glycosides, bitters, alkaloids, volatile oils, minerals, and vitamins. These components have potent therapeutic action on different body system and function including inflammation, membrane stability, lipid peroxidation, immune mediated disorders, cancer and in nervous, cardiac, pulmonary, liver and kidney diseases.

Number of herbal formulations contain some flavonoids, which have wide range of actions including anti-inflammatory, anti-tumor and antioxidant properties. The flavonoids also help in maintaining circulation and strengthen capillary wall. Arjuna *(Terminalia arjuna),* astragalus *(Astragalus membranaceus)* buckwheat (*Fagopyrum esculentum),* eucalyptus *(Eucalyptus globulus),* lemon *(Citrus lemon),* tulsi *(Ocimum sanctum),* etc possess flavonoids, which may be responsible for their significant medicinal value including antioxidant activity. Intake of food rich in flavonoids such as g-rutin and luteolin has been reported to alleviate side effects of anti-tumor agents thus improving the quality of life. Many plant species such as turmeric (*Curcuma longa*), wintergreen *(Gaultheria procumbens*), thyme *(Thymus vulgaris)* and white willow *(Salix alba)* contain phenols as their active ingredients. Besides antiseptic effects, phenols are also potent anti-inflammatory agent and antioxidants. Curcumin, a phenolic substance found in *Haldi*, is stronger antioxidant than vitamin E. The strong antibacterial action of turmeric is also attributable to curcumin.

All plants produce tannins in greater or lesser amount. Tannins draw tissue closer and thus improve resistance to infection. Being astringent, tannin rich plants such as catechu (*Acacia catechu*) and Oak bark (*Quercus robur)* are mainly used in antidiarrhoeal preparations. Mucilaginous plants such as slippery elm (*Ulmus rubra*), maize (*Zea mays*), sweet flag or Bacc (*Acorus calamus*) protect mucous membranes of the digestive tract, throat, lungs, and urinary tubules and are used in herbal prescriptions meant for ailments of these organ systems. Alkaloids contain pharmacologically active amino molecule (-NH2) and are present in several medicinal plants. Some well-known drugs such as vincristine and atropine are alkaloids derived from *Vinca rosea* and *Atropa belladona*, respectively. Chiretta or chirayata (*Swertia chirata*) used extensively in traditional medicine for treatment of digestive disorders, fever and hicups, also contain appreciable quantities of bitter substances including iridoids (amarogentin) and alkaloids.

Volatile oils constitute another important phytotherapeutic group. These are extracted from plants to produce essential oils. Tea tree (*Melaleuca *alternifolia*), clove (*Eugenia caryophyllata*) sweet flag and garlic (*Allium sativum*) contain appreciable quantities of volatile oils. Medicinal plants such as clove, neem (*Azadiracta indic*a), garlic (*Allium sativum*), aloe (*Aloe vera*), ginger, ashwagandha (*Whithenia somnifera*), Amla (*Emblica officinalis*), gudhuchi (*Tinospora cordifolia*), brahmi (*Centella asiatica*) with wide range of therapeutic uses, contain more than one active ingredients.

Tips in Herbal Methodology

In the beginning, most herbs were collected from wild sources. However, with increasing demand, the wild resources started dwindling and cultivation of herbs was started to maintain sustainable supply. Some of the herbs such as opium, cinchona, poppy, cardamoms, ginger, garlic, onion, etc. have been cultivated since time immemorial. The cultivation post harvest care geographical sources, climate, plant morphology, etc. have significant bearing on the medicinal value of the herb. *Charak Samhita* clearly defines various factors that affect quality and efficacy of herbal drugs. Some of the important parameters, which need attention for harvesting, collection, preservation and preparations, are listed below.

- The herbs should be preferably harvested in a non-contaminated land and use of pesticides, chemical fertilizers and agro- chemicals should be avoided.
- Skilled persons with basic knowledge of herbs should be employed for collection of medicinal plants.
- Seasons of collection greatly influence quality Anthroquinones are completely absent in Rhubarb in winter.
- Age of plant influences the phytoingredient composition even in 24-hr cycle. Collect leaf samples just before beginning of primordial, and flower samples before they are fully bloomed. Underground samples should be collected immediately after the disappearance of aerial parts.
- Never collect dew covered and discolored herbs. No collection should be during rain.
- Shade drying or slow drying is recommended for majority of herbs. Clove, cardamoms, cinnamon, etc can be open air-dried.
- Generally leaves, flowers and whole herbs are dried between 20°C and 35°C and roots and bark between 30° and 60°C
- Extraneous matter such as dirt, plant debris, adulterants, etc. should be remove and rhizomes, tubers, bulbs root, etc. should be washed thoroughly to remove contaminants.

- Long storage is not generally advisable, and herbs should be kept in moisture free and dark place. Drying is a very useful preservation of herbs.
- Stored herbs may be infested by pest/insect. Periodic cleaning of drug storing places, good ventilation and temperature regulation (at 15°C) can check infestation and infested herbs should be removed immediate. Fumigation with ethyl oxide may be used in infested herbs.

Options, Challenges and Solutions

Vast knowledge of traditional medicines exists in India from ancient time. The country has plethora of ITKs, basically consisting of use of herbs for treatment of animal diseases in local areas. Of the 70 million flowering and non-flowering plant species in the world, 45,000 (6.43%) occur in India. Majority of these plants possesses medicinal properties and about 2000 of the plant species figure frequently in literature, and traditional healers employ nearly 750 of them. Despite early origins and long history of usage, the traditional knowledge in heathcare of animals as well as human received official support and consequently little attention from practitioners and researchers during the past two centuries. The traditional healers became a rarity even in villages and number of medicinal plants and knowledge of their usage was pushed to the brink of extinction. This not only has adversely affected animal and human health in rural areas resulting in significant inimical impact on rural and national economy.

There is a common perception that herbal medicines are quite safe, cost-effective, easily accessible and non-toxic. These can be taken at high doses and for longer duration and even with allopathic drugs without any possible side effects. These beliefs are unfortunately not always correct. Not all plants used in ethno- medicines are non-toxic and of the hundreds of plants used in the ethno-veterinary medicine, only few have been tested for their efficacy and safety. There are incidences where use of medicinal plants has caused mortality in animals. Moreover, some natural supplements and herbs may interact adversely with allopathic drugs intensifying their action or even producing dangerous side effects. For example, garlic may intensify action of anticoagulants including aspirin and overuse of *Aloe vera* juice can cause loss of potassium.

In United States of America medicinal plants used for human medicine are registered with the Food and Drug Administration and as per USDA regulations medicinal plants used for livestock must meet the same stringent requirement as the other veterinary drugs. Countries like Australia, New Zealand also enforce stringent regulations for complementary health products and dietary supplements. However, there are no such regulatory provisions in India and only fewer of the mushrooming 'Veterinary Herbal Pharmaceuticals Companies' in the country have R& D facilities to test their herbal products for quality, efficacy and safety. Also formal education and training on ethno-medicine or herbal system of medicine to veterinary professionals is lacking. Thus the challenges for traditional medicines may be summarized into following category:

- National policy and a central apex body with regulatory organization
- Identification of educational and training needs of the traditional system
- Collection, documentation and validation of traditional medicines for their safety, efficacy, and quality
- Standardization of traditional practices and their transmission to similar agro-geo-climatic areas through effective extension system
- Promoting herbal gardens to have easy accessibility to medicinal plants
- Development of database on livestock population, veterinary infrastructure including NGO, private sectors, private veterinarians and ethno-veterinarians

Validation of Novel Ingredients and Ethnoveterinary Medicine Practices

Novel ingredients, such as herbs and nutraceuticals, have had a major role in human and veterinary medicine and despite availability of the modern allopathic medicines, herbal medicines are still used on a very large scale through out the world. In many developing countries including India, which possesses a rich treasure of medicinal plants, majority of traditional medicines is plant based containing one or more herbal components. Despite the resurgence of interest and impact of the products, their use is controversial, and is complicated by issues regarding their safety, efficacy and manufacturing.

Ethno Veterinary Medicine?

The word '*ethno*' means traditional or the ' folk' or 'indigenous to local people'. Thus the Ethno Veterinary Medicine may otherwise refer to the application of Indigenous Technological Knowledge (ITK). ITK refers to unique, traditional, local knowledge, existing within and developed around the specific conditions of people indigenous to particular geographical area.

Ethnoveterinary medicine (EVM) is commonly defined as a system of folk beliefs, skills, techniques and practice relating to the healthcare of animals that is transmitted orally from generations to generations. In the Indian context, EVM is the part of the traditional knowledge system that comprises two distinct forms (i) the formal codified system of knowledge of disease and healing for both human and animal, whose principles and practices were formulated and codified in the form of *Ayurveda, Sidhha* and *Unani-Tibb* and (ii) informal systems which evolved over thousands of year through innovation and experiences of communities and passed from generations to generations mainly through oral preaching. Yet, there are many similarities between these two forms and both the traditional knowledge may be classified as 'Ethnoveterinary medicine'.

Indigenous medicine mostly comprises of drugs of plant origin. Herbal medicine is unique that differs from biomedicine with respect to adverse effects. Increasing global importance of herbal medicine has been witnessed in the recent years because of its many beneficial effects over biomedicine. Herbal medicine often complements conventional medicine providing safe, well tolerated remedies for a number of diseases, especially chronic ones. Moreover, they are inexpensive, easily available and locally accessible. Medicines prepared from plants or commodities of plant sources are used both in livestock feeding as well as health care management.

Herbal medicine plays a pivotal role among the remedies employed in treatment of different ailments of livestock in India. The wealth of knowledge on herbal medicine was originally confined to a few individual and transferred from generation to generation as family tradition. The compilation of information on herbal medicine was of interest to the researchers. Presently, there has been worldwide interest in research and development of herbal medicine, especially on their scientific validation. Hence, large number of native indigenous medicinal plants has been screened for various pharmacological properties mainly to develop products for the treatment of human diseases.

Gur, methi, rice gruel, gundi grass are fed to animals for getting more milk. Herbal treatment is also advocated in case of diarrhoea, wound healing, abscess, yolk gall, fracture, tympany, prolapsed uterus, snake bite, arthritis, ulcer, , respiratory diseases, ecto- and endo parasitism, urinary problems, food poisonings maggot infestation and infectious diseases like Foot and Mouth Diseases, mastitis, etc. The crude preparations obtained from single plant or a mixture of different plants is commonly used for the treatment of different cases. They work exceptionally well in non-infectious or dietary disorders.

In India, and its neighbouring countries like China, Nepal etc., Ayurvedic medicine dominated the medicinal practices. The name '*Ayurveda*' derives from Latin word ' *Ayur*' means life and '*Veda*' means knowledge or science, and it is more than a system of medicine. Ayurveda is an integral part of Indian culture.

Importance of Herbal Medicine

- Herbal medicine is positive, and heart of traditional healing. They are safe, cost effective and eco-friendly.
- They are locally available and easily accessible.
- They restore natural function and vitality of the body.
- They are easily absorbed and integrated into the cells and tissues of the body.
- They reinforce body's own healing mechanisms and do not suppress the way that many of the chemical drugs like antibiotics and cortisone do.
- The polyherbal formulations like Bramha rasayana, are said to exhibit immuno-restorative property and can be used against auto-immune diseases.
- Some indigenous drugs do possess immunomodulatory and antioxidant properties,
- They have multi-system effects and contain vitamins, minerals that make them beneficial to be used for supportive therapy.

Usage of Indigenous Drugs

Indigenous drugs can be used alone or as polyherbal formulations. They can be used directly i.e., crude forms in which the various plant parts viz. roots, leaves, flowers, and barks can be collected and dried. It can be used in the form of powder, paste, decoction, infusion, etc. The active components viz. carbohydrate, glycosides, tannins, lipids, alkaloids, mucilage, etc. can be separated by various processes viz. Thin Layer Chromatography (TLC) and High Performance Liquid Chromatography (HPLC) and can be employed as medicines. astringent, smoothening, protective, refrigerant, laxative, and antioxidants. Immunomodulatory properties of the herbal medicines are being exploited for their uses as medicine.

Indigenous Preparations in Diarrhoea

Diarrhoea and dysentery of varied etiology is a major problem of great clinical concern for both physicians and veterinarians. The treatment of diarrhoea with chemotherapeutic agents is disappointing in majority of cases, if supportive therapy for correction of fluid, electrolyte, acid –base balance as well as energy deficit is not given simultaneously. Plants and their products have been used for its management. Leaves of *Morinda umbellate*, dried aerial parts of *Andrographis paniculata* (Kalmegh or Bhunimba), dried stem and bark of *Tinospora cordifolia, Cimmiphora wightii, Streblus asper, Xeromphis spinosa*, seeds of *Annona squamosa* and bark of *Ficus bengalensis* have been widely used for the management of diarrhoea and dysentery mainly in man. However, these plants have also been used in the treatment of various other animal diseases. *C. wightii* have been claimed to have anti-amoebic properties. Fresh unripe fruit of *Aegle marmelos* (Bael), dried unripe seeds of *Plantago ovale* (Ispaghula), dried aqueous extract of leaves of young shoots of *Uncaria gambir* (Kath), *Accacia catechu* (Raktasar), *Berberis aristata* (Daruharida), *Holarrhoea antidysenterica* (Kutaj), and young twig excrescence of *Quercus infectoria* (Oak) are in common use for the control of diarrhoea in man and animals. The latest trend of utilization of herbal medicines and indigenous preparations along with modern (allopathic) therapy has added advantages over use of allopathic drugs alone.

Dalbergia sissoo (*Shisham*) has medicinal importance, and is being used extensively by rural folks in India for the treatment of animals suffering from nonspecific diarrhea. The bark, roots, leaves and mucilages of shisham has astringent and homeostatic properties and can be given at a dose rate of 70-105 g per 100 kg body weight orally twice a day for 3 days for control of diarrhoea. *Aegle marmelos* (Bael) is used in both human and animal medicine. The half-ripen bael acts as an astringent and reduces irritation in digestive tract and has been used for the treatment of diarrhoea and dysentery. The full-grown fruits when begins to ripen is the best time for its use as medicine. The fruit pulp contains reducing sugar, tannin and marelosin and the later is the most important active principle of fruit. Unripe fruit of bael exhibits astringent, digestive, stomachic and laxative activity. Liquid extract of bael prepared from dried slices of unripe fruit is given @ 1-2 drachms. Powder of dried pulp kept in an airtight bottle is administered @ 20 grains to 2 drachms. In cattle, it is used generally @ 16-24 g per 100 kg body weight orally twice a day for 3 days. Half ripen bael fruit is minced and dried to make powder which is considered to be an excellent medicine for children with chronic diarrhoea and dysentery without rise in body temperature.

Oryza sativa (Rice) starch and *Hordeum vulagare* (Barley) flour have been used to correct diarrhoea. Rice gruel helps in restoring fluid-electrolyte balance in noninfectious diarrhoea. It is given @ 200-300g twice daily for 3 days in calves. Becknor, a herbal formulation with anti-diarrhoeal potency has pivotal role in reducing severity of diarrhoea in young calves. It contains *Acacia nilotica,* Aegle marmelos, Tinospora cordifolia and Cyperus rotundus (Ali et al. 2001).

Indigenous Technical Knowledge in Combating Diarrhoea

Linseed plants or soaked gram or thorn apple or arharwood mixed with ash, salt, water can be given to animal passing loose stool. Clay soil has been used in goats suffering from diarrhoea. Barks of *Butea monosperma, Mahewa latifolia* and *Accacia catechu* mixed with water is first heated, then cooled and kept overnight as such. Next day it is strained and the filtrate is fed to diarrhoeic animals. Pulp of ripened tamarind (*Tamarindus indica*), sap of guava (*Psidium guajava*), barks and roots of sensitive plants (Mimosa pudica, sap of banana (*Musca pardisiaca*), leaves of bamboo tree (*Bambusa arundinacea arundinacea*), neem (*Azadirachta indica*) and red water lily (*Nymphaea nouchali*), pine apple (*Anarus comosus*) juice, bark of sal tree (*Shorea robusta)* are amongst few practised by the villagers in cases of diarrhoea in cattle and goats etc.

Some Polyherbal Formulations used in Gastrointestinal Disorders

There are large numbers of polyherbal formulations manufactured by different companies for use in animals for correcting the gastrointestinal disorders. They are Neblon, HB strong, Rumbion, Herbasol, Appevet, Digestone, Digesovet, Himalayan Batisa, Rumenton powder etc.

Techniques for Evaluating Side Effects of Medicinal Plants

Adverse or toxic effects of herbal preparations are required to be studied before being used in large-scale practice. The following criteria should be taken into consideration while assessing the herbal preparation. The general appearance of animal and behavioral changes should be monitored during treatment. The chemical biochemistry such as carbohydrate, protein and lipid profile test, organ function test for liver, kidney, thyroid, mineral and vitamin status, blood hematology like haemoglobin, Total Leukocyte Count (TLC), Total Erythrocyte Count (TEC), Differential Leukocytes Count (DLC), erythrocyte sedimentation rate, packed cell Volume, MCV, MCHC, are some of the tests that should be carried out to assess the toxic potential of the preparation.

Limitation in Herbal Medicine

It is still obscure as to how they act on the body. Their active principles are seldom identified. The quality, evaluation and standardization of finished products should be ensured before marketing. Scientific rationale and chemical validation is highly required. There should be mass production of herbal formulation with reliability, therapeutic efficacy, safety, etc.under GMP and TQM (Total Quality Management) norms.

The availability of scientific tools for quality control and standardization of ethnoveterinary practices have added a new dimension to overall acceptability. The following points require attention for better exploitation of herbal preparation for use in animal health practices

- Pesticide free cultivation of herbs
- Isolation and analysis of the active principles and causes of their seasonal variation, efficacy, and appropriate method of storage pertinent to individual plants
- Mechanism of their action in the body
- Creation of infrastructural facilities to process extraction of herbs, much-used in Ayurveda.
- Validation of the existing formulations

The scope of herbal medicine in enhancing health and production of Indian livestock is very bright. However, collective efforts are needed with a multifaceted approach involving traditional physician, medical chemist, veterinary pharmacologists, clinicians and veterinary pharmaceutical industries. Efforts should also be directed towards quality control and standardization of herbal formulations.

Index

E

F

G

H

W

Z